A NURSE'S STORY

WINCHELL

A NURSE'S STORY

LIFE, DEATH, AND IN-BETWEEN IN AN INTENSIVE CARE UNIT

TILDA SHALOF

M&S

National Library of Canada Cataloguing in Publication

Shalof, Tilda
A nurse's story : life, death and in-between in an
intensive care unit/ Tilda Shalof.

ISBN 0-7710-8086-7

1. Shalof, Tilda. 2. Nurses – Canada – Biography.
3. Intensive care nursing – Anecdotes. I. Title.

RT37.S53A3 2004   610.73'092   C2003-907296-7

We acknowledge the financial support of the Government of Canada through the Book Publishing Industry Development Program and that of the Government of Ontario through the Ontario Media Development Corporation's Ontario Book Initiative. We further acknowledge the support of the Canada Council for the Arts and the Ontario Arts Council for our publishing program.

Typeset in Sabon by M&S, Toronto
Printed and bound in Canada

This book is printed on acid-free paper that is 100% ancient forest friendly
(100% post-consumer recycled)

McClelland & Stewart Ltd.
The Canadian Publishers
481 University Avenue
Toronto, Ontario
M5G 2E9
www.mcclelland.com

1   2   3   4   5   08   07   06   05   04

CONTENTS

To nurses everywhere

PREFACE

This book is the story of my life as a nurse. In writing it,
I have culled from my twenty years of professional experience, almost all of it caring for people who have
catastrophic and life-threatening illnesses, in a number of hospitals in Toronto and other cities. Although the stories are true and
based on first-hand experience (either my own or, in a few cases,
that of my colleagues), I have changed the names and descriptions
of all individuals in order to protect their privacy. A few of the
characters portrayed are actually composites of two or more real
people. The time frame of this book is the early eighties to the
present; however, some chapters take place over days, others
encompass years. I have expanded and telescoped time in order to
describe trends in nursing and the health-care system, rather than
to document specific political or historical occurrences.

My work is critical care and where I work is the intensive care
unit – the ICU. Sometimes, even after all these years, I hear those
initials as words – I See You. They remind me of the privilege that
nurses have to see deeply into our patients' lives as we accompany
them through some of their most private, difficult, and vulnerable
moments. But when I explain to people that my patients are

critically ill and that some are likely, or even certain, to die, they often ask me if I find my work upsetting. I tell them that yes, at one time I did and now, I don't, but I know they find my answer hard to believe. "It must be so depressing," they say. I struggle to explain why I don't find my work sad, but they remain unconvinced, because *they* certainly find it so.

This book is my attempt to explain why I do not find my work either depressing or distressing – why, in fact, I find it inspiring, challenging, and endlessly fascinating. Nursing has given me the opportunity to master technical skills, achieve a degree of maturity as a person, come to terms with my own emotional vulnerability, and, above all, to work with other women and men, who, in my experience, have been generous and devoted friends and extraordinarily accomplished practitioners of our profession.

No, I do not find my work upsetting or depressing, yet I believe that many nurses do at times, and I have tried to give voice to their concerns. Not only that, but I know many nurses who are disenchanted and disheartened by what they feel is a lack of recognition or respect from the hospital, the public and politicians. Many nurses are exhausted from the burdens of shift work, impossible workloads, and severe staffing shortages. In addition, there is another, and to my mind, equally serious and pervasive stress: the constant exposure to the suffering and despair that grave illness can bring. Perhaps even more disconcerting is that as nurses deal with these known and familiar stresses, we are now faced with brand-new risks that may put our health – even our lives – in jeopardy. These risks take the form of new and more virulent infectious diseases and hazardous work environments.

It may not be fashionable to say so, but even after all these years, I still love being a nurse. Sometimes I worry about the future of my profession. Recently, on a summer evening, at a barbecue dinner with friends, I asked the mother of teenagers how she would feel if her kids went into nursing.

"Not pleased. I'd do everything possible to steer them in a different direction."

I asked her fourteen-year-old daughter if she'd ever considered nursing as a career.

"No way! Why would I go into something that all I hear about it is how difficult it is, like how all nurses hate it, like how the government is cutting back on health care? I'm going to be a stockbroker."

I decided to bring my informal survey closer to home and asked my own children. Max, my six-year-old son, said, "No, not a nurse. I am going to be an artist and a doctor." (I have come to believe that this happens to be an excellent combination.) But perhaps there is a glimmer of hope because when I asked Harry, my eight-year-old son, he answered, "First, I want to play in the NHL, and then I'll be a nurse."

However, this book is intended neither to entice young people to enter this profession nor to dissuade them from doing so. Nursing is not for everyone, but I can honestly say that now I have learned some of its challenging lessons and I am very grateful to have chosen nursing. Nursing has been very good to me.

A few years ago I attended an old woman's funeral. The rabbi spoke of her generous nature, how even throughout her long and difficult illness she continually put aside her pains and worries and made time to listen to her children and to play with her grandchildren.

"She was a woman who conquered herself so that she could serve others," the rabbi said.

I sat up suddenly. That sentence set my mind on fire. In a moment I understood what I had been trying throughout my life and career to do. I have had to conquer many personal fears, anxieties, prejudices, and insecurities. I have had to learn basic fundamentals of taking care of myself in order to become the kind of nurse that I aspired to be. I happened to stumble into my profession, but now I walk proudly. I used to wait outside a patient's door, hesitant and tentative, trying to build up the courage to go in and do something helpful. Somehow, I propelled myself into the room sideways, hoping not to be noticed, to get through my shift without harming anyone. As far as I know, I have never harmed anyone. There were many patients I have cared for over the years that I could have given more to had I been taking better care of myself and had I known what I know

now, but it took me a long time to learn all of these things.

This is the story of many stories. It is what I've learned from my colleagues and my patients over the years. It is my journey of learning to conquer myself so that I could serve others. It is my expression of gratitude to nursing and to the nurses I have known and have had the privilege to work with. They have given me the best of nursing care and it has made all the difference.

ACKNOWLEDGEMENTS

Thank you to Douglas Gibson and Jonathan Webb of McClelland & Stewart for believing that a nurse's story deserved to be told, and to Wendy Thomas, Kong Njo, Elizabeth Kribs, and everyone else who contributed to the editing, design, and production of this book.

To the patients and families I have cared for, I will always feel honoured that they have entrusted me with their lives.

Faced with the impossible challenge of acknowledging all the nurses who inspired this book, I have had to compromise with this short list. My apologies to those I've unavoidably missed: Lesley Barrans, Georgia Barrett, Dawn Barretto, Stephanie Bedford, Karen Bennett, Polly Ann Boldt, Patricia Bone, Allyson Booth, Richard Bowen, Bryan Boyachuk, Judy Brooks, Stacey Burns, Christine Caissie, Anita Chakungal, Paula Chen, Suzanne Chiasson, Dallas Christian, Sherrill Collings, Sharon Cudck, Ingrid Daley, Penny and Helen Damilatis, Blonie Deza, Belle Dhillon, Maureen Falkenstein, Barbara Farrell, Debbie Finn, Marcia Fletcher, Jo-Ann Ford, Gary Frazer, Roberto Fuerté, Catherine Gadd, Cheryl Geen-Smith, Elizabeth Gordon, Dorota Gutkowski, Janet Hale, Kathy Haley, Lynda Hattin, Rosie Healy, Helena Hildebrandt, Claire Holland, Grace Ho-Young, Linda Hunter, Tammy Hutchings, Anita Jennings,

Isabel Jordão, Lori Karlstedt, Chris Kebbel, Sandi Keough, Anisa Khan, Nydia Khargie, Meera Kissondath, Connie Kwan, Cathy Landry, Kwai Lau, Edna Lee, Marianne Leitch, Murry MacDonald, Shona Mackenzie, Isabella MacLeod, Kate Matthews, James Mazgalis, Bridgette McCaig, Kathleen McCully, Margaret McGrath-Chong, Robert McGregor, Moira McNeill, Carolyn McPhee, Julie Millar, Amanda Moorhead, Sue Morningstar, Denise Morris, Kerrie Murphy, Sue Nash, Cecilia Neto, Patricia Nunes De-Sousa, Linda Nusdorfer, Carol Oyerzabal, Janet Patterson, Kate Pettapiece, Winsome Plummer, Jennifer Post, Jonathan Pridham, Sharon Raby, Wendy Radovanovic, Cheryl Ramsden-Lee, Juliet Ramsay, John Remington, Katie Reposa, Terri Ritter, Karyn Robinson, Theresa Robitaille, Karen Roche, Elizabeth Romano, Les Rusland, Carla Samuels, Maureen Samuels, Kathleen Saunders, Jackie Spandel, Paula Spensieri, Rosemarie Stangl, Janice Stanley, Marilyn Steinberg, Adrella Suban, Kelly Sundarsingh, Oliver Tadeo, Claire Thomas, Jasna Tomé, Stacey Toulouse, Angela Tozer, Brenda Twa, Amber Verdoni, Jenny Vian, Sue Wegenest, Paulette Weir, Tanya White, Theresa Zamora, Denise Zanus, Mugs Zweerman, and the late Jane Jackson, who deserves a book of her own.

There are many other dedicated professionals who are a part of this book. To name but a few: Jimmy Arciaga, Trisha Barnes, Carolyn Brunette, Laurie Campoverde, Gary Corney, Roger D'Amours, Hanwar Dilmohammed, Sister Teresa Forma, Mary Georgousis, Fernanda Gomez, Gail Henry, Billal Jehangeer, Ludwika Juchniewicz, Brenda Kisic, Urszula Kolomycew, Wade Morey, Cyndy Rahm, Cecilia Reblora, Rosa Ricciardi, Sandy Rothberg, Loretta Savage, Roman Schyngera, Lola Troper, Gary Wong, and Zeinul Velji.

I feel enormous gratitude to these dear friends who are also colleagues, for nurturing me and my dreams, with love and patience over the years: Judith Allan-Kyrinis, Karen Calverley, Ann Flett, Cecilia Fulton, Lisa Huntington, Mary Malone-Ryan, Linda McCaughey, Julia Piercey, and Sharon Reynolds.

Thank you to Marlene Medaglia for mentoring me and for being the kind of nurse I am still striving to be and to Maude Foss, whose unwavering support has been invaluable.

With appreciation to these fine physicians from whom I have learned so much: Richard Cooper, Wilfred De Majo, John Granton, Laura Hawryluck, Margaret Herridge, Brian Kavanagh, Neil Lazar, John Marshall, Janet Maurer, Joanne Myer, Tim Winton, and the late Bill Mahon.

I am deeply grateful to Dr. Mark Bernstein for his encouragement, generosity, and for throwing open the door.

Thank you to Rabbi Elyse Goldstein for her wise counsel.

Thanks for the steadfast and enthusiastic support from the families of Tony and Daneen Di Tosto, Desmond and Michelle Hirson, and Alan and Rivi Horwitz. Thank you to Larissa Ber, Méira Cook, Elise Dintsman, Vanessa Herman-Landau, Mara Koven, Annie Levitan, Ella Shapiro, Dawn Sheppard, Anne Werker, Rhea Wolfowich, Bob and Marcie Young, and David Zitzerman for friendship and advice. Thank you to Joy Friedman-Bali, my sister of the earth, and to Robyn Sheppard, my sister of the air.

A huge debt of gratitude to Barbara Turner-Vesselago, friend and teacher who gave me the courage to write and taught me to go "fearward" and mine the vein. I thank fellow free-fall writers for reading my early drafts and sharing their writing with me: Karen Alison, Malca Litovitz, Ann McLurg, Faith Moffat, Sue Reynolds, Monique Shebbeare, Cathy Shilton, and Susan Zimmerman.

I am grateful that I had the good fortune to have many parents. First, my own, the late Harry and Elinor Shalof. Also, Alec and Leah Lewis; Jerry and Bernice Friedman, Dr. Shlomo Katz and the late Dr. Shirra Katz, Dr. Robert and Norah Sheppard; Florence and Richard Weiner, and Rita Young. Thanks to Robert and Stephen Grant, and Tex and Bonnie Shalof for being my brothers and sister.

Thank you to Harry, Max and Ivan Lewis – especially, Ivan. Although he's never read a word I've written, without him I couldn't have written even one.

I

TREATING THE NUMBERS

I t's night shift. I jot down a series of numbers onto my patient's twenty four-hour flow sheet and then prepare to read them out loud to the medical resident who is standing with me at the patient's bedside, waiting to hear them.

"Everything is out of whack," I say: "7.26, 68, 76, 14."

That's a losing lottery ticket. No one can survive such a deranged acid-base balance, sky-high carbon dioxide levels, and plummeting oxygenation and bicarbonate ions.

"Those numbers are not compatible with life," the resident says.

"Not life on *this* planet, anyway," says Lynne, the nurse who's kneeling by the door, packing up her knapsack, getting ready to leave. She was on the day shift and is the only one in the room who's smiling: she's going home. "I'm outta here. I'm going home to have sex with my husband." Lynne has finished giving me report on Mr. DeWitt, all the facts and the numbers, what's high, what's low, what's rising, and what's falling. Now it's up to me to carry on throughout the night.

"Have fun," I say as I'm thinking about something else. "You know what, Lynne? I think we should call a family meeting. Does his wife know how bad the situation is? Has anyone told her? I'm going to call her. I think she needs to come in."

"She just went home," says Lynne. "She's been here all day and was exhausted when she left. What makes you think he might not make it through the night? He's been spiralling downward for weeks. You could probably get him through the night."

Together we stand there, Lynne just outside the door, me just inside, surveying the body of the middle-aged man stretched out in the bed, surrounded by machines and monitors, tubes and wires, bags and drains that expose all the secret fluids of the body.

"I see your point, though," Lynne said. "When you take a minute to step back and really look at it all, you do start to wonder sometimes. But do you really think it's going to be tonight?"

"I have a feeling." I have learned to trust my feelings.

I consult with the medical resident and together we decide that I should call Mrs. DeWitt and ask her to come in. I tell her that unfortunately, her husband is not doing well. His blood pressure is very low, I say. It is dropping, I add, as gently as possible. He is on powerful intravenous medications for his blood pressure, inotropes we call them, but we have had to add another drug because of the serious heart irregularities that he developed today. Another problem is that his urine output is dropping off. Perhaps she would like to return to the hospital and we can talk about it further? Is there someone who could drive her?

"FAMILY MEETING" IS the term we use to gather all the people closest to the patient to provide them with an update on the patient's condition. Sometimes we call a family meeting to discuss the death and how we will let it happen. A family meeting is rarely called if the patient is improving.

We convene in a shabby, cramped room called the "quiet room." It is a tiny room with buzzing fluorescent lights, no windows – I would never take anyone in there if they suffered from claustrophobia. It has the feel of a bunker in a war zone, but aesthetics aside, it seems to be the only room in this huge, bustling, overcrowded, downtown hospital that could be made available for this purpose. The quiet room! It is probably the most *disquieting* place in the whole hospital. Bombs are detonated in here.

We turn our attention to Mrs. DeWitt. She is the one who knows Edgar DeWitt best. She is the person who will speak on his behalf, as he is no longer conscious and cannot tell us himself what he wants us to do. She perches on the chair, frail, but tensed up. She knows why we're gathered here.

"What would Mr. DeWitt have wanted?" the doctor asks his wife.

"To live! That's what he would have wanted." She sobs into her hands.

Of course. Isn't it obvious? Isn't that what anyone would want?

"We understand," the doctor says, "but, given his deteriorating condition and his irreversible medical problems, if we continue with the life-support measures that we have in place, we are merely prolonging the inevitable."

I watch Mrs. DeWitt and I can see that in her panicked state, she finds comfort in the simple fact that the doctor is talking, because all the time the doctor is talking, her husband is still alive.

"We do not believe that we can reverse his medical problems. Perhaps the time has come, that we should very gently, slowly, when you are ready, of course, remove the ventilator, all the life supports, and let nature take its course?"

She sits weeping into the cave of her two hands. I offer her a new box of tissues and pull out the first one to get it started.

"Did you ever discuss this situation with him?" I press gently. "Do you think he would want all this to be done?" My words are like sticks, poking at a fire, making it flare.

"Who *would* want all this done?" she asks.

The doctor and I smile at her response, so true and honest.

"I don't know what to do," Mrs. DeWitt says. "Whenever we had a big decision to make, Ed and I always made it together."

"There's no need to decide anything this minute," I say, "but his condition is very critical. Anything could happen tonight."

Whatever happens, it will be a long night for all of us.

The family meeting is over and we return to Mr. DeWitt's room.

Frances peeks her head in the door and whispers, "Do you want to order in food, Tilda?"

Frances is one of my pals – we've worked together for years. Tonight she's the nurse in charge and her duties include organizing transfers in and out of the hospital and discharges and admissions to and from the ICU, making rounds with the doctor to check on how the patients are doing, and finding out if any of the nurses or doctors want to order snacks or meals from the sheaf of menus we keep on hand – Greek, Thai, pizza. It never sits well to eat this heavy food late at night – it's already 9 p.m., or 2100 hours, according to the twenty-four-hour clock we use – but we often do because we're always hungry. I order a veggie sub with hot peppers and a bottle of Grape Beyond juice and return to my patients, who are, in equal measure, Mr. and Mrs. DeWitt.

Mrs. DeWitt smiles at her neighbours from the street she lives on; they have joined her at her husband's bedside. They stand there, looking uncomfortable. These helpful people drove her back to the hospital when she received my phone call. Mrs. DeWitt's smile reflects the required gratitude of someone who has no relatives or true, trusted friends to call upon and must rely on favours from acquaintances. Friends you choose, family you're born into, but neighbours are random and have no obligation whatsoever. What they offer is truly a gift.

"I don't want my husband to die on March 5," Mrs. DeWitt says.

It's not like booking an airline ticket. Or is it? I look up at the clock on the wall near the door and note that it is 2200 hours on March 5, 2004. In two hours it won't be March 5 any more. Can we keep him going until then? Anything can happen. There are no guarantees. Of course I'm curious to know why she's made this request, but I've heard stranger ones. I wait for her to tell me, if she wishes.

"It's Greta's birthday," she says, pointing to her neighbour, and this gesture brings a tear to Greta's eye. "I don't want Ed's death to ruin her birthday. Good neighbours are hard to find."

We all stand around Mr. DeWitt's bed and I do my work of measuring and monitoring, watching and waiting. Together we keep the vigil.

I am instilling drops of lubricating fluid, called artificial tears, into Mr. DeWitt's swollen, bulging eyes. The medical term for this condition is scleral edema, but sometimes, among ourselves, we refer to them as "jelly eyes." We see eyes like this all the time in the ICU.

"Why is his face so puffy?" asks Mrs. DeWitt.

Anasarca, massive edema, third-spacing, fluid shifting . . . how to explain it to her? It is so upsetting for her to see him like this! "When there is overwhelming infection throughout the body, the tissues don't hold the fluids inside the cells and it leaks out and causes swelling, known as edema," I explain.

"So why are you giving him more fluid?" She points at the bank of electronic machines pumping fluid into his veins.

"That fluid contains powerful medications to help his blood pressure."

"Why is his blood pressure so low?"

"Because of the infection in his blood. The infection releases substances called endotoxins that cause the arteries to expand."

"Why is there an infection in his blood?"

"Well, his diabetes put him at risk, and the surgery he had last week. . . ." I reiterate explanations that we have all gone over many times before, but bear repeating. "The disease itself and the treatments, too, can cause all these problems."

One thing leads to another. . . .

"Why isn't the infection getting any better? Isn't he on antibiotics to fix that?"

"Yes, but the antibiotics don't seem to be working."

"Why aren't the antibiotics working?"

"They don't always work in these situations . . . of overwhelming sepsis. We may add a new one."

"A stronger one?"

"Yes."

"Is it a better one?"

"It may work better for him. In his case."

"Is it better?"

"It may be, for him."

"Well, then, why hasn't he been on that better one all along?"

I fall silent. I have no more answers because these are not the real questions she wants to ask. For those questions there are no answers, certainly none that I have. She scowls at me and I return to the patient, to listen to his heart, his lungs, his stomach. I study his heartbeats on the cardiac monitor and make notes in the chart.

"Getting all this down, are you?" she asks. She is standing beside me, peering down over my shoulder, as I write in the chart. "Is my husband an interesting case for you?"

She doesn't like that I am writing notes, but she kept notes, too, for a long time, especially in the beginning of her husband's long stay in the ICU. One day she left her notebook behind on the bedside table, and a nurse found it. She had written comments about all of us and kept a list of the "good" nurses and the "bad" ones; the ones she wanted, the ones she didn't. She recorded the names and dosages of the drugs we gave each day and what percentage oxygen he was receiving. How unnerving it was to all of us to be so closely scrutinized.

She has a hard, bony face and she is making it difficult for me to feel warm toward her, as I try to do under these circumstances. I stand up, face her, and find it in myself to put my arms around her and envelop her in a hug. With this hug, I am trying to offer an answer to Mrs. DeWitt's questions. I am trying hard to like her, but even though I don't, I have learned that I can still do my job well. I hold her in my arms and she sobs and I let her.

The unit is quiet now. Only a few, necessary lights are on now, the rest have been dimmed. The earlier swirl and turmoil of activity in a patient's room across the hall where a fresh lung transplant was admitted a few hours ago has now settled; the room has cleared out and calm has been restored, so I know the patient has been stabilized. A few nurses are gathered at the nursing station sipping coffee and chatting quietly, their voices a familiar and pleasant murmur.

In my room, I can feel the growing distress brewing in my patient's wife and I remind myself to stay calm. For it is only if I remain calm and centred that I will be of any help to Mrs. DeWitt tonight. She stands at her husband's bedside, telling him she's there, knowing all too well by now not to expect any response from him. I see her legs in droopy stockings and faded sandals that were probably once jaunty and colourful, but at this hour, under these weary fluorescent lights and these dismal circumstances, they look pathetic. She wipes up the countertop with a dirty towel and dumps it into the laundry basket. She takes a clean face cloth, wets it under the tap, and presses it to her husband's sweaty, bloated face. By now, after so many weeks of her husband's illness, she makes herself at home here in her husband's room. It's her room as much as his, and certainly more hers than mine.

I busy myself with paperwork. It's almost midnight – 2359 hours – and the new date involves a lot of extra documentation. It seems quite irrelevant, especially at a time like this, but it must get done.

Then a horrible stench fills the air and we know instantly what this is. Mr. DeWitt has lost control of his bowels in the bed and Mrs. DeWitt flees from the room.

Later, when she returns, he has been cleaned, his linen changed, and I have managed to make the room smell more pleasant with a floral spray and an air deodorizer. Fresh air is an impossibility as the windows are hermetically sealed throughout the entire hospital.

"If we were to let him go," she asks me as if it's a test question for which she knows the correct answer and wants to find out if I do, too, "what would the cause of death be?"

Each time she asks a question, it is as if she has never received any information, no one has told her anything. Even though we've spent weeks providing her with information, sitting with her every day to go over everything and answer her questions, she still feels as if she's been kept in the dark.

I decide to go where she is leading me. She wants information.

"Multi-system organ failure," I take a breath before the list of Mr. DeWitt's medical problems: "Overwhelming sepsis, disseminated intravascular coagulation, pancreatitis, renal failure, and complications of diabetes."

"Oh."

I sense she's looking for wrongdoing: there must be someone to blame for the condition her husband is in. Someone must have made a mistake. Surely there were things that could have been done that weren't; things that were done that shouldn't have been. Something must have been missed. I see accusation on her face. Perhaps she still finds some comfort in our conversation. For all the time we are talking, mortal decision making is delayed and her husband is, more or less, alive. Technically speaking, anyway. Legally alive. In biological terms, that is.

She holds herself in her two arms, close and tight, doing it for herself as if she already knows that her husband will not be doing this for her ever again.

IT'S 0100 HOURS and a new admission has just arrived. Without even going out of my room, I can feel the buzz, the energetic spring into action of the other nurses, a few doctors, and the respiratory technicians. Frances has gone in the room to help and another friend of mine, Tracy, steps forward to cover for me while I go check out who has arrived. Tracy has been reading my telepathic messages for years. She probably senses I need a short break from Mrs. DeWitt's gaze and the hopes she has pinned on me to save her husband.

"It's a pink hamburger lady," says Laura, another nurse I've worked with for years, referring to her new admission. Laura looks concerned about her patient, a young woman, thrashing in the bed. One leg is right over the side rail. Her body looks healthy, an even tan all over, no bikini lines, and silver nail polish on her toes. She is babbling incoherently, calling out to people she sees, voices only she can hear.

"Only twenty-two years old. She's been seizing, her eyes are bulging out from intracranial pressure, and, I think – she might be going" – Laura milks the urinary catheter tube for a few more drops of amber-coloured urine – "into kidney failure."

"All from eating rare meat?"

"Yup, can you believe it?"

"She looks pretty sick. You must be busy."

"It's steady," she admits. "But I'm glad to be busy. The night is flying by. So, how's Mr. DeWitt doing?"

"I think he's going to die tonight."

"He's been circling the drain for weeks." Laura shakes her head. "Mrs. DeWitt can't let go."

The resident on call tonight rushes in, still chewing the last bite of her submarine sandwich. Meningitis has to be ruled out, so she's preparing to perform a lumbar puncture on Laura's patient. She pulls her long, dark hair back and tucks it into the collar of her white lab coat that is not so white any more. Her eyes sparkle in anticipation of this procedure. She told me earlier that she was looking forward to performing it and hoped for a "champagne tap." That's when you just get the clear cerebrospinal fluid, no red cells, and no white cells. It's supposed to look like water. CSF comes straight from the brain and is the cleanest, purest bodily fluid, the hardest to come by.

"DO YOU REALLY think he's going to die? Is there any chance at all that he might make it?" Mrs. DeWitt asks as I re-enter the room to resume my sentry post at her husband's bedside.

I look at her long and hard. "I hope I'm wrong," I say. I would like to remind her that it's not up to me. We have failed you, I think, by encouraging you to believe that we can cure anything and everything.

The night grinds on. Most rooms are settled and there is a feeling of calm in the ICU. There is an unspoken understanding among all the nurses: we will get through this night together.

It is now almost five in the morning, well into the day of March 6. Mrs. DeWitt looks exhausted and I offer her a blanket and a pillow, but she refuses.

I have now added two more potent medications to boost Mr. DeWitt's blood pressure, but his urine output has petered out. His body is shutting down, organ by organ, and even Mrs. DeWitt can see where we're heading and that what we are doing no longer has any purpose. She is beginning to see, too, how it detracts from her husband's dignity to have all this inflicted on him. She decides it is time to let him go. He is already so close to death that as soon as I cut off the flow of just one medication, his blood pressure drops and his heart goes into a slow, erratic pattern.

"What's that called?" After all these months, she's learned to recognize significant changes on the cardiac monitor screen and she knows that every configuration has a name.

"Do you mean the heart rhythm?" I ask.

"Yes."

"It's called the dying heart."

That's the truth. That's the name of that particular configuration. Textbook.

The resident is having a busy night with other patients but comes into the room. She is obligated to make a difficult request and she approaches Mrs. DeWitt now to put it to her.

"Would you be in agreement for us to perform an autopsy?"

"Is there a question about the cause of death?" Mrs. DeWitt's raised eyebrow conveys renewed suspicion as she makes one last rally to apportion blame. "What would you be trying to find out by doing an autopsy? Are there unanswered questions?"

"It is not an investigation," I cut in to explain. "It will contribute to medical knowledge. Science. Even in cases like this, your husband" – and we pause to look over at him as I speak – "even in cases like this where the cause of death is known, the information that we will obtain from the autopsy and will pass on to you, may help you come to terms with . . . it."

"Can he donate his organs? Ed signed his organ donor card." She brightened visibly at the thought.

"Unfortunately, there is too much disease and infection for organ donation."

I see she takes this as a personal rejection and is miffed. "Very well then, autopsy, with the remains to be returned to me for cremation."

NOW THERE IS just an occasional blip and then long, smooth, green lines on the monitor screen. I turn off a button at the back of the ventilator and it stops pushing air into his lungs. I close the clamps on the intravenous fluids and shut off the pumps that are pushing those fluids into the body of Mr. DeWitt.

"How low could the numbers go?" she asks.

She keeps her eyes trained on the cardiac monitor.

"To zero," I say. "It could go right down suddenly, or drift gradually. Why don't I just turn off the monitor now, since we're not treating the numbers any more, right?"

She nods. It seems that only when I push the "off" button on the cardiac monitor – the "TV screen" that played a constant movie of her husband's heart for so many days – and the fluorescent green lights zap off and the screen goes black, only then does Mrs. DeWitt believe that her husband has died. To her, the heart monitor had been the proof of life, especially when there were no other signs, and only now, turned off, is she forced to face what it means.

"So, is he . . . he's gone now?"

I think she needs time to tell herself the answer, so I keep quiet.

I close off all the IVs and turn off the other machines. Once, it all held such promise and now, in a moment, it has become useless paraphernalia. Junk. Much of it disposable.

Then I turn to her husband's body and, like an old-fashioned country doctor, take out my stethoscope from my lab coat pocket. It comes down to this. How strangely reassuring and quaint it seems to use this basic piece of equipment. It's based on a principle as simple as two pop cans connected by a string to carry the voices of kids across a backyard. I stand over my patient's body and listen to his heart with my stethoscope for a long time so that there will be no doubt in anyone's mind that his life has ended. The stethoscope has long since replaced a feather under the nostrils, or a mirror held up to see if there is moisture from a breath on the glass, or fingertips pressed to the neck. Yet it does the same thing. I keep on listening. There are no signs of life. Legally, this diagnosis will have to be confirmed by the doctor, but I am confident enough of my findings to tell her myself.

"Yes," I say. "He's dead. I'm very sorry." For her, I really am.

Some of the other nurses who had gotten to know Mr. and Mrs. DeWitt over this long hospitalization come to offer comfort and say goodbye.

WHEN I WALK in the door in the morning after my shift and my husband, Ivan, who's sitting at the breakfast table, looks up and asks, "How was work?" I say, "Fine, no problem."

"Busy?"

"Yes," and we leave it at that.

Should I tell him the truth? That I helped a man die, that I comforted his wife who sobbed in my arms, and that no, I am not upset about it. This is what I do for a living as a nurse in the intensive care unit.

When my husband asks about work I almost always answer the same way. I rarely go into too many details. He might regret he asked if I did. He would stare into the newspaper. His coffee would go cold. It might make him worry about me – or about himself – and I feel protective of him. Another reason that I don't go into details about my work is for the sake of our children, who might be within earshot and become frightened. They are very young and beginning to wonder about the world. Sometimes they see a still, squished bug and other bugs that are alive, busy creatures, and that's the closest thing they've ever seen that has anything whatsoever to do with the work I do. Not that everyone dies where I work, but some do, and there are a lot of close calls.

Now I will eat a bowl of Cheerios and go straight to bed, because even though it's early morning, the sun is up, and most other people are starting their day, I need to sleep.

2

FIRST, TAKE YOUR OWN PULSE

The stopcock terrified me.

Before I became a critical care nurse, I worked on a variety of medical and surgical wards in many different hospitals and I had acquired a lot of experience with veins. Veins trickled, oozed, or dripped. One of the big differences of working in the ICU was that, for the first time, I was confronted with arteries. Arteries spurted and gushed. After all, they are the vessels that pump blood directly from the heart. The stopcock is the gateway to the world of the artery.

In my early days of working in the ICU, the arterial stopcock – that little nub of hardware – taunted and haunted me. It was a mere half-inch piece of white plastic, and its mechanism was simple, yet its implications were immense. Each and every ICU patient had an "art line" in place (inserted in the radial artery in the wrist or femoral artery in the groin) to give us easy and instant access to the patient's circulation. The art line allowed the nurses to monitor patients' blood pressure and procure the many blood samples – most importantly, the arterial blood gases, ABGs we call them – without disturbing the patient.

With the stopcock positioned in the upright direction, we could monitor the patient's blood pressure. We made sure to set the alarms to upper and lower parameters for the systolic (contraction of the heart) and the diastolic (relaxation of the heart) measurements. As long as the numbers stayed "WNL" – within normal limits (something I was expected to be able to ascertain at a moment's glance) – all was well.

Problems could occur. Sometimes, a stream of blood crept up backwards and went along the tubing in the wrong direction and I was supposed to troubleshoot the problem. It could be a loose connection somewhere in the system or insufficient counter-pressure. Sometimes, the waveform on the monitor was dampened or had an overly high amplitude. Then I would have to flush the system, re-calibrate the transducer, heighten the sensitivity, or merely check the module and cables.

In order to obtain a sample of arterial blood to send to the laboratory to test the oxygen, carbon dioxide, and bicarbonate levels (substances that had to stay within a narrow range or else the patient would be in life-threatening danger), I had to turn the stopcock to the left – which meant the artery was wide open – and then move swiftly to attach a special tube that withdrew a sample of bright red blood from the pulsating stream. Then I had to flush the line clear of blood, reset the stopcock to the upright position, and close it off, all the time keeping everything absolutely sterile.

For other procedures, I had to turn the stopcock to the right. In that position, a flat green line would suddenly appear on the cardiac monitor and an urgent, piercing alarm would sound. If family members were present, they would jump, especially when their loved one was being cared for by a novice nurse – something they seemed to sniff out moments after meeting me. However, the alarm could also go off if the patient rustled the sheets or moved in bed, in which case the alarm was caused by "artifact." Most importantly, the alarm could signal the "real thing" if the heart went into a sudden lethal arrhythmia. It was my responsibility to know the difference.

As if the stopcock wasn't daunting enough, I also had to deal with the transducer, which connected to the monitor, cables,

computer module, and the oscilloscope. Those, together with
the electrodes, waveforms, and amplitudes, were just some of the
vocabulary of a brand-new language in which I had to become
fluent. In addition to all that, I had to add on the lexicon of critical illness, such as multi-system organ failure, congestive heart
failure, and hepatic or renal failure. Then there were the shocks:
anaphylactic, hypovolemic, cardiogenic, and the worst shock of
all: septic shock. All failures and shocks.

I HAVE ALWAYS been a big reader, and as a child I devoured the
Cherry Ames stories – *Cherry Ames, Cruise Nurse*; *Cherry Ames,
Dude Ranch Nurse*; *Cherry Ames, Ski Patrol Nurse*; and *Cherry
Ames, Department Store Nurse*. I had dreamed of being like her,
one of those compassionate, selfless people who did generous
things for people in need. The glamour and exotic adventures that
nursing seemed to offer were appealing, too. All in all, nursing
seemed like a good way to do all that and make a living at it, too.

In some ways, my career choice of nursing felt like a fallback onto
something familiar. In my family, I had always been the caregiver. I
was one of those little girls who could spot the one person in a crowd
who wasn't feeling well, the one who needed a chair or an arm to
lean on. Early on, I figured out that to help someone who is unsteady
on their feet, you offer your arm, rather than take theirs in yours.
Without anyone telling me, I would run off to fetch an aspirin and a
glass of water if someone had a headache or a pain somewhere.

I often wonder if other nurses come from homes where they
learned to be the caregiver, where that was the role handed to
them or the one they took upon themselves. It was at home, where
my parents were older than most, and where there was so much
illness, that I first honed my nursing skills. My mother had
Parkinson's disease and manic depression; my father had diabetes
and heart disease; and one of my brothers, schizophrenia. Doling
out my mother's pills, monitoring my father's blood sugar, and
coping with my brother's paranoia and verbal outbursts occupied
my free time as a child. To the best of my ability I took care of
them all until my parents died and my brother and I lost contact.

My two other brothers left home to escape the madness, and who could blame them?

Nursing was a logical, if ironic, choice for me: those very skills that I had developed at home in my family provided the vehicle that transported me away from that house of sadness. They provided my means of escape and became the tools of my trade. However, when I first told my self-educated, working-class father and my uneducated, yet cultured mother my choice of career, it took them aback.

"Jewish girls don't go into nursing," my father said when I told him what I was thinking of studying. It was the early eighties and I had just finished high school and was casting about for something to do. There would always be sick people and nurses would always be needed to take care of them, I reasoned. Surely I could do that; I had been doing it for years.

"I never heard of a Jewish nurse, have you, Ellie?" He turned to the couch where my mother lay. My mother knew a lot about opera, but very little about anything else.

"She'll be Florence Nightingstein," my mother said in a voice muffled by a giggle and her arm, flung back across her face.

"I wonder why there aren't many Jewish nurses," my father mused. The question seemed to interest him, as did most everything. "It is one of the oldest professions, although by no means the oldest one, mind you. We all know what that is, of course, heh, heh. Perhaps it is because the noble vocation of ministering to the sick is, somewhat – how shall I put this?"

"Icky," offered my mother.

"Well, Ellie, now that you mention it . . . but it's not just the menial work, it's also that nursing is not very, well, it's not the most –"

"High class and refined. Not at all," my mother said, with a melodramatic shudder of disapproval behind her arm and her now-closed eyes.

"Surely, Tilda, you could choose a profession that doesn't involve such selfless, back-breaking labour and long hours for such meagre remuneration. What are your girlfriends going into?"

It was true that none of my friends had even considered nursing. Natalie was off to study social work in New York. Allison was going to do a liberal arts degree at the University of Toronto, but first a year of backpacking through Europe. Stephanie was an aspiring actress.

"Your mother and I always hoped you would go to university," my father said wistfully. I knew he regretted that he had not had that opportunity when he was my age.

"Maybe I could study nursing at university," I said, wondering if I'd even be accepted with my ho-hum academic performance in high school.

"I see," he said slowly. I knew he was trying to come around to supporting me, as he did in most everything else. "Whatever you decide," he said finally. "In life, it's not about doing the work you love, it's about loving the work you do."

I had no idea what my mother thought. At any rate, she had no further comment, as she had risen from the couch and was busy being Madame Butterfly in the kitchen.

FOR THE NEXT four years I stumbled, bumbled, and fumbled my way through university lectures and clinical assignments in hospitals throughout the city. Somehow I got through it all but I began to have qualms about my choice. There was something about my personality that seemed unsuited to being a nurse. Nurses were by and large practical, sensible people, oozing with confidence and common sense. I was nothing like this. There was also something about my temperament (too mercurial) and my constitution (too sensitive) that made me ill suited to be a nurse. Yet, at the same time, I still felt passionately committed to the noble idea of service to human beings in need. I longed to be a bona fide member of the "helping profession."

I drifted along in my first two years of university in a state of dreamy distraction. Then, during my third year, my father died suddenly. I barely had time to register the shock, so busy was I caring for my mother, who was in the advanced stages of her disease and overcome with grief and depression. It was just before my final exams and my professors advised me to drop out and defer my studies for a year, until things settled down. But I was in so much of a hurry to get out and be free that I didn't take their advice. Somehow I managed to finish that year and then the next, all the while counting the days until I could escape my home and family, and most of all, myself. Somehow I got through it all. I managed to graduate with a Bachelor's degree of Science in Nursing and a Certificate of Competence to practise nursing. I was familiar with abstract theories and had read lots of research studies, but the rigorous discipline and practical skills of basic nursing practice eluded me.

The dean of the Faculty of Nursing shook her head sadly at me on graduation day. Prim and starched as Florence Nightingale herself, she wore a dove-grey suit with a white blouse and the requisite coral cameo at her throat. I had scraped by with a 66 per cent average. Who would want a nurse who knew only 66 per cent of the material? I knew I was a liability out there, but I promised myself I would be very careful, double-check everything, and try to stay out of the way of patients.

"You do have potential, dear. If only you had applied yourself, you could have made the Dean's List," said the dean herself. "Maybe you should go into research or administration. If you repeat courses and improve your marks, you could apply to graduate school. Have you considered that?"

I had thought about it, briefly, then quickly put the idea out of my mind. I was too impatient to get away from home – and to work, to travel, and to have fun and adventures – to pay much attention to her suggestion.

"She's a good nurse," I heard the dean telling the other professors afterwards at the graduation party. "Competent, but a bit scatter-brained."

UPON MY GRADUATION, full-time nursing positions were scarce. That didn't particularly perturb me, as I was not ready to settle down in one job, anyway. I joined a nursing agency and took on a variety of placements, such as private-duty nursing for imperious, rich old ladies recovering from hip replacements in their homes. Over the next few years, I did freelance medical writing for a pharmaceutical company; computer work for a doctor; and lots of part-time gigs in hospitals around town, never going more than a few times to the same place. I thought of myself as a "freelance" nurse.

In my travels, I discovered that many nurses were suspicious of degree nurses. Sure, they know lots of theories and research, they said, but can they cope with the demands of the job? In my case, they had reason to be concerned.

I recall one of my first days on a general medical ward. The doctor ordered a naso-gastric tube to be inserted into my patient's stomach after surgery.

"There's the clean utility room," said the nurse in charge, waving in one direction and running in another to receive a fresh post-op patient who was coming off the elevator on a stretcher. Over her shoulder she called out instructions. "Get a size 10 or 12 tube, a large syringe, and a basin of ice. Make sure you auscultate the gastric bubble to check for proper placement. Once you get it started, connect it straight drainage – no, better make that low Gomco – and replace the hourly losses with saline. While you're at it, his potassium is low, so you'd better change the IV to 20 mille-quivalents of KCl per litre and run it at 100 cc per hour. When you're done that, insert a Foley catheter and measure his hourly urine output. If this is your first time, you lucked out, 'cause males are a lot easier to catheterize than females. Got all that?"

I had read about these things, even seen one or two, but had never actually done any of them before.

"Oh, you university grads!" she said when she saw me floundering. "We need *real* nurses around here."

The littlest things could trip me up. One day, on a postpartum ward, I was assigned to take care of five new mothers and their babies. One new mother, exhausted and in discomfort after a Caesarian delivery, needed my assistance with a bed bath, but something was wrong with the curtains around her bed. I tugged and pulled, but they were stuck and didn't slide along the rails on the ceiling. I yanked at the curtains but they wouldn't budge. I went off to find the nurse in charge to report the curtain problem. I advocated for the client's right to privacy. Patients needed personal space within the vast public territory of the institution that they can call their own, I argued, recalling a lecture I had once heard on the subject. Patients have an inalienable right to autonomy, and with their permission, we may enter their domain.

"Call housekeeping," the nurse said, pushing the laundry cart into a patient's room. "Probably just needs some more rods and hooks. That and a spritz of WD-40 should do the trick."

"You're right," I conceded. A few rods and hooks, not a paradigm shift. I went back to work.

Even though the agency sent me to different hospitals around the city, and I rarely returned to the same ward twice, after just a few months, wherever I went, they considered me "senior staff" on the team. But "team nursing" was beginning to be considered old-fashioned and on the way out. Nursing theorists were promoting the virtues of "primary nursing." In primary nursing, nurses were responsible for all aspects of the care of a small group of patients to whom they were assigned. Whereas in team nursing, the work was divided and each nurse focused on a few tasks – say, vital signs or dressing changes – and did those tasks for all the patients in that ward, sometimes up to as many as forty patients.

From the patients' point of view, team nursing was "off-the-rack" shopping and primary nursing was personalized service; it was assembly-line production versus a made-to-measure, custom job. As so-called "senior staff," working with a team, I might be the one to administer the meds for all the patients in the ward or pair up with an orderly and make rounds turning patients in bed, giving baths, changing the IV bags. It was a big responsibility, but my role was clear and straightforward.

I loved making beds, especially an "occupied bed," when we turned the patient from side to side and did everything for the person who lay there helpless. As we went from room to room, I worked with a nursing assistant and we moved together wordlessly in concert with the sheets and blankets, making corners and pulling up the linen, folding it down, and making it smooth all over. Presto: the finished product, so crisp and inviting. Those beds we made would be a gift to any feverish patient.

Team nursing also gave me a fleeting sense of belonging to a group, even though I never stayed anywhere for long. Team nursing assuaged my loneliness and gave me a sense of family, something I craved, but then wanted to escape from. From the nurses' point of view, team nursing was an efficient way to work. It even occasionally allowed for time at the end of the shift to sit and drink coffee together at the nursing station while we finished up our charting. Although team nursing was convenient for nurses, I could see that for patients it fragmented the care they received into separate tasks performed by different people coming and going at various times. However, at that stage in my career, patients were the least of my concerns.

In those days of adjusting to the realities of my profession, one of the hardest things for me was waking up each morning for work. The luminous green numbers on the face of my alarm clock glowed in the darkness when I woke up long before it rang, after a night of broken, restless sleep. During those nights before work, I couldn't afford to abandon myself to the deep sleep that allowed for dreaming. The hours of the night were a countdown. My alarm clock was set for 5:00, but bells were ringing in my head at midnight, around 1:30, at 2:00, again at 3:14, around 4:00, at 4:33, until I finally shut it off at 5:00, before it had its chance to do its job. I lay there in disbelief that it was so early and that there was so much ahead of me that day. Would this be the day that would break me? I wanted to go back to sleep, not because I was tired, but because I was afraid. Duty propelled me forward. I put on a tape of Glenn Gould performing the Bach Concerto in E Major. His deliberate and forthright interpretation helped drown out my apprehension. The music fortified me to go on.

At 6:00 I left the house and rushed through the deserted streets to the subway. At that time of the morning, the moon is still out, as well as the bright headlights on the few cars in the city streets. When I reached the hospital, I entered the chrome-walled elevator and rode it to whatever floor I was assigned to that day. I strode through dark, disinfectant-smelling corridors, opened the heavy door of the ward or department *du jour* and reported for duty like a soldier.

The work was hard and I was busy every minute of each twelve-hour shift. Mostly I was running, fetching, pushing, hauling, lifting, carrying, and pulling. There were lots of opportunities to use my mind, but there was little time for it; the work required a Trojan's stamina and stopping to think only deterred me from completing all the tasks that were required. I was beginning to realize that the best way I could excel as a nurse would be to invest in a good pair of running shoes and a gym membership. I had to get in top physical shape for this line of work.

Nursing also required close attention to detail, quicksilver problem-solving abilities, and strict time management. Often, I fell short. Once, I increased the rate of a patient's IV, not even noticing that it was not properly connected, and fluid and medication had dripped into her slippers. On another occasion, on an ophthalmology floor, I reported that my patient's pupils were wide and unresponsive to light. Could he be having a stroke? Should I call for a neurology consult? When the nurses gathered at the nursing station stopped laughing, they told me that the patient's widened pupils were due to the drops the doctors instilled to dilate the pupils, a standard procedure prior to an eye examination.

At least I always tried to be empathetic. I had been taught that empathy was the most important quality a nurse had to offer. In fact, it was the hallmark of the professional nurse. However, in my case, some common sense and maturity would have helped, too.

One evening on an Oncology floor, a man with advanced stages of cancer silently ate his dinner. The news was on the TV, but he paid it no notice. The room was filled with flowers and boxes of unopened candy, but there was no family at his side. His disease was progressing rapidly, and at times he endured excruciating pain.

He pushed away his half-eaten dinner, leaned back against the pillows, and sighed deeply. I noted his "flat affect" and reminded myself to document that later in his chart in the "emotional/psychosocial" category. "Oh," he let out a long sigh. "What will be?" He shook his head and covered his face with his hands. "What will be?"

Finally, my chance to be empathetic had arrived. I pulled up a chair to his bedside.

"Tell me how you are feeling, sir. Are you perhaps worried that the cancer has spread?"

He looked up and noticed me. "No, my dear." He patted my arm. "This Mulroney government is ruining everything. Oh, for the Trudeau days. Now there was a leader!"

I HAD A tendency to take patients' reactions too personally. Toward the end of a busy evening on a Cardiology ward, I brought a plastic med cup of pills to a patient. I gave her the pills along with a glass of water with a bent straw in it.

"Which pills are these?" She sat up in bed to examine them.

"Please don't sit up yet, Mrs. Jones." I put my hand gently on her shoulder. "You have to lie down and keep that sand bag on your groin. You're at risk for bleeding after your angiogram."

"These aren't my pills." She took her glasses from the bedside table, shook them out, and put them on to examine what I was offering.

"Yes, they are," I insisted.

It was my last med round of the evening. I pushed the unwieldy metal wagon ahead of me like some pharmaceutical ice-cream vendor, dispensing a rainbow of pills, capsules, liquids, elixirs, and suppositories to thirty-six cardiac patients. I glanced at my watch. An hour to go and I still had ten more patients' pills to give out. Call bells were ringing. A mountain of uncompleted charts was heaped up at the nursing station.

"What are these pills?" she demanded.

"The blue one is your water pill, the white ones are digoxin for your heart rhythm. The little yellow football is for your blood pressure and the tiny white one, that's for your nerves."

I was going to need one for *my* nerves too, if she kept this up.

"That's not what my nerve pill looks like," she said.

"But Mrs. Jones, that's your Ativan. It's 1 mg of Ativan."

"Ativan is bigger than that. I know Ativan! Ativan is oval, not round. You're giving me the wrong pill."

"Here's the bottle. You can see for yourself what Ativan looks like. Here, have a new one," I offered.

"No, you're not going to give me anything. I want a different nurse. I know what you're up to. You want to knock me out so that I can't report you."

I was finished. My shift was almost over. I pushed the cart to the next bed.

WITHIN ONLY A few years, the trend in the nursing job market was completely reversed. The public's need for nurses was just as great as always, but now a new provincial government had been elected with the promise to pay for them. Suddenly, nurses could choose which hospital they wanted to work in. Attractive signing bonuses and educational benefits were offered. Almost every department in each hospital was advertising nursing positions. The only problem was that now, there was a nursing shortage. Enrolment in nursing was down and the previous "surplus" of nurses had forced many nurses to move to the United States to find work. Splashy newspaper advertisements and job fairs proliferated to try to lure them back to Ontario hospitals.

I applied for a job at a big downtown hospital. It was the same hospital where I had been a candystriper as a teenager, where I had once worked in the patient lending library as a summer job, and where I used to accompany my mother to appointments with her specialists for her various, mysterious ailments.

"A degree from the University of Toronto? Mmm." The nurse recruiter who reviewed my file looked pleased. Not many nurses had a university degree in 1986, and it was definitely the way of the future. In fact, nursing leaders were predicting that by the year 2000, all nurses at the bedside would have their degrees.

"Which specialty area do you prefer?" she asked. "We have openings everywhere."

I was hard-pressed to choose. I didn't have a particular loyalty to any specific organ, like the brain (neurology) or the heart (cardiology). At that moment, I happened to look out the window and saw a sign that had arrows pointing to the various departments in the hospital. There was Admitting, Radiology, and a sign that said Intensive Care Unit – the ICU – fourth floor. The reputation of ICU nurses was that they were the elite squad. To work there was an achievement many nurses aspired to attain. There, the patients were the sickest of the sick and the nurses wore serious green scrubs (which I thought might be more flattering to my fair complexion than the white or soft pastels I wore on the wards), stethoscopes slung around their necks, and got a lot of respect. As I stared at the letters, I sounded them out in my head and found myself hearing the words as "I see you," beckoning me to take on this challenge.

"ICU," I said. "I'd like to work in the intensive care unit."

"Normally, we prefer a nurse to have acquired at least a year of experience in one specialty area of acute care before progressing to critical care," the recruiter explained, noting my spotty employment history, "but we're desperate for staff in every department. I have so many openings to fill." She paused. "With your university degree, I'm sure you'd catch up in no time. You will have to go on a special course first, would you be agreeable to that? Tuition will be paid, plus your salary for eight weeks. In return, there will be a commitment from you to stay with us for at least a year and work in the Medical-Surgical ICU. The patients there have critical illnesses such as major surgeries or complicated medical problems – and we are now starting to perform lung and liver transplants. You will find it a very interesting place to work."

"Good, no problem. Where do I sign up?"

ROSEMARY MCCARTHY WAS the nurse manager of the Med-Surg ICU. She was short, round, and serene. It was calming to be in her presence, something I tried to be, whenever possible. She wore the same green scrubs that the staff nurses wore, and over that, a white lab coat. On her bookshelf she kept a graduation picture of herself in a navy blue cape, wearing a nursing cap – a high, starched one with a black velvet ribbon. To me, it looked ridiculous. I had learned that the cap was an obsolete symbol of the subservient role of nursing and of nurses' subordination to doctors – and practically everyone else. We had come a long way from those days.

For the first few weeks of my orientation to the intensive care unit, they buddied me with Frances. Only a year older than I, Frances was already an experienced ICU nurse who had acquired her "training" (as she called it), "back home" (as she referred to it), in a small town in New Brunswick. She had learned on-duty from nuns, who were nurses in the local Catholic hospital, but since there were no jobs available for nurses when she graduated, she left her hometown to seek work in Toronto.

Frances was patient and didn't seem to mind taking me on. *Orientation* was a good word for what we did together, because *dis*oriented was exactly what I was. Disoriented and discombobulated. The first thing she did was help me overcome my fear of the stopcock by giving me an unused arterial line set-up that I took home to practise with privately, in a strange-looking pantomime of drawing blood.

Frances watched me closely my first time drawing blood from a patient. I knew that if I didn't do it exactly right, the person could lose a lot of blood very rapidly. Litres of blood would pump out in few moments and if I wasn't fast enough, or didn't pay proper attention, the patient could hemorrhage and slip into unconsciousness. That degree of blood loss could lead to iatrogenic anemia, exsanguination, and death!

"Probably not," said Frances, "but it sure would make a mess."

AT THE START of every day shift in the ICU, the overhead fluorescent lights were turned on, one by one, as if to simulate sunlight and daybreak. However, I quickly realized that this was truly an illusion as there was very little natural light, and for most of these patients, there was no real sense of differentiation between day and night; they were sick around the clock.

In each room, the weary night nurses moved around the beds, finishing up their work and preparing to give report to the fresh

and well-rested incoming nurses who bounced into the room, energetic and eager to start their day. They would nod and listen to the
night nurses' report, wish them a "good night," and then start their
day with their own assessments of their patient. They would make
their own interpretations, adjust the plastic tubing and wires the
way they liked them, and take charge of the flow of fluids draining
in and draining out.

We started work at precisely 0715 hours when we went to our
assigned patient room and received report from the night nurse.
Since all the patients were critically ill and unstable, we were rarely
assigned more than one patient at a time. Each one required our
complete and constant attention.

Frances decided that I should take full responsibility for my
patient's care, and she would be there as backup, only if I needed
her. By then, I had completed the critical care course that the hospital had sent me on and was soon expected to be out on my own,
to have my own patient assignment, and do everything myself. I
was just about to start my initial assessment of my patient when
Laura, one of the other nurses who always worked with Frances,
came by to offer me advice.

"Don't panic. If there are green lines moving along on the
monitor and no alarms ringing, everything's okay, for now. Sit
down and have a coffee. Relax."

My stomach was churning. "I think I'll run to the washroom,
first, before we start."

"No. That's not allowed," Laura said sternly.

I was too stressed to notice the twinkle in her eye. "What? I
can't go?" I gasped.

"Of course, silly. Just kidding."

We were never supposed to leave a patient in the ICU unattended.

"NURSING ISN'T FOR everyone, don't you know," said Frances to
me as we sat in the staff lounge, eating our lunch. She said it
kindly. "You remind me of this girl in our class back home. She
had to run to the bathroom all the time, just like you, before

she gave an injection, before she changed a dressing. She dropped out of nursing and became a nun. Some people can't take the pressure, especially here in the ICU."

"I might very well turn out to be one of those people," I said grimly, "but I want the chance to find out."

"That's good on you!" she said.

I WORKED HARD to learn the routines, to stay on top of the hourly vital signs, to perform the ventilator checks, to give the medications on time, do the treatments, participate in team rounds, arrange for X-rays and ECGs, and assist with tests and procedures. There was something to do every minute. I noticed how Frances did not only the task at hand, but also two or three other things at the same time, all the while, preparing for upcoming tasks that she anticipated.

"Where did you do your training?" Frances asked me one day.

I was standing there, watching her draw a blood sample from my patient's arterial line. She flipped the stopcock to the right, attached a test tube, and then flipped the stopcock open to the left. As she waited for each tube to fill, she smoothed her patient's ruffled hair and checked his heart rhythm and blood pressure on the cardiac monitor. When the test tubes were full, she flushed the tubing, took a moment to hold up a tube of blood to the light to admire its bright redness – an indication of good oxygenation – and praised the patient for his progress. All the while, she was listening for my answer to her question.

"My training?" I was embarrassed by my university education, paid for by my parents. The other nurses in the ICU with their college diplomas were, in many cases, still paying back their student loans. Not only that, but they were the competent ones, and I was the disoriented and discombobulated one. I mumbled my answer.

"And where did you work before coming to the ICU?" Frances asked.

"Oh, here and there," I said. "A little of this and a little of that."

We started every shift by performing a head-to-toe assessment of our patient. "Head" meant to talk to the patient, but it felt awkward to talk to patients who couldn't talk back because of the tubes they had in their mouths or because they were sedated or unconscious. But I did as Frances had shown me. I approached the bed and greeted my patient who, on that first day, was a sixty-eight-year-old man, two days post-op major surgery to repair a ruptured aortic aneurysm.

"Hello, Mr. Stavakis. My name is Tilda and I'm your nurse today. Can you squeeze my hand? Can you give that a try?" Then I started to go through, in a systematic fashion, the tests of a patient's level of consciousness. First I checked his pupils with a flashlight to assess their reaction to light. I gave him simple commands, such as "Open your eyes" or "Wiggle your toes." When he passed those tests, I proceeded to the higher cortical-level functioning tests to determine if he was oriented to person, place, and time. I checked his reflexes, handgrips, and his response to painful stimuli such as pressing on his nail beds and rubbing his sternum.

"When a patient is fully conscious, you don't have to go through *all* the tests, Tilda." Frances gave me a nudge and whispered in my ear. "Move on."

Of course.

I turned my attention to auscultation of the patient's heart and lungs with my stethoscope, and then assessed the condition of his skin and incision. I checked all the equipment and examined his heartbeats on the monitor and measured each one with my brand-new pair of calipers. I palpated his stomach, measured the amount of urine in the Foley catheter, and peeked under the sheets. *No problems there. Well,* I congratulated myself, *so far, so good. I might make it here, after all!*

After I finished my assessment, I decided to say something to my patient that I had heard Frances say to her patients. Sweet words that were the essence of nursing itself. I silently praised myself that here I was, ready to say them to a patient, and so soon in my career as a critical care nurse.

"Mr. Stavakis? I'm your nurse and I'll take good care of you. You don't have anything to worry about because I will be with you all day. I will take care of all your needs and make sure that you're comfortable. Okay, Mr. Stavakis?" He squeezed my

hand in agreement (what choice did he have?) and gave a weak
smile around the tube in his mouth, a tube that went into his throat
and down into his lungs.

Maybe if I said the words and went through the motions, that
feeling of confidence, of being the capable ICU nurse that I dreamed
of being, would follow? I had read somewhere that orthodox Jews
advised skeptics to go through the actions of keeping kosher, light-
ing the candles and observing the Sabbath – even if they didn't yet
fully believe: do the deed and the faith would surely follow. But
even as I performed the correct actions, so much of the complex
information that I was learning in the ICU remained a bombard-
ment of separate, concrete items. I still couldn't put the whole
picture together. I tried to imagine the complicated drugs I was
giving and what each one was doing. This one is contracting
the heart, this one is expanding the lungs, this one is carrying the
oxygen molecule, I told myself. But the images were like cartoon
pictures in my mind.

As we came to the end of the long twelve-hour shift, I emptied
all my patient's drains and measured their contents, changed the
IV bags, tallied my fluid balance, made my final notes in the chart,
smoothed the bedsheets and pillows, made sure Mr. Stavakis was
comfortable, and prepared to give report to the night nurse. By
then it was evening and so I dimmed the lights in my patient's room
to create a peaceful atmosphere at the end of the day.

Frances said, "You're doing great, Tilda."

I beamed. Yet I was exhausted from the heightened state of
alertness I had been in all day, listening for and responding to the
ringing of alarms. As I walked out the door, I felt the weight of
responsibility unfurl from my shoulders, as physical a sensation as
shedding a heavy winter coat on a spring day.

MR. STAVAKIS DETERIORATED during the night. The next morning
when I came in I saw that his colour was dusky and he was sweaty
and restless. He wasn't responding to my questions; he didn't
squeeze my hand. I tried to ignore what I saw and pretend it wasn't
happening. I didn't feel ready to cope with an unstable patient.

Frances came over. She took a look at my patient and her eyes
went straight to his chest. She studied the rise and fall of each
breath for a few moments and pointed out to me that the two sides
were not symmetrical. "How long have his saturations been in the
80s?" She glanced at the monitor. "Look how fast he's breathing."
She called for a bag of ice upon which to place the sample of arterial blood that she was busy drawing for testing of his gases. "He
may have blown a pneumothorax." I knew that meant a possible
collapse of the lung. Frances cranked up the ventilator to deliver
100 per cent oxygen but the patient's saturations kept falling – they
were now down to 78 per cent – and then grabbed the oxygen bag
off the wall and began ventilating him herself, with fast, strong
pumps of the bag. She unwound her stethoscope from around her
neck and listened to the patient's chest. She suctioned his lungs,
listened again to both sides of his chest, and then looked up to me.
"There's no air moving in there."

She yelled out, "I need help in here!" and then told the ward
clerk to page for a chest X-ray and call for the doctor and the respiratory technician to come immediately – "STAT."

All these events took place in a matter of moments. I stood watching and wondering what it was that I was supposed to be doing.

"He needs another IV line. Start one in his antecubital space,"
Frances said. "Use a large bore needle – at least an 18 gauge – and
run it with normal saline at 50 cc an hour."

Quickly, I found the equipment I needed. The old man's veins
looked so easy to get, but as soon as I stuck the needle in, the vein
collapsed and I watched in horror as a big blue lump popped up
like a plum under his skin.

"Elderly veins can be tricky," Frances whispered from across the
bed. She came over to my side and slid the needle into another vein
on the patient's arm, taped it up, and pushed the clamp open to let
the fluid flow in, all in a matter of seconds. "We got it," she said.

Frances went out to the waiting room to bring the patient's wife
to her husband's bedside. "He's hanging in there," Frances assured
her. Both Mrs. Stavakis and I breathed a sigh of relief.

But the patient worsened as the day went on. He became agi-
tated and delirious. We put in a chest tube but his oxygenation still

kept falling, and once again, Frances went back out to the waiting room to bring the wife in. Frances, together with Dr. Daniel Huizinga, one of the staff physicians of the ICU, explained that her husband's condition had worsened and he was now very critical. We would have to give him medication that had a drastic side effect. It would render him unable to move.

"Paralyzed," Dr. Huizinga explained, in his curt but not unkind manner. "It's a temporary measure. We have to paralyze him so that we can get more oxygen into his cells. Pavulon is the neuromuscular blocking agent that we use to decrease his metabolic requirements."

"What?" cried the wife in alarm. "Paralyzed?"

Mrs. Stavakis watched in horror as her husband gasped for air. She did not have to be convinced that something had to be done immediately, but this? A drug-induced paralysis? It must have sounded like a nightmare to her.

"We sometimes paralyze patients, Mrs. Stavakis, for a short time," Frances said, putting her arm around her. She made paralysis sound like a desirable thing, perhaps even a pleasant experience. "It will probably be for only a few days, and then we will stop it and he will move again and wake up. It will make him more comfortable with the breathing tube. See how he's fighting the ventilator? Right now he's not getting the oxygen he needs. This drug will help him."

Frances and I prepared the infusion of the paralyzing drug, and after the doctor administered the first dose, it was up to me to continue it and monitor the patient closely. Frances reminded the resident not to forget to order sedation, too.

"Sometimes the doctors overlook the fact that the patient might still be wide awake," Frances explained to me. "Paralysis without sedation is cruel. Can you imagine you can't move, but you're mentally intact inside? It's called 'locked-in' syndrome and it's my biggest fear. Pavulon is a scary drug, but it really helps patients. Some nurses even call it Vitamin P."

BEFORE SETTING ME loose on my own, Frances kept a close eye on me and made sure I had gone through all the important experiences – that I had transferred a patient to the floor, received a fresh post-op patient, cared for a lung transplant and a liver transplant. She made sure I had given and received report to and from the other nurses and that I knew how to make a concise presentation of my patient to the team during morning rounds.

"You need practice helping the doctors with procedures," she said on one of my last few days of orientation to the ICU under her supervision. "Go give that new resident a hand putting in a pulmonary artery catheter. He doesn't know his ass from his elbow."

Frances came to check on us later and brought a few extra catheters and sterile green towels, because he was having difficulty cannulating the vein that led into the artery. "Give him these," she said, tossing them on to the bed for me to hand to him. "Looks like he might need a few tries." She adjusted the height of the table where he was working and lowered the bed to make our work more comfortable. "Body mechanics can make such a difference," she said. "We have to protect our backs."

Justine, another nurse who seemed to be a regular part of Frances and Laura's group, showed up at the door to see how the procedure was coming along. She pretended to take aim with an imaginary dart and shot it into the room, ostensibly directly into the patient's internal jugular vein.

"Bull's eye!" she crowed. "I could get that line in from here."

WORKING IN THE ICU reminded me of an animated short from the National Film Board I had seen as a child in school. It started with a boy rowing a boat on a lake. Then it zeroed in on a mosquito stinging the boy's arm. Down the camera went from the skin, into the layers of epidermis, then into the blood cells, the nucleus of the atom, the electrons and protons. Then, zoom, the camera went back out to the boy, the boat, the lake, the country, the world, the galaxy, and the universe. That's how I felt: tossed between the stopcock and the complicated world of the ICU; zooming in between drawing blood from an artery and helping to withdraw life support on someone's dying mother.

"You'll get the hang of it," said Frances. "You'll figure out what's big and what's small, what's urgent and what can wait. There are some nurses whose main goal is to settle the patient, make them look nice, tidy up the room, so they can sit down and read a magazine. I have a feeling you're not like one of those."

IT WAS THE last morning that I would be buddied with Frances. My orientation was over.

"Are you okay?" she asked. "You look a little green."

"Yeah, fine, thanks." I peered down into my coffee cup to avoid her eyes.

The truth was, I was having problems sleeping, problems getting up in the morning, and still, the constant churning in my intestines.

"Are you sure nothing's wrong?"

"Not a thing!"

"Well, that's good, because we're going to have a busy day today. A patient came in during the night and she's really sick."

I listened to report from the night nurse.

"Andrea . . . a twenty-three-year-old . . . just graduated from law school. She and her husband were scuba diving in Lake Simcoe and she was caught in a strong undertow. She panicked and rose to the surface too quickly. She dislodged her mask and oxygen tank and aspirated a lot of cold lake water. Too bad they weren't in the ocean, seawater would have been a lot less damaging to her lungs, poor thing."

The patient's healthy, muscular arms were a startling sight against the white sheets, the cage-like bed with its metal rails, and the bottles and tubes attached to her body. I squinted at her and tried to imagine her in jeans, her wedding dress, or a wetsuit, anything but the faded blue hospital gown she had on over her naked body. As I recorded her vital signs, I noticed some occasional but worrisome beats on the cardiac monitor upon which a teddy bear presided as a sentinel. Around one side of her bed, machines and equipment huddled like a team of robotic consultants. A group of real consultants huddled on the other side.

On the patient's bedside table was a clipboard. I knew how private and intimate were the notes that patients wrote and had no choice but to leave them out in public for all to see. I couldn't help but read the shaky scrawl that trailed off the side of the page:

Don't blame yourself. I came up too fast. You gave me your O_2.

On another page, *How sick am I?* was followed by, *Go easy on Mom and Dad. Edit a bit. I Love you.*

She must have written those notes during the night when she first came in and since then had deteriorated fast. Now she was unconscious, probably due to air bubbles, called emboli, in her brain.

"No eye opening, no following commands, no response to deep pain, no response to voice," I reported to Frances.

No response to the Mozart symphony on the radio that her husband had placed beside her. No response to his touch, no awareness of his presence when he came in the room.

"She'll probably need a CT scan of her head," said Frances, planning the day ahead. "Make sure that all the alarms are on. She's having some premature ventricular beats – see there goes one – but right now let's wash her hair."

I looked at her, surprised that the patient's appearance would be a priority now.

"I know she's sick," Frances said. "But whether she makes it or not, I'm sure she'd want to look nice for her husband when he comes in."

Frances prepared syringes of various emergency drugs and lined them up along the counter like ammunition. "Just in case," she explained. "I don't have a great feeling about her."

As the day went on, I stayed focused on the tasks at hand, but all of a sudden, late in the afternoon, while Andrea's husband was visiting, something made Frances glance up at the cardiac monitor, seconds before the alarm even had a chance to sound. "She's gone into V-tach! Get the crash cart!" she shouted at me.

Ventricular tachycardia! Here it was, the real thing! If I didn't act fast, it could lead to ventricular fibrillation!

Frances pulled the husband out of the way as the room quickly filled with people. He shrank back against the wall. I thought of reaching out to him, but didn't. I didn't know what to say, anyway.

Laura, Justine, and two other nurses, Tracy and Nicole, appeared out of nowhere and they helped Frances lift Andrea and place a hard board under her back. With that board now in place, Frances climbed up onto the bed and started doing vigorous chest compressions while Nicole hooked up the patient to the defibrillator to prepare for shocking her with electricity to get her heart going again.

Tracy injected an ampoule of epinephrine into an IV that went directly into Andrea's heart.

Justine thrust her fingers into the patient's groin to feel for a pulse. Nothing. She nodded at Frances to resume compressions.

Within a few moments, a doctor arrived on the scene and took over directing the resuscitation efforts that the nurses had already begun.

I stood frozen to the spot. Unable to move. Unable to think. Unable to recall accurately even one of the resuscitation logarithms I thought I had memorized: *If the victim is without a pulse and unresponsive, then shock with 200 joules. If patient does not convert to sinus rhythm, repeat shock with 300 joules.* Or was it 360?

"Here," said Tracy, shoving the arrest report at me. "Record the arrest."

How could she have known? Paper and pen had always been my refuge.

THEY MANAGED TO bring Andrea back. Meanwhile, I went to the med room to prepare a drip of a powerful new drug called amiodarone, which we were going to use to try to stabilize Andrea's still-erratic heart rhythm. It was taking me a long time to get the medication ready. Six glass vials were lined up on the counter and I was struggling to crack them open – already, I had a cut in my thumb from the first one, which had shattered in my hands.

"Leave that for a moment," said Frances. "Do you want to know the first thing you do in an arrest? Take a deep breath. Then take the pulse. Your own, I mean. Then, take the patient's. Do everything slowly. Don't run for anything. Don't let anything or anyone rush you. Ever." She turned to go back to Andrea's room. "By the way, there's a trick to those vials. Let me show you. They break with light pressure. You can't break them if you push too hard."

Easy, not hard. Light, not heavy. Slow, not fast. Relaxed, not rushed. How was I going to learn all this?

Later that day, Andrea arrested again and that time, she didn't make it, which was the way Frances put it gently to the husband. He knew, but needed to be told. He slumped into Frances's arms and sobbed in the comfort and safety she offered. I wanted to enfold myself in there, too. Frances's arms were wide and strong enough for a lot of sorrow and I knew she could handle his and mine, too, and still be intact herself.

Andrea's death affected a lot of the nurses who identified with someone so young and newly married, someone so full of life and promise. Some stopped by to console the family, to take one last look at her lovely body lying in the bed, still attached to the machines that had now fallen silent and useless, disconnected from the electrical outlets, their screens gone blank. Some of the nurses even cried, and I could see that their tears touched the family. The family probably knew that the nurses couldn't always cry over their patients, so that when they did, they were especially grateful that their grief was shared.

I pulled myself away. It was the end of my shift and the others would carry on. They would wash Andrea's body and prepare it for the morgue. They would tidy up the room and soon it would look like no one had ever been there. It would be made ready for the next patient.

I hung up my lab coat and walked out the door. I was completely spent. I had nothing more to give. Many hours had gone by, but I had no sense of the passage of a day; it was just a jumble of events and experiences to be sorted out later. I wondered if I had enough steam to get myself home, take a shower, and fall into bed.

When I stepped out into the cold, rainy evening, the cool mist felt good on my face. My boyfriend was waiting for me in his warm car with the engine running and I slid in beside him.

"So, how did it go?" Ivan asked, but I was at a loss how to answer.

We drove in silence, but when we got home, I pulled him into my bedroom. Suddenly, I was seized with the desire to have sex, to make love all night, to chase death out of my body.

3

THE VEIN, THE ARTERY, AND BEYOND

I t got better.

Like an actress, I memorized my lines; like a dancer I learned the steps.

"How's the patient doing?" the doctors would ask when they breezed into the room, and I could rattle off all the numbers they wanted to hear: "Pulmonary artery pressure 38 over 22; wedge pressure 16; mean arterial pressure 72 to 78; sinus rhythm 110; blood pressure 118 on 72; pressure support of 20 with a rate of 8 at 80 per cent; positive end expiratory pressure 7.5. Blood gases 7.34, 41, 88, and 22. Urine output 30 to 50 cc per hour."

The more numbers, the better!

(I made sure to first find out the specialty of the consultant I was talking to, so that I would not uselessly go into details about the patient's kidney function to the cardiologist, or start telling the thoracic surgeon about the liver enzymes. They weren't interested, anyway.)

The chaotic noise of the ICU began to make sense to me. The ringing of the alarms was no longer a maddening cacophony,

creating a constant state of expectation in my mind. I could differentiate between the ominous gongs of the ventilator, the melodious
chimes of the IV pump, the insistent buzz of the cardiac monitor.
Most importantly, when an alarm went off, I checked the patient,
then the equipment.

It was a serious place, and I appreciated the atmosphere of
scholarly inquiry and the dedication to erudition and research.
Late one night we had to summon the security guard to unlock the
library in order for a resident to retrieve a back issue of the *Journal
of Immunological Disorders* that had an article about an obscure
disease of one of our patients. It was exciting to work in a place
where the pursuit of knowledge could be a 911 emergency. And
yes, I mastered the arterial stopcock and was soon flipping it right
and left, drawing blood, monitoring the blood pressure, and trou-
bleshooting the equipment.

I started to relax and even began to look forward to going
to work.

The ICU had twenty beds and each nurse was assigned to one
patient. Sometimes we doubled up if a patient was stable enough to
do so. Sometimes, even when the patient wasn't stable enough, if
staffing was short, we had no choice but to double up. At times, that
was a concern.

On each shift there was a nurse in charge plus an assistant nurse,
so there were always twenty-two nurses on any given shift, day or
night. We all worked twelve-hour day or night shifts, starting in
the morning at 0715 hours and finishing at 1915 hours, when the
night shift nurses came in to relieve us. They would then work
all night until 0715 hours the next morning.

A small group of us – Frances, Tracy, Nicole, Laura, Justine,
and I – worked together and soon came to be dubbed "Laura's
Line." Possibly it was because of the easy alliteration of the Ls, but
more likely it was due to Laura's commanding presence, formidable intelligence, and consummate skills. Her sassy attitude and
high jinks became legendary, too.

Although each nurse was extraordinary in her own way, Laura
was arguably the best nurse of all. She was the nurse you would
want in any situation, good or bad. As rude and irreverent as she

was privately, behind closed doors, she was equally respectful and kind, dedicated and compassionate to patients and their families in person.

She made everything she did seem effortless. I remember her running off one day to help with a patient who was arresting. When she came back an hour later, she looked not in the least bit flushed or exhilarated after saving someone's life. She looked distant, even a little bored, as if she was in need of a coffee to perk her up.

On another occasion, Laura admitted a patient, examined him, and went ahead and wrote all the doctor's orders, including medications, X-rays, and tests. Later, when the doctor came to admit the patient, he was taken aback that everything was already ordered, but he agreed with everything she had done. He even admitted that Laura had picked up on things that he hadn't noticed himself. He co-signed the orders she had written.

We all wondered if one day she would go too far.

The schedule we worked, when I think of it today, was so gruelling, so unhealthy, and fundamentally insane, I wonder now how we managed to do it. On Monday, Tuesday, and Wednesday we worked three nights in a row. Then we came back on Saturday and Sunday for day shifts, then returned on Wednesday, Thursday, and Friday. Then we were off that weekend and back again on Monday and Tuesday for days. Then we worked four nights in a row, from Thursday to Sunday night. By Monday morning, the group of us planned to go out for breakfast, but more often than not, by the time that fourth morning came around, we felt too cranky and out of sorts and cancelled it. Each of us then staggered home to sleep the day away. We'd lounge around sluggishly for a few days, recovering from work and preparing to go back. We followed this schedule for years.

Some of us still do.

There was a lot of death in the ICU, but for the first few months, Rosemary, the nurse manager, took care not to assign me very sick or dying patients. She probably did this because of the reputation I was developing – Laura kept telling everyone that I was "too sensitive" and predicted I wouldn't last long in the ICU. Perhaps

Rosemary was also protecting the patients from a nurse who was still gaining clinical skills in caring for stable patients, but who didn't yet have the ability to handle complex and delicate situations.

If we could arrange it, the group of us tried to take our morning break at the same time. We went to the cafeteria together in the elevator, except for Laura, who took a circuitous route around the back of the hospital and down the stairs. She avoided walking past the waiting room with its smell of tension and sweat, full of families waiting and worrying. She claimed the families begrudged us taking breaks.

"I never tell them I'm going for breakfast. I say that I'm going to a meeting. Their loved one's life is in the balance, and they think all we care about is whether to have the pancakes or the French toast."

But I believe she couldn't bear to face their eyes, which scanned ours for scraps of hopeful news. She needed that separation.

We always said we wouldn't talk about our patients – we told each other we needed a break from it all – but we always did, and it was usually Laura who started off.

"I have Mrs. Wong," she said one morning. She was careful to keep her voice low to ensure confidentiality. "She's a thirty-eight-year-old Chinese woman who was found collapsed in the supermarket yesterday evening. She's unresponsive but the neuro-surgeons are in there now examining her to see if she's operable or not. Anyway, Mrs. Wong had a massive cerebral bleed and is likely going to be declared brain dead soon. Then the *vultures* – I mean the *surgeons* – will flock down for her organs, if the family agrees."

I watched Laura's pretty face, its indignant expression and fine, delicate features. Her attractive appearance was so at odds with the harshness of this story. It seemed that none of this shocking information stopped Laura from enjoying her coffee and toasted English muffin with peanut butter. But then, I asked myself, why should it? She has to eat breakfast. Who would want a hungry nurse?

I had passed Mrs. Wong's room earlier that morning and guessed now that the two teenagers I had noticed standing outside her door must be her children. The boy wearing a denim jacket and an absent expression must be around sixteen or so. The girl in a school uniform with a tiny knapsack on her back looked about twelve.

"One day they have a mother, and the next day they don't?" I said.

"Well, it's not over yet. She might make it, if the bleed is localized, but it's a slim chance," said Laura with a grim expression.

She sounded like she was the patient's doctor, not nurse. But what was a doctor? What was a nurse? These roles all seemed to be changing, especially in the ICU.

So, Mrs. Wong is hovering, I thought, suspended, neither here nor there, in such an uncertain place: neither dead nor alive. No wonder the children's bewildered eyes.

"What really got to me," Laura went on, "was when I opened the locker where we stored her personal belongings. I pulled out plastic shopping bags full of grapes and rice and bok choy and gave them to the kids to take home. Imagine, a mother's last actions, buying food for her family."

"Was Mrs. Wong previously healthy, no past medical history?" Tracy asked as she munched on her signature bacon, cream cheese, jam, and ketchup sandwich — salty, creamy, sweet, and sour.

By her wry smile I knew a joke was coming.

"Yeah, aren't they all?" retorted Laura. "They're all healthy before they get sick."

"Then something must have gone *tewibbly wong*," said Tracy.

As we were going up in the elevator, we stood in front of two surgical residents and we couldn't help but overhear their conversation.

". . . What a trip that was, harvesting the heart! But by the time I scrubbed and got in there, it was too late, they'd lost perfusion. They opened her up after things got really bad, but by then they couldn't get control. . . . Man, when things go wrong, they go really wrong."

"*Weally, weally wong*," Tracy whispered and we burst out of the elevator laughing our heads off.

How long could I remain sad about everything? I asked myself. I relished the relief that laughing brought. Besides, I couldn't be part of this group and always be standing off to the side, always the sober, observing one, could I? These nurses found laughs in everything. Even if something wasn't funny, they made it so. I was trying to hold in my mind simultaneously all the contradictions of my new work – respect and irreverence, humour and sadness, hope and despair, compassion and detachment.

"What's so funny?" Ivan asked me when I told him about some of the amusing things that happened at work. "I can't understand how you guys can laugh so much. It sounds pretty sad to me."

I did have a lot of fun at work. What was stranger still was that the sicker the patients – the more unstable they were, the worse their conditions – the more fun we had, and the more we laughed – always behind closed doors. How could that be possible and at the same time be true that we were kind and caring nurses? We had all chosen nursing as our life's work, and our specialty, critical care, was the business of suffering and sorrow. Even if the outcome was good, there was still a great deal of suffering along the way.

I had to laugh. Laughing with the nurses assuaged a despair that had lodged tenaciously in me for many years. It was a despair that I tried to keep secret, yet friends told me they saw it ingrained in my face, in the slope of my shoulders, in the droopiness of my eyes.

GRADUALLY, ROSEMARY BEGAN to assign me more challenging patients. For the most part, I coped with whatever came up, but I noticed an uncanny phenomenon that I never figured out. Whenever I was getting out of my depth, or not sure about something, one of them – Laura, Frances, Nicole, Tracy, or Justine – suddenly appeared. They seemed to know just what was needed, usually without asking me. They each had their own patients and were busy too; how did they know I needed help?

A lot of patients died in the ICU, but so far since my orientation with Frances, no one directly under my care had died.

My introduction to death came from one of my favourite night nurses. Valerie was a dark black woman from St. Lucia who had lived in England for many years. She could be intimidating because, while she carried herself with the air of sophistication and elegance like the royalty of her adopted country, she was at the same time blunt in her way of communicating. She came to work with a briefcase that she gripped in a hand that was always beautifully manicured with scarlet or fuchsia fingernail polish. In that briefcase she kept handwritten manuscripts of Victorian mysteries that she worked on downstairs in the dimly lit cafeteria during her break.

"Your patient is dead," she said by way of greeting as I walked in to start my shift. She ripped off a strip of heavy-duty cloth tape from her table, rolled it up into a ball, and tossed it into the wastebasket. On it she had jotted her "nag list." This was what she called her list of point-form notes of concerns she had about her patient and issues she had wanted to raise with the doctor during the night. They were obviously no longer relevant.

"What ventilator settings is he on?" I asked.

"I told you, Tilda, he's dead."

"Meds? IVs?"

"No meds. He's dead. Got that?"

But there was a person in the bed and the equipment was running; green lines marched across the cardiac monitor. From where I sat with Valerie, I could see that the patient, a young man, was in a normal sinus heart rhythm, which meant that his heart was functioning properly. The ventilator was pumping air into his lungs, which were rising and falling, and a steady drip of urine flowed into the urometer. These were all the vital signs of life, as I had learned them.

"I'm not too sure what you mean by dead," I ventured.

"Two staff doctors have declared him brain dead, legally and medically. The family just left and they have refused organ donation. All you have to do now is disconnect everything, wrap him up, and send the body to the morgue. If you don't get another admission, you'll have an easy day. You can float around and help the others."

"Please, Valerie, I don't understand. Surely he's not dead." *He looks great.* "I want to get this right. I can't disconnect life support on a man like this."

"I know, it's very sad. He's a young man, only thirty-six. Seems he was having sexual intercourse with his wife and suddenly, in the middle, had a heart attack. Tragic. But don't worry, Tilda, you can't do anything wrong, because he's dead."

"But . . ."

"Read the doctor's report of brain death yourself. Pupils fixed and dilated, absent reflexes, and a failed apnea test. It's all there. You'll be out of a job now," she said.

For a moment, I thought she meant I would lose my licence.

"Need a hand?" asked Tracy, her tall, lanky form suddenly appearing at the doorway.

AS I BEGAN to be assigned to more and more complicated cases I could see the others trusted me and so I began to trust myself. But then, one day, something happened that made me think of giving up. If it hadn't been for the support of my group – Laura's Line – I might have.

"How was your night, Casey?" I asked as I came into the room one morning.

She was a heavy-set, grey-haired older nurse who worked her fair share of nights. She always complained that she was tired, but it was hard to believe her because she spoke with such verve, rarely went on a break, and never took shortcuts with patient care. She always gave a colourful and entertaining report, and I got ready to listen to it.

"A-OK. I've been flying on cruise control, but I'm glad you're here, Tilda. I'm really beat."

Casey had already changed out of her uniform and into her street clothes. This was clearly going to be a straightforward report. A cut to the chase.

"She looks good, Casey," I said, glancing over at a tiny white-haired lady in the bed. She had an oxygen mask on her face and it was on maximum flow. Her breathing was rapid and shallow, but she looked well taken care of and perfectly aligned in the bed. The covers were smooth and the room orderly.

"Grab a chair, darling, and I'll give you the scoop. Mrs. Templeton is an eighty-six-year-old woman who lives at home with her grown-up son. Congestive heart failure, emphysema, and now pneumonia. She's been trying to die for a few days, but he won't let her. He wants her intubated and ventilated, the whole nine yards. We're treating him, not her. Anyway, she was stable during most of the night. At one point she was trying to climb out of bed and pulling at her tubes, so I had to restrain her and give her a whiff of sedation. Anyway, I've got her all buffed, puffed, and fluffed for you. Make sure you grab a coffee before the charming son comes in. He's been here all night and apparently stays all the livelong day, too, if you let him. He'll be in here soon, breathing down your neck, asking you a million questions. Doesn't believe that visiting hours apply to him. Well, that's the story, that's the glory."

"Maybe someone should have talked to Mrs. Templeton before she got so sick, when she could still express her wishes," I said, thinking out loud.

"Woulda, shoulda, coulda – do you ever watch *Judge Judy*? – oh well, it's too late now."

She pulled her knitted poncho on over her head. "I'm outta here."

"Thanks, Casey. Good night. Sleep well. See you tonight."

I began to go through the chart for a more comprehensive medical history. When I looked up, I saw a tall man glaring down at me through thick glasses. For someone who had likely slept overnight on a couch in the hospital waiting room, he was immaculately groomed and dressed. His plaid shirt was tucked tightly into dark trousers that rode up high on his waist, cinched tightly with a leather belt.

"Who is my mother's nurse today? Is it you?"

"Yes," I said and introduced myself.

"Are you aware of Mother's condition?"

"To be honest, I've just started my shift. I'm about to start my initial assessment."

"I'll just wait here while you do that and then you can tell me what's what."

I wasn't used to having an audience, much less a likely critic of my work. It made me uncomfortable to perform my head-to-toe assessment under his watch. Some nurses made family members wait outside until they were finished their work, but I was afraid to ask him to leave.

"She's struggling with her breathing and very weak, but her blood pressure is good," I told him afterwards. "She has a fever, but we hope that the antibiotics will take effect soon and she won't need to be intubated and go on the ventilator."

"Well, whatever she needs, she should have. She's a fighter. We want everything done to save her life."

"You know, Mr. Templeton, the doctors and nurses – plus the rest of the team – would like to have a meeting to talk with you about the situation," I said gently. "In the event of –"

He cut me off with a scowl. "I know what you're getting at, and there is nothing to talk about."

By then, a crowd had gathered in my patient's room. Dr. David Bristol, one of the staff physicians, and Dr. Jessica Leung, the senior ICU fellow, accompanied by the residents under her supervision, along with Rosemary, the pharmacist, and respiratory therapists and other nurses who were able to attend, arrived for morning rounds.

"Mr. Templeton," I said to him, "the team is here to discuss your mother's case. She's stable and in no immediate danger. Would you like to go to the waiting room?"

He scrutinized me with hostile eyes and folded his coat over his arm. "I want Mother looked after immediately. I'll wait just outside the room. I'm not going anywhere. I have a number of questions for the doctor." He didn't leave right away, however, but fussed with his mother's pillows and blankets for a few minutes more before going out the door to stand in the hallway.

Justine had just finished transferring her patient to the ward and came over to join us on rounds. Short and pretty with flaming red hair pulled back in a ponytail, she was oblivious of her attractiveness, yet always highly aware of her intelligence and sharp wit, which she could use like a weapon at times. Justine was our union representative, and we knew that our concerns were well taken care of. Over her loose-fitting ICU scrubs, she wore a baggy white sweatshirt emblazoned with "Nurses Care But It's Not in the

Budget" in red letters. Purple socks, running shoes, and earrings in the shape of tiny flowerpots, finished off her get-up. She stood with her hands on her hips, watching the son tend to his mother before he left.

"What's with this guy? He needs to get a life. Is he still on the breast?" She tried to whisper, but I think Justine was constitutionally incapable of lowering her voice. Her *sotto voce* was heard by other members of the team, who tittered at her comments.

"Shh," I hissed at her, but couldn't help but laugh a little, too.

"In the absence of advance directives from the patient herself, and given the inability of the patient to speak on her own behalf, due to her decreased level of consciousness," Dr. Bristol was saying, "we will be advised of the patient's wishes by proxy. The son is her substitute decision maker and will represent her wishes. Has he been spoken to?"

He had been, by me, and I volunteered what I knew.

"He wants everything done. She is to be a full code – inotropes, intubation, cardiac compressions, and defibrillation – in the event of an arrest. Whether those are his or his mother's wishes, I can't be sure."

"Well, continue then we must. It would be a shame to intubate her as she'll be difficult to wean off the ventilator, but it doesn't look like we can hold off much longer," Dr. Bristol added, as he glanced at the deteriorating numbers and failing lab values recorded on the flow sheet. "Her work of breathing is considerable." He paused. "Sometimes it's easier not to start things at all than to withdraw them later," he mused.

Mr. Templeton confronted us in the hall as we came out of the room. "I want to understand." The team moved on with Dr. Bristol at the head, but Dr. Leung stayed behind to answer Mr. Templeton's questions.

"The problem is her lungs," he said. "What if I sit with her and remind her to breathe, won't that help? What about the pneumonia? Is it just in her lungs or is it anywhere else, too?"

"Yes, her respiratory status is the primary system affected." Dr. Leung spoke slowly and carefully, to avoid misinterpretation. "But she is frail and debilitated and eighty-six years old, with a chronic, irreversible disease. She doesn't have the recuperative powers of –"

"She's eighty-five. Who said she was eighty-six? I want that corrected."

I came forward and assured him it would be.

Later that day, during the shorter early evening team rounds, Dr. Leung got right to the point.

"The nurse and I spoke again with the son about withdrawing care and he was –"

Dr. Bristol interrupted her. "We never withdraw care. In certain circumstances we may withdraw *treatment*, but never *care*."

"You're right," she agreed.

I looked at him with huge respect. I loved working in a place where words mattered.

"WHAT ARE YOU giving her?" Mr. Templeton jumped when he saw me drawing up medication in a syringe.

"A small dose of morphine. Your mother's breathing is laboured and she's in respiratory distress. It will make her more comfortable."

"No, I don't want her to have it. She won't be able to fight. It will make her too groggy and she won't recognize me. No, I don't want her to have morphine or any sedation. Nurse, why are there bubbles in the IV tubing? What about that moisture in her oxygen mask?"

I flicked the bubbles out of the tubing and wiped out the condensation from his mother's breathing mask.

One of the junior residents came to tell Mr. Templeton that she was going to put in a special intravenous line called a pulmonary artery catheter. Its purpose was to measure the various pressures in the chambers of the heart. The son looked pleased with this plan, even after hearing that there were risks involved, such as blood clots, air emboli, and infection. He glanced over at me, as if vindicated.

MRS. TEMPLETON WAS restless, flailing her arms about in the bed as the doctor tried to insert the line into a deep vein in her neck.

"You're going to have to tie her arms down," the resident said in frustration. "I can't get this line in with her moving all over the place."

Maybe she's trying to tell us something.

"Maybe she's trying to . . ." I started to say, and then stopped myself.

Soon there was blood all over the bed and clots hanging off the doctor's gloved fingers. The patient will need a blood transfusion after this, I thought. The doctor carelessly squirted blood from a syringe in the general direction of the wastebasket, spraying it out in all directions, dangerously close to me, where I stood at the side of the bed.

"Hey, watch out," I said, stepping back.

"Sorry. Did I get you?"

"Have you done this procedure before?"

"Once."

"What are we trying to accomplish here?" I asked, knowing I might be getting on her nerves. She had a job to do and I was distracting her with my questions.

"We need more information about her right and left chambers so that we can differentiate between pulmonary edema and possible cardiac failure. Fluid management will be guided –"

"I know what the textbook says, but do you think we should be doing it? It seems kind of, well . . . cruel. She clearly doesn't want it." I hated having to hold down Mrs. Templeton's frail arms as she struggled to get away from what must have felt like an assault.

"It's hard to say for sure. She can't tell us. Her son is the next of kin."

I helped the doctor with the line insertion.

For Mrs. Templeton, I could not fathom how there could be any benefit in performing this painful, invasive, and risky procedure, other than academic. Sure, a more exact diagnosis could be made and medications adjusted accordingly, but I did not believe that the outcome would be any different. Perhaps the only good that could come of it was that the resident was gaining much-needed practice

that would one day benefit other patients. How else could I continue restraining her arms and offering her useless, reassuring
words, as she struggled to get away from what we were doing to
her, if I didn't rationalize it in some way or another?

It made me recall a night shift I worked once on a geriatric floor
in another hospital. A patient had died and the porters hadn't yet
arrived with the gurney to transfer the body to the morgue. As I
passed by the dead patient's closed room later in the night, I
noticed a light under the door. That was strange. I opened the door
to find the medical resident and his intern putting in a central line
in the corpse. In a second the expression on their faces flared from
guilty to self-righteous.

"Dean has to learn this procedure," the resident explained.
"He'll be a resident in a few months and has never put in a central
line. He has to learn. Isn't it better to practise on a dead patient
than on a live one?"

His protestations were wasted on me. We all knew that what
they were doing was wrong in all ways – legally, morally, and eth-
ically. However, I could also see they had a point. Was it possible
that something could be wrong, but also have benefit? If no one
was harmed or hurt, was there really a problem?

"Take it easy, guys. I'm not going to report you," I said.

We all knew that they would be in trouble, seriously repri-
manded, or even worse. I didn't even stop to think if knowing and
not reporting them implicated me, too.

Justine sauntered over while the resident and I were still
working on Mrs. Templeton. "If I ever get like this," she said
loudly, not caring who heard, "shoot me."

"We need to find out what's going on with her," said the resident defensively. She was still having difficulty threading the
catheter into the superior vena cava.

"I'll tell you exactly what's going on with her," Justine said.
"What's going on with her is that she is trying to check out. In the
olden days, before all this high-tech stuff, they used to call this
'dying,' plain and simple. That's what it's called."

"But the son is calling the shots," answered the doctor. "He
wants –"

"Does he really think we can turn back the clock, offer her the fountain of youth? Tell him there's no cure for old age. Poor thing, she was trying to die and we won't let her. Someone should tell her that's not allowed around here." Justine took the old woman's wrinkled hand in her strong grip and shook her head in disgust.

After the line was in, the son came back and pulled up a chair beside his mother. I lowered the bed rail so that he could get closer and hold her hand.

"Thank you, nurse. I'll sit here, give her a little ginger ale, and she'll get her strength back, you'll see."

The resident returned to review the situation with him one more time.

"Mr. Templeton, the question here is whether to intubate or not. If we do, your mother will be back on the breathing machine. She will be in some discomfort, which we could manage with sedation, but we cannot offer any guarantee whatsoever that we will be able to wean her off the ventilator."

"I want everything done for Mother," he said.

The resident shrugged her shoulders and rushed off as her pager was beeping.

I sighed and faced him alone. "Mr. Templeton, it must painful to see your mother in this condition, but try to imagine what it is like for her and what she would want. Would she want us to keep her alive on a ventilator with an intravenous, urinary catheter and feeding tubes? Her mind is deteriorating and she suffers from an incurable lung disease. How much time does she have left and is the suffering worth it? Is it possible she wants to die?"

"Are you saying she is dying?"

Now the word had been uttered.

"Are you suggesting giving up on her, just like that? Pulling the plug? I'll take you all to court! I want a second opinion. If you're not going to do everything for her, I'll take her somewhere else."

I drew a deep breath to calm myself. "Mr. Templeton, nothing will be done against your wishes. We will do what you decide. We just want to make sure that you understand the implications of putting her back on the breathing machine. Think about what is best for her. What would she want?"

He was aghast at my apparent cruelty. "There is nothing to think about. I want everything possible done to bring her back. How can you ask me to put an end to my mother's life? Give her all the life support available!"

It occurred to me that once you call it "life support," how *could* one justify withholding it from anyone? Who could ever withdraw it?

I reached out to touch his arm to comfort him, but he pulled away and got up from the chair to confront me. "You're trying to kill my mother! Do you know who this woman is? She was Miss Georgian Bay, 1923. She sews award-winning quilts. Just last week she walked to the hairdresser, and we had lunch together at Eaton's. You think these other people have more right to live than an old woman?" He waved in the direction of the other patients, then pointed a long finger at me. "How dare you give up on her! Are you the Angel of Death?" Spit flew from the corners of his mouth.

I became small, and shrank away from his accusations. Was I just supposed to do what I was told and not think? Was I just there to carry out orders?

I escaped for a moment to the nursing station and sat staring at the central cardiac monitors that displayed all of the patients' heartbeats by remote view. I pressed my hand to my forehead, which seemed to throb along with the beep . . . beep . . . beep of the patients' heartbeats. The various alarms ringing in the different rooms and the ventilators whooshing in and out played on, like a never-ending soundtrack.

Rosemary came over and sat down beside me. "I'm worried about you, Tilda. Maybe you need a change of assignment. Maybe you're not ready –"

"Of course not, Rosemary. I'm fine." Did she think I wasn't coping? Did she think I was – Laura's epithet – *too sensitive*?

"Come on, Angel of Death, it's time for lunch." Justine came over and pulled me along. "I asked Pang-Mei to cover for you. I'm going to get you a T-shirt with a skull and crossbones, or a black gown with a hood, like the Grim Reaper."

I followed Justine to the cafeteria where we joined the others.

"We're trying to be helpful, compassionate, and we get this kind of insult?" I complained over lunch. "The Angel of Death! It's the exact opposite of why I'm a nurse."

Frances said, "I remember in nursing school, back home, they used to tell us, 'When you come to work, leave your self at the door.' It's probably the best advice, if you can do it."

"Dying is a natural process and they used to let it happen to the elders of our society, for God's sake!" said Justine, eager to resume her rant. "The public buys into this belief that everything can be fixed, that even dying can be reversed. And the doctors themselves like them to think that way so that they can be God. I said to Dr. Bristol this morning, do you know what's the difference between God and a doctor? *God* knows he's not a doctor!"

"Listen, Tilda, don't take the son's anger personally," said Nicole. "It's like, families need to express these feelings and it's easier to take it out on the nurses – they'd never talk like that to a doctor. It's hard when they say hurtful things, but you have to rise above it and not blame him for it."

"Oh, I blame him. He's nuts." Justine stabbed her fork into a huge slice of lemon meringue pie. "Why should we have to take this bullshit? We have a right to be treated respectfully. Besides, this guy has got to be told to let go. The time has come. It's cruel what we're doing. Does he actually believe that his mom is going to walk out of here, come home and cook him a meatloaf? Her lungs are like empty paper bags. There's nothing left to perfuse. But he wants to have a breathing tube, the size of a garden hose, shoved down her windpipe, and we have to be the ones to carry out the torture. She's eighty-six, for God's sake, and not exactly the picture of health."

"Ah, make that eighty-five," I said. "For the record."

"But she's a young eighty-five," said Tracy mischievously. "She has the lungs of an eighty-year-old!"

"Doesn't look a day over eighty-three!" added Justine. "How long does the public believe that people actually live? By the way, does anyone ever consider the costs to the health-care system that this type of situation creates?"

But by then we were doubled over, trying to contain our howls of laughter.

"But what if we're wrong?" I asked. "Is it possible that she really would have wanted this done? Is it possible she could pull through this?"

"If someone really knew what all of this entailed, I mean really knew the truth, the details, if they knew what nurses know, not just the way they show it on TV, who would want this?" asked Laura. "If there's a reason to believe there's some benefit, that's another thing."

"It's like the Bruce Cockburn song." Justine sang out in a startlingly lovely alto voice, "They're all waiting for some miracle to come along."

But was all this indignity and discomfort that we were inflicting on Mrs. Templeton worth it, for the long shot of a miracle? If Mrs. Templeton did make it, if she did survive this ICU admission, it wouldn't be a miracle, it would be an oddity, an aberration, an anomaly, an exception, a blip, a delay of the imminently inevitable.

"Well, what about miracles?" I asked. "Have you guys seen any?"

"Not unless you count a child's smile or a rainbow," said Laura in a syrupy-sweet voice.

"I believe in miracles," said Tracy. "But I've never seen one around here."

"What about Mr. Collacutt?" Frances reminded us. "He had a miraculous recovery."

"You mean Mr. Cold Cuts?" said Justine.

"Yes, Mr. Collacutt was on a ton of meds, three or four inotropes, and the next day he was off everything, don't you remember?"

"Yeah, that's because he died, Frances. You were off that day."

"He died?" said Frances. "I thought he got better."

"You're slipping, Frances. Haven't you been keeping up with the obituaries?"

We all knew that Frances made a habit of reading the newspaper memorials to search out ones for our patients who had died. She blushed at having her morbid hobby exposed.

"Haven't we all heard stories of people who were thought to be irretrievable, who were in a deep coma, and then suddenly woke up?" I said. "Those stories give a lot of people reason to believe that it could happen to their loved one, too."

"Yeah, but not someone so old, with so many serious, irreversible medical problems," said Laura, shaking her head.

"It's not just that he wants her to survive, he wants her to get up, and come home and be his mother. We all want to go back to the dream of being a child again," said Nicole in a way that made me think she might harbour that dream herself.

As we headed back upstairs, I decided what I would do. I just needed to find a few minutes alone with my patient.

We returned to the ICU and since there was no sign of the son anywhere, I went over to Mrs. Templeton, lowered the side rail, sat down beside her, and took her dry, papery hand in mine. I looked at her wrinkled face and bony chest and I caressed her soft white hair. Her chest heaved and rattled like an old furnace. I put my hand on her damp forehead and brow in a way that I hoped was soothing.

"We want to do what *you* want, Mrs. Templeton," I said. "Do you want all of this, what we're doing here, or is it enough? Are you ready to die? Give me a sign if you can."

I willed her to speak. I explained about the breathing tube, the ventilator, the IV in her neck. She turned her face to the window where her cloudy blue eyes seemed to meet with the cloudy blue sky. I had no idea if she understood a word I said.

Laura appeared at my side and shook her head sadly.

"She needs a ticket on the Morphine Express but unfortunately, we can't give her that ride."

We felt certain in our belief that she was dying. The way she pulled at the tubes and her IVs, the way she shut us out with her eyes, and the way she turned inward and away from the world, made us feel sure about this.

There was something else that was making me feel uneasy and I was trying to shake off the question in my mind. How would I be able to work here, if these cases affected me so much? I tried to switch off, tune out, go under, and close off my heart from what was happening. I looked at my watch to see how many more hours of my shift were left. I could wander out to chat with Frances and have a few laughs with Tracy or Justine.

Then I remembered morning rounds with Dr. Bristol and the distinction he had made between treatment and care. While I didn't agree with the treatment in which I was obligated to participate, I felt wholehearted about the caring, which was the essence, if not the very definition, of nursing itself. I knew what nursing was all about – I had seen the best of it in Frances, Laura, and Tracy and Nicole, even Justine, too, in certain moments. I knew what I had studied, from Florence Nightingale to all the modern nursing theorists: Watson, Rogers, Parse, and Leininger. Nursing was about pain relief, hygiene, nutrition, comfort, spirituality, kindness, and empathy. All those things I could still offer Mrs. Templeton.

I saw the son striding past the nursing station toward his mother's room and I met him halfway.

"Mr. Templeton, you know your mother best. You know what she wants."

"You people just don't realize how strong my mother is. She's going to make it. When will the doctor . . . ?"

4

A DAGGER IN THE BED

I peered deep down into my cup of coffee. It was a ritual of mine, a thing I did at the beginning of every shift in the ICU, just before going into my patient's room.

"Oh, you lucky dog," said Laura. "You're going to have a busy day. You've got that leukemia patient they admitted during the night and he's sick. I see the whole family have moved in with him."

"Yeah, that's good. I haven't had a busy patient for a long time." I pretended that I, too, was a seasoned veteran and craved action like the others.

"It's busy when they're dying. That's usually the busiest," said Laura.

We put up with Laura's sarcasm because she was such an astonishingly good nurse. I had recently watched her stand at the foot of a patient's bed and pronounce: "Congestive heart failure. This man needs Lasix, 40 mg, IV." Not only that, but she went ahead and prepared the drug and told the doctor what she planned to do.

"Yes, I agree," he said. "I haven't had a chance to take a look at the X-ray."

"I have and it's 'wet,'" said Laura. "Signs of early pulmonary edema."

"I've been meaning to come and write that order . . ."

Laura had stalked off, muttering something about his incompetence.

"What makes you think that patient is going to die?" Frances said to Laura, returning me to the day ahead. "You're so negative. Lots of leukemics do well these days."

"C'mon, it's time to get to work," interrupted Tracy.

Pamela was the nurse on nights and I knew she'd be annoyed if I was late getting in there, even by a minute, so I hustled off to relieve her, my coffee cup still in hand.

There were very few windows in the intensive care unit, none that opened. The small one that was in my patient's room looked out into a narrow alley that led to another wing of the hospital. Even though it was morning, the patient's room was still as dark as night. There was only a small ceiling spotlight that illuminated the patient in the bed, like a spotlight on centre stage.

Outside, in the long hallway between the rooms, nurses were turning on the overhead fluorescent lights, one by one, nudging the day to take over the night.

Pamela gave me report.

"Manjit Gujral is a twenty-six-year-old male, diagnosed a few weeks ago with acute myelocytic leukemia," she said, pausing to yawn. "He's septic, with a fever of 39.5, elevated white count, and fulminant infection in the blood. He's on every bug drug, anti-fungal agent, plus chemo, too. The works. He had a bone marrow transplant from an unrelated donor from Sweden, but it looks like rejection. Oh, and the family – they've moved in here. By the way, his brother is an orthopedic surgeon and asks lots of questions."

"Thanks, Pamela. Go home. Sleep well."

She stood up to pack her knapsack, something we all use to bring our stuff to work in. "They're nice enough but they're here all the time, and it really can get on your nerves to have them watching everything you do, you know what I mean? Say, are you going to the Christmas party? One of the respiratory therapists is selling tickets, if you want any."

"Maybe. Thanks, Pamela. Good night," I said as she ended her day and I started mine.

In my patient's room, an old woman stood at the bedside, her eyes gazing heavenward, deep in prayer. She must be his mother, I figured, and I went over to stand with her for a few minutes. We nodded at one other because we did not speak each other's language, at least not the language of words. We looked down at her son's long, husky body, mostly covered with a blue cotton bedsheet. All around him was the tangled spaghetti of plastic tubing, wires, and electrodes. Green numbers and lines marched across the monitor. The ventilator whooshed in and out as oxygen was pushed into his lungs, and then released. Tubes were running in to his body delivering fluids, nutrients, medicines; other tubes were running out of his body, directing the flow of urine, stool, and other fluids into tidily hung bags or bottles around his bed. The patient was at the intersection; his body was the meeting point. What a person can withstand, I stood at his bedside thinking – the onslaught of illness, plus a counterattack with our weapons of chrome, metal, plastic, and chemicals.

This is war. This place is a war zone and this man's body, our battlefield.

His heart rhythm was stable, so I sat down at one of the small tables on wheels that we keep in the unit. Our patients can't sit up and eat meals in bed, so we use these portable tables for our charting purposes. I wheeled it over to within an arm's length of the foot of the patient's bed.

"Are you Manjit's nurse today?" asked a pretty young woman with a mocha complexion. She came from behind me and approached me tentatively, as if not wanting to disturb me. Perhaps she was trying to determine my reaction to her early presence, unannounced and long before the official hospital visiting hours. She probably sensed that not every nurse was friendly to families. Each nurse had his or her quirks. Some kept their distance and wanted space to do their work; others were more relaxed and welcoming. Would I be one to open the way for the family or would I be another obstacle for them to overcome? Would I be one of those nurses who keeps them in the waiting room, closes the curtains, and bars them from the room, or would I be an ally?

"Come right in," I said. "I was just going to do my initial assessment, but you're welcome to visit Manjit. You are his wife?"

"Yes, I am," she said with a smile. "My name is Jatinder." She wore a wrinkled purple T-shirt over black stirrup pants and carried herself with the grace of a dancer.

"Have you been here all night?" I asked as I recorded Manjit's vital signs and noted that his fever had spiked to 40.0°C.

I could plainly see that she had. The dark circles under her eyes told me the whole story of her night in the waiting room on one of the lumpy, narrow couches. I lowered the side rails and beckoned her to move closer to her husband. I drew the curtains around his bed and examined him from head to toe, as I had been taught.

As I did this, out of the corner of my eye, I watched Jatinder caress Manjit's sweaty bald head and his swollen face. He was intubated and heavily sedated, so he could not communicate to her in words, but she seemed satisfied merely to be near him. Later that morning, we bathed him together, and she rubbed his back. I began to wonder how a person as sick as Manjit could get better. Perhaps it was simply a limitation of my imagination. Perhaps I was not religious enough to believe in miracles. Perhaps because I had such misgivings, I was not the best nurse to be caring for this patient.

I turned my focus to his body and noted that he looked pale. He had lost a lot of blood in the operating room where he'd gone to have an abscess removed and he was bleeding from his wound and from sores in his mouth and in his lungs. I logged on to the computer to check his hemoglobin just as Laura poked her head into the room. She said, "Your hemoglobin's down to 64, so I've cross and typed him for two units of packed cells."

"Thanks. I'll call a porter to pick it up."

"I sent one already," she said and was gone.

THE SECOND DAY that I took care of Manjit, his blood pressure was even lower, and he was on a few additional intravenous blood pressure medications (inotropes) to support it. The ventilator was on even higher settings to take over more of the work of breathing for him.

I went about performing my various tasks and made notes in the chart. Then I stepped back and let the family administer their homemade medicine of loving words, caresses, and prayers.

"Keep that heart beating, buddy," said the brother, Deenpal, into Manjit's ear. "You're going to get through this, man." He picked off some flakes of dried skin from his brother's fingers, and then held the mottled hand in his warm one. The two hands joined like that looked like one. Even their stainless steel bracelets, symbols of their faith, seemed to be intertwined.

In her real life, not this new nightmare life she was living, Jatinder was an aerobics instructor and Manjit was an executive at Canadian Tire.

"The fall is usually his busiest time. Just before Christmas," Jatinder explained to me. She showed me a letter from Manjit's boss at head office:

> Your amazing courage and fortitude will get you through this, big guy. Just as you always give your best to the company and never give up when the going gets rough, you will pull through this.

At lunchtime the family brought me warm chapattis, eggplant with coriander, and fresh samosas.

They placed a dagger in a leather sheath in Manjit's hand by his side.

His mother asked for my help to put on his special ritual under-garment, underneath his hospital gown. She placed a small wooden comb on the bedside table.

They pinned a clear plastic bag containing a small, thick prayer book to the pillowcase under his head.

His father placed photographs, credit cards, and a few dollar bills in a wallet and put it in his hand.

"For my son to use in the next life, should his time come to go there," he explained to me with a slight bow of his turbaned head.

Jatinder and Deenpal rocked the bed vigorously to stimulate Manjit's blood pressure and make him know that they were there, at his side.

"Let's take a walk," Jatinder crooned into his ear. "Let's go away from this place. Please, Manjit, come with me. Deenpal and I are with you. Feel our energy. We are here. Use our energy. Take it. You have given everyone else so much. Keep on going. If anyone can do it, you can. Absorb that oxygen, Manjit. You are so strong. We can feel it. Your body is full of energy."

The next day, if it was possible, Manjit's face was even more misshapen, his neck even more swollen around the endotracheal tube. Jatinder and I wiped away the blood clots that were spilling out of his mouth. Clear fluid dripped out of his nose. The air in the room was stale, unmoving, and at times foul odours came off him. The odours were the vaporized residue from the chemotherapy he had received, combined with the decaying smell that often emanates from bodies that have not been exposed to fresh air for weeks. His skin sloughed off in sheets and the brother collected it and disposed of it.

"I know you are in there, Manjit." Deenpal took up Jatinder's loving litany whenever she faltered. "You're going into the home stretch, man. All of us are here with you. Don't worry about anything. Your blood pressure is good. Keep it up. You missed the Santana concert with cousin Suresh, but there will be another. Everything is taken care of at work. Come on now, you're scaring us. Just get better. Concentrate on the fight. Once this is over, we'll get out of here together. Here's cousin Suresh. He came in from Vancouver to see you. We're going to keep talkin' your ear off. Get that oxygen into those cells. You do the work on the inside and we'll do the work on the outside. We're nowhere else but here with you. Keep fighting. Don't be tired. Be strong. You'll rest later. Keep focusing. Remember we set this year aside so that we'll have the rest of our lives together. Keep beating those odds. Mind over matter. Use this energy to clean out the bad stuff. We're here, with open arms. Let's go through this together. We're brothers for another sixty-seven years together. It is written.

We have all the time in the world. Sponge up that oxygen. Don't be afraid."

I fell into a trance from the sound of their loving incantations that was broken only when Dr. Leung came to tell them that she wanted to do a CT scan of Manjit's head. His pupils were dilated and unresponsive, and she was afraid there might be swelling or even bleeding in his brain.

As a professional courtesy to Deenpal, who was a doctor, we allowed him to come into the darkened viewing room to see the various views of his brother's brain on the computer screen. He stood, blinking at the images before him. I could see the twelve pictures reflected in Deenpal's glasses. He saw what even a first-year medical student could see. Massive hemorrhage with clotted blood blocking the vesicles and passageways. There was no circulation in his brother's brain, therefore no oxygenation, and no activity.

"Massive global infarction of the left and right hemispheres" was the radiologist's diagnosis as he looked over at me. I could read the message in his eyes: *Even if he survives, what kind of condition would he be in?*

I knew Manjit was going to die. Surely Deenpal, a doctor himself, realized that, too?

Later, when we returned to Manjit's room, Jatinder told me that Deenpal felt guilty at having persuaded his brother to undergo the bone marrow transplant.

"But what option did we have?" she asked as if I had objected, too. "It was that or for certain he would die. But we don't want to be the instrument of destruction to his next life. We have many bodies. That is our belief."

She pulled out a picture of their wedding ceremony to show me what a handsome man her husband had been. I could allow myself only a fleeting glance at it, out of politeness, and then had to look away. I knew that if I looked at it, I'd be drawn in too deep. I glanced sideways at the photograph of the beautiful couple, Manjit, handsome as a king in a black tunic, Queen Jatinder in a red gown, and elegant Prince Deenpal at their sides. I couldn't reconcile that image with what I saw before me, the grieving young woman, the distraught family, the unconscious, bleeding man in the bed.

"I wish you could have met him," she said, "and got to know him as he really is."

I pulled out a roll of surgical tape from my lab coat pocket and took the photograph from her hand. "I'll put it up on the wall, for everyone to see."

"Thank you." Palms together, she bowed slightly to me. "How can we ever repay you?"

When they left the room for a short break and fresh air, I tried to keep up the one-sided conversation with Manjit, as I had learned from Frances. I tried to always make it part of my practice to talk to unconscious patients, but at times I found it awkward. It was like leaving a message on a telephone answering machine; you're not sure if it will be received, but you go ahead and speak, anyway, on faith.

"You have a lovely family, Manjit. They're all rooting for you. I'm with you now. I'm Tilda, your nurse, today," I said. "Tomorrow, too," I added, a little tentatively.

My words were sincere but came out tersely. Somehow I couldn't carry on with the healing chorus that the family was providing. I held myself back from entering their loving circle. It was more than I could bear.

LATER THAT NIGHT, at home, I couldn't sleep. I wanted to call the ICU to find out from the nurse in charge how Manjit was doing. I knew it wasn't a good idea. I probably should make that break, keep more distance.

I picked up the phone and called.

"How's Manjit doing?" I asked.

"Hanging in there," the in-charge nurse said, "but the family is losing it. You back tomorrow?"

"Yes."

"Do you want to go back in there or do you need a break from them?"

"Put me back in there, please."

"Oh, I see here that Rosemary left a note saying she thought you should have a change of assignment. She thinks you're getting too emotionally involved. Are you?"

"Of course not."

I LAY ON my bed and thought about them until late into the night. If such a tragedy could strike such a loving, close family, what hope was there for anybody in this world? I imagined having to resuscitate Manjit with Deenpal standing by, watching to make sure I was doing everything correctly. I fantasized that when Manjit died, as it seemed inevitable he would, Jatinder could marry the equally handsome older brother, Deenpal. That way there could still be a happy ending. I worried how Jatinder would go on and how the mother and father would cope with their loss.

"Death is not the end," the father had whispered to me, but I wasn't convinced.

I stared up at the ceiling, at my alarm clock, at my wristwatch that lit up in the dark at the touch of a button. I mulled over all the sadness and suffering at work and couldn't wait to get back in there.

THE NEXT MORNING, when I walked in, the family members were dressed in long white gowns, the men all with white turbans on their heads, even Deenpal and cousin Suresh, from Vancouver. They were immersed in their Olympic marathon of devotion. Their hands swarmed all over Manjit's body in frenzied caresses.

The mother massaged his bladder to try to push out a drop or two of urine, but his kidneys had shut down.

The cousins kneaded his limbs to stimulate his circulation.

The father stumbled around the room, chanting his prayers, but in a daze.

Deenpal told his brother off-colour jokes to try to rile him up. Then he poured forth relentless commands into his brother's ears.

"Kick their butts, Manjit! Break the door down! This is our last fight. I'm going with you all the way, my brother, my baby. C'mon.

Hang tough. Get that oxygen into the blood. Think about Umma, how much she needs you. Think about Jatinder, how much she loves you. It's Deen, your only brother. Your right-hand man. No time to relax now. Keep running like an athlete and don't think about the finish line yet. You are going to do that MBA, you hear me?"

It seemed to me that their words were medicine, just as important as the Vancomycin, ceftazidime, and Levophed that I was injecting. The family's voices, the dagger at his side, and their offerings to their God were just as effective – perhaps in this case, even more so – than the treatments I was giving or the procedures I was performing.

Their heads were bent over him, their arms clasped in prayer. The mother was prostrate over his body. I feared she might faint, collapse in her grief.

Deenpal pulled me outside into the hallway. "Tell me. How do you think he's doing?"

I looked at him, a little surprised. He's a doctor, surely he knows the score?

"Prepare yourselves for the worst."

"Do you think so?" he asked, just like a brother.

"It must be hard being a doctor and a brother," I said.

UNBELIEVABLY, MANJIT HUNG on for another few days.

"It takes a lot longer for the young ones to die," said Frances. "Their hearts are strong."

When Manjit died, the mother collapsed. Frances gave her oxygen and Tracy called for a stretcher. The mother's wailing could be heard throughout the intensive care unit.

The father shook his head in disapproval at the mother's keening. "The soul never dies," he told me, "so there is no mourning."

"You've been a wonderful Umma," Deenpal called out to her as they carried the mother away. Then he turned to his brother's body, looked over at me and I thought he was going to smash something. Only Jatinder was peaceful.

"It is God's will," she said, closing her eyes. "Once his mind was gone, I knew it was over. I don't want his body if I can't have his mind, his smiling eyes, his incredible personality."

Frances came in to help me and together we removed the tubes and wires, and pushed to the side the heavy machines that surrounded his bed like ugly, hulking monsters. She went out to invite the family to come back in to see him, if they wished to do so. Only Deenpal and the cousins came back. I was glad at least they got the chance to see Manjit, who looked so much better dead than alive, so much more like himself without our trappings. In his face at rest, one could see something of that proud handsome groom on his wedding day.

The other nurses congregated in the room to comfort first the family, and then me, too. Frances and Nicole put their arms around me.

"Are you okay?" Justine asked. "You're shaking."

"No, I am not. Shaking, I mean."

"Well, you don't look too good."

Rosemary told me to "take some time off, Tilda. You need a rest from work."

In the locker room, Laura, Frances, Nicole, Tracy, and Justine pulled me toward the door.

"C'mon," said Justine. "We're taking you out for a drink."

5

DECOMPRESSION

I was beginning to wonder if it was all too much for me: the suffering, the death and dying. Even getting up so early in the morning at times seemed like an inordinate burden. Who needed it? Surely I could find work that was less demanding, that took place during normal hours, that wasn't so full of misery? I had been a nurse for a few years and was finally able to see beyond my own personal problems and begin to appreciate the pain of others. However, my emotions threatened to overwhelm me. My patients' suffering was becoming mine.

One morning when I drove to work, I listened to a radio talk show on which callers described their jobs. A young woman gushed about working at Disney World and how she loved "making children happy." A florist rhapsodized about creating beautiful bouquets for brides and other people in love. Even the description the computer programmer gave of sitting day after day in his quiet office moving a mouse around and staring at a blue screen sounded appealing.

I knew I might make a good librarian, but the old-fashioned kind who advised people what to read and stayed hidden among shelves of dusty books. I could give piano lessons to children, but didn't think I could make a living from that. Being a lifeguard at a pool was another option. I was a strong swimmer and could gaze into the water most of the day and just jump in when needed.

Yet I did want to do something that helped people, and as sad, and at times disturbing, as my work in the ICU was, it was also fascinating and exhilarating, and I remained determined to master it.

On days off from work, I lay in bed after I woke up, stared up at the ceiling and relived whole scenes from the hospital, as if I were watching a movie. Then, over the next day or two, I began to prepare myself to face it all over again.

Ivan and I were planning to get married, but for the time being, it seemed just as well that I lived alone. I wasn't too much fun to be with and most people tended to recoil when they heard about my work. I tried not to impose it on others.

Our group, Laura's Line, all worked the same schedule, so we were also off on the same days, too. Sometimes we met for lunch at Hannah's Kitchen, Fran's, or the Daily Planet. Each time we vowed that we wouldn't talk about work, but inevitably and within minutes, our conversation drifted in that direction. Who else knew what we had seen, what we had experienced? To whom else could we unburden ourselves? Who would want to hear? Who would understand?

"The problem with you is you're too sensitive," Laura kept saying whenever I moaned about whatever tragedy was currently taking place in the ICU.

It was true. It was something I had struggled with all my life. Yet somehow, I wanted to believe that I could find a way to turn that liability into an asset, that I could find a way to use it to help people.

"Try not to think about it so much," advised Frances. "I know it can get to you, but when you leave work, put it all out of your mind. Now, what are we having for dessert?"

"I know," said Nicole. "Sometimes it gets to me, too. No one likes to think that terrible things could ever happen to you or to someone you love. That's how you do this work. How about the chocolate cheesecake and a bunch of forks?"

But we all knew that something terrible *had* happened to Nicky. Her mother had died of cancer. My own mother had died, my father too, and I was estranged from most of my family. Coupled with my own problems, the sadness of my work felt like a lot to bear, especially because I did take it so seriously and personally. Yet I couldn't leave now. I was six months into the yearlong commitment I'd made to Rosemary, our head nurse, to stay in the ICU. Even more important to me than keeping my promise, however, was the dread of leaving in failure and starting over somewhere else.

It wasn't only the death and dying that made me wonder if I could be good at this work. It was the inadequacy I felt when I didn't know what I could offer patients, other than my rapidly expanding repertoire of technical skills. I was still so far from possessing the critical thinking, the intuition, and the courage of so many nurses that I admired, and not only the ones within my tight circle.

There was Valerie, the night nurse with the beautiful fingernails and the British accent, who on more than one occasion stayed long past the end of her shift to hold the hand of her dying patient.

"No one should ever die alone," she said as if enunciating an axiom.

There was Nell with her unreliable attendance and dubious, outlandish stories, who was always calling in sick at the last minute, just before the start of a shift. But when she did come to work, she gave exquisite care to her patients and they loved her. It didn't bother her in the least, for instance, to create chaos in the room and to mess with the monitors and machinery in order to turn her patient's bed around to face Mecca as he was dying.

It was Nell who stood up to Dr. York, a senior hospital administrator, when he asked to see the chart of a patient who was a prominent government official, recovering from an aortic aneurysm in our ICU.

"No," said Nell, holding on to it. "You can't have access to the chart. You are not his doctor."

"I am a doctor." He reached for the chart in her hands.

Nell held tight. "You are not *this* patient's doctor."

"Do you know who I am?"

She smiled, almost laughed. "Of course," but didn't deign to tell him who he was.

"He's an asshole, that's who he is," she told us later, to our delight, in the lounge at lunchtime. It was fun to see that word come out of her pretty, lipsticked mouth. "When I wouldn't give him the chart, he stormed off in a huff, saying he was going to report my insolence to Rosemary."

It was a breach of patient privacy, something we were there to protect. We all knew what had happened to the curious nurse who had gone into the computer chart of a prominent journalist who was a patient in our hospital. It had sobered us to learn that she had been fired over her thoughtless invasion of patient privacy.

Murry was another nurse I admired. He was an artist, and his patients' bodies, his canvas. They became his masterpieces. He took impeccable care of them, cleaning the wax from their ears and whatever dripped from their noses. He applied patients' favourite creams and lotions and gave them massages. Once I watched him tenderly wipe away drips of menstrual blood from between a young woman's legs and then made her feel clean and well-groomed with a perfumed bath and a manicure and pedicure before her boyfriend came to visit. Murry talked to her all the while, treating her like the lovely young woman that she was, despite the fact that she was completely unconscious from raging bacterial meningitis.

Murry's nursing care was not merely cosmetic: he could read an electrocardiogram like a cardiologist.

Of course, it wasn't all just nurses. The ICU was teeming with many other professionals and the doctors, too, from interns to residents, senior fellows and researchers, specialists of every organ of the body, consultants, students and visitors from other hospitals, and from countries as far away as Bahrain, Ecuador, and Norway, who came to share what they knew and to learn from us. But anyone who spent any amount of time in the ICU readily admitted that it was the nurses who ran the place. Sure, the doctors made the diagnosis and ordered the tests and treatments, but the nurses did just about everything else.

The residents were full-fledged doctors who had finished their internship and were specializing in internal medicine or general surgery or a sub-specialty, such as cardiology or urology. They came for a week or a month and then moved on. The Medical-Surgical ICU was one of many of their rotations throughout the hospital. A few of them went on to specialize in critical care medicine and they spent a longer time with us as "fellows." Their next step would be vying for a staff position somewhere. A small group of permanent staff physicians, called "intensivists" and who had specialized in critical care medicine, were the medical directors of the ICU, and they rotated with each other on a weekly basis. We nurses always checked the board when we came in to find out who was the attending staff physician on that week. By the name on the board, we knew how things would be handled; whom we could count on in the middle of the night; who would pass the buck on making tough decisions; who respected what the nurses had to say and who didn't.

Dr. Daniel Huizinga was a cowboy. He often told us about his travels with his wife and family to Third World or war-torn countries to volunteer his expertise. Daniel – we were familiar enough with him to call him Danny – wore a black leather jacket and black Reebok running shoes, which he needed, as he was always on the go. He smirked and guffawed at whatever anyone – nurses, patients, or families – said. He knew best. Yet everyone who could see beyond his gruff, rough manner grew to love him.

"Thank you for coming in," I said to him gratefully at 0300 hours one morning. Laura was in charge, and she had called him at home to tell him that my patient was crashing and that the resident on call that night was out of his depth and not coping.

"I'll always come in," he said, "especially if the patient is young."

"That's very caring of you," I murmured as I watched Justine sticking her finger down her throat to tell me to quit sucking up to him.

"Nonsense," he said with a shrug. "In court when they ask me if I examined the patient, it won't wash with the judge if I just say that my resident described him to me over the phone. That's why I come in."

I told him that my patient's blood pressure was dropping, his urine output, low. "He was stable up until an hour or so, when –"

"You call that stable? He looks like crap, and why is this saline bag half closed?" he bellowed at Laura, who had come in to help me. He flipped open the clamp on the IV so that the fluid would pour in, and when that wasn't fast enough for his liking, he squeezed the IV bag with his whole fist. "I said on the phone to give him a bolus. When I say bolus, I mean give the fluid as fast as possible," he muttered.

I had been the one who had set the rate too cautiously, but Laura told him, "Relax! Look at it this way; it's also half open. Look on the bright side!"

He grinned at her and at me, too.

"Send off a bunch of lytes, minerals, and a lactate, too," he said, but Laura had already done that before he arrived and had the results ready to show him.

"I've seen guys like this go sour in a few minutes," he said, pacing around the room, keeping his eyes on the patient.

"What do you mean?" I asked.

"I remember a guy just like this. He was sitting up in bed eating a hamburger and less than two hours later, I was draining pus out of his belly in the OR."

"Yeah," said Justine, who had come in to lend a hand. "It's that cafeteria food."

If I saw Dr. Huizinga in my patient's room when I came on at the start of my shift, it meant the patient was sick. All the patients were sick, but if the nurses said a particular patient was "sick," it was cause to worry. They were the ones that Daniel hovered over, anytime, day or night.

That night, while he was there working alongside me at my patient's bedside, I got flustered and accidentally disconnected the "jet" ventilator, a high-powered breathing machine that delivered up to 150 breaths per minute. It was one of the things we brought in as a last resort for the sickest patients.

Laura stepped in and calmly began to hand-ventilate my patient with 100 per cent oxygen, while Dr. Huizinga plugged the machine back in and re-calibrated it.

Justine began to sing the song about leaving on a jet plane to tease me.

"Don't worry, Tilda, he's okay," Nicole said when she saw my stricken face.

Laura came in to tell Daniel about a phone call she'd just received from a doctor at another hospital who was looking for an ICU bed for a very sick patient.

He wanted the details, quick and to the point. "What's the story?"

"She's a forty-one-year-old woman, two days postpartum, thirteen previous pregnancies –"

"Has she got rocks in her head?" he growled.

"Hold on." Laura put up her hand to stop him. "She's bleeding, unconscious, already lost about two litres of blood during the delivery. She's intubated –"

"Bring her in," he barked, "right away."

"Bow-wow to you, too," said Laura.

There they were, the two of them pretending to be Rottweilers, when everyone knew they were both spaniels.

It didn't take me long to figure out there was nothing about Dr. Huizinga to be afraid of. Even though he could be intimidating and demanding and was a brilliant, world-renowned specialist in the complex relationship between oxygen and hemoglobin molecules in microcirculation and in the biochemical reactions involved in lactic acidosis, he was actually very approachable and enjoyed teaching us all that he knew. He could be preoccupied at times and disinterested in the minutiae of the daily management issues of the ICU. On morning rounds he often perched up on the counter in the patient's room and became engrossed with his clipboard, upon which he tinkered with mathematical equations and scientific formulas. Once there was a lengthy discussion between two of the residents about which antibiotic to choose for a septic patient. Should it be one that protected against anaerobic microbes or a more broad-spectrum one that would cover a possible hospital-acquired pneumonia? Should we wait for the results of the cultures, or should we proceed with an antibiotic on spec?

"What do you think, Dr. Huizinga?" Dr. Leung asked.

"About what?" He looked at her blankly. "I wasn't listening."

One day Justine caught him perusing the *Cosmopolitan* magazine she had tucked under her patient's chart.

"Are you checking out Hot Sex Tips on page 87?" she asked him in front of the team. "I've tried them all and my boyfriend likes number 32 the best."

Later, when she was on lunch, I noticed him return to her patient's room and open the magazine. He blushed, put down the magazine, and glanced around to make sure no one saw him. I didn't let on that someone had.

Hot Sex Tip No. 32: Guaranteed to drive your man wild: Gently pull down on his balls as you are sucking on his cock.

"THIS UNFORTUNATE GENTLEMAN choked on a piece of filet mignon," said Dr. Leung one morning as she began to review a patient's history during team rounds. She was a senior fellow, just a year away from completing her specialization as an intensivist. She had confided in me that she hoped to be offered a staff position at our hospital, but believed her chances were slim. She was pregnant, early on so she was still able to hide it, but would soon be unable to actively engage in the research projects that the hospital expected.

We loved working with Jessica, whose soft voice and sweet words could make even choking sound elegant. She wore her long dark hair in a ponytail, pulled back. She told me that although she loved clothes, she always wore green scrubs – some families mistook her for a nurse – to bolster her credibility with the other doctors. She was entrancing to watch and listen to, because of her intelligent face and her articulate way of speaking. I once observed a large noisy family, overcome with shock over the death of their father, become momentarily distracted from their grief by Jessica's beauty, which in itself seemed to offer comfort. If someone this angelic, smart, and kind couldn't save their loved one, maybe it *was* God's will, they seemed to reckon.

Once I heard Jessica deliver bad news, and even she sometimes stumbled over the words in these difficult situations.

"Despite all of our best efforts – and I want you to know that we did everything we could, the doctors – and the nurses too," she added glancing at me, "did absolutely everything we could, but unfortunately, there has been a negative outcome for your mother."

"Do you mean Ma is out of it? She's *comatoast*?"

"Unfortunately, your mother has expired."

So had a carton of milk in my refrigerator.

But surely that was better than Laura's short form: DAD – Dead As a Doornail – not that she ever put it that way when a family member or patient was anywhere within earshot.

I had started accompanying doctors to family meetings during which they told upsetting news. The family members were often hunched over and tense, but I made sure to keep my pose and posture more in keeping with the doctor – straight-backed and in control. I always came equipped with a small box of tissues in my lab coat pocket to have at the ready. Although I wanted to contribute helpful comments, I usually couldn't think of anything to add, so I kept quiet and listened.

It was in that tiny, airless, windowless, grey-walled room – the quiet room – that even those well-spoken, well-educated, and brilliant doctors ended up resorting to clichés. After they'd offered elaborate explanations of physiological and pathological processes, delivered in arcane medical terminology, after they had expounded on the complicated legal ramifications and temporized with lofty philosophical disquisitions about the patient's condition, they all ended up saying things like the patient was "not out of the woods," or "might not make it"; that we were "doing everything we could," but that he had "taken a turn for the worse," or that we had to let "nature take its course."

The most disturbing cliché, the plainest and the most rarely uttered was "There is nothing more we can do."

The families listened carefully and tried to follow the logical reasoning. They occasionally asked questions or wept softly. However, I knew that all they really wanted to know was, what does this mean? Will he make it? What are his chances?

After the meeting, the family and I would return to the patient's room. It was there that the families pored over all the details of the quiet room discussions with us, the nurses. They felt more at ease with us to go over the details and ask questions that they had been afraid to put to the doctor.

THE SKILL AND confidence of the nurses impressed me, but how they occasionally covered for the doctors astounded me.

"Watch out for that one," whispered Laura, pointing at one of the new surgical residents. "Make sure you go over every order she writes. Yesterday she ordered Dilantin 900 milligrams IV to be given as a loading dose. Can you imagine? She's scary."

Thankfully I knew that the usual loading dose was 300 milligrams, but what if I hadn't known? What if I had given the amount that had been ordered, almost a gram of Dilantin? What would have happened was that the patient would have arrested and died.

"Adenosine," I said to one of the foreign medical residents when my patient suddenly went into a rapid atrial arrhythmia. "I'll go get it, draw it up for you, but you'll have to give it."

"What?" He started flipping through the spiral-bound ICU handbook he'd pulled from his lab coat pocket.

"You need to diagnose the underlying rhythm," I explained "Adenosine will slow down the heart rate in order to differentiate between a supraventricular –"

I scanned the unit for Frances or Laura to come and explain all this to him, but there was only me. Clearly he was struggling with English, with the ICU, but most of all, he was struggling with the basics of medicine.

"They don't pay us enough for what we do," said Laura, enjoying the role of the unsung hero.

DR. DAVID BRISTOL, in his well-tailored dark suits, with his intellectual, esoteric language, spoken in a strong British accent, droned on endlessly with abstract theoretical discussions and kept us all at a distance with his slender Mont Blanc fountain pen. He stood outside the patients' rooms during morning rounds and talked to us from behind that silver pen, which he used as a pointer to highlight numbers and lab values on the patient's flow sheet.

"I don't touch patients," he said when Laura hid his pen from him. He was at a loss without it.

"How about windows? Do you do windows?" Justine inquired, but it was very hard to get a laugh out of him.

Dr. Bristol liked to expound on the ethical arguments involved in each case and often gave spontaneous lectures about the deontological framework of Immanuel Kant and his Moral Imperative versus John Stuart Mill's Utilitarian philosophy of the greatest good to the greatest number. Every patient became a jumping-off point for a discussion about the allocation of precious resources, withdrawal of life support, and his all-time favourite topic, the supremacy of the hallowed concept of "patient autonomy."

He upbraided me one morning because I was not forthright in answering his question about whether the thoracic surgeons had been by to see my patient.

"What did they tell her about her prognosis?" he asked.

"Well, um, I, er . . . they were here, yes . . . and they did see the patient, yes, but . . ." I hesitated. "They didn't really go into . . ."

The problem was that my patient was sitting up in a chair and fully conscious. I didn't think she knew about the cancer that was rapidly spreading through her lungs, but was this the way to tell her?

"Come on now, Tilda, speak up! We don't keep secrets around here. We give full disclosure and respect patients' rights to all information pertaining to their condition. Good morning, Mrs. Lawson," he called out to my patient from where he stood in the hallway. "Did the thoracic surgeons mention to you if your cancer had spread or not?"

Had she even been told she had cancer in the first place, much less that it had spread? The notes didn't say. She was a frail woman, lovingly tended to by her husband, who had stepped out during rounds. I felt certain that she would want him by her side, if she were to be told such news. Fortunately, she hadn't heard Dr. Bristol. She merely waved at him and didn't answer.

"I'm not trying to hide information from my patient," I said in my defence, "it's just that I don't know what she *has* been told. This doesn't seem the kindest way to tell her."

"Nonsense, Tilda," he scoffed. "You're being paternalistic. Your patient has the right to know the truth about everything. She is entitled to have all the information that we have about her condition."

"All the information she can handle," I answered back, thinking that my motive was more *maternal* than paternal.

"Which is everything," he countered.

"But her emotional state is fragile, and sometimes news like that could cause a setback. It might make her feel less motivated. Maybe the truth is too much for her to handle right now, especially all at once."

"And who are we to judge for her what she can handle?"

Later in the day he came back to see Mrs. Lawson to tell her himself that the cancer had spread and that it was inoperable, but she was in bed, sleeping.

"Why is she back on the ventilator?" he asked me. "I thought we were weaning her."

"She was tired. She said she didn't want to do any more weaning today and asked to be put back on the vent. Given her prognosis, I didn't think that weaning her off the ventilator was top priority," I explained.

"Since when does the patient make a medical decision?" He was kind enough, at least, not to wake her up then and there, but he was completely oblivious to his contradictory moral stance.

"Why didn't you call him on that one?" demanded Justine, her hands on her hips.

"I only thought about it after he left" was my lame reply.

"MORAL COURAGE IS what's needed in these situations," Rosemary told me many times. "We're here to do what's right for the patient. That is your ultimate guide."

From time to time Rosemary invited me in to her office to check on how I was doing and to give me a pep talk. She always had soft classical music playing. Her cubicle was a peaceful refuge, even though it was littered with Post-it notes, "to do" lists, and framed sentimental cross-stitched sayings such as The Serenity Prayer and Desiderata, that she hadn't got around to hanging up on the wall. Messy piles of nursing journals, policy and procedure manuals, and memos spilled onto her desk.

"How is it going?" she asked with her serene smile.

Why not be honest with her? She knew the score.

"It's still pretty stressful, Rosemary." I drew a deep breath. "I keep having the feeling that there is so much to learn and that I don't know enough. To the families, sometimes I just don't know what to say. I want to make it to the end of my year here, but I'm not sure."

"It's the nurses who raise these questions that I never worry about, Tilda. It's the ones who have all the answers that concern me. Let me tell you something that may help put your mind at ease. Do you remember when Harriet – one of our most senior nurses – her brother was in our unit for a liver transplant? You were one of the nurses she asked me to assign to his care."

There was no greater praise than that, I knew. Perhaps I had arrived as a critical care nurse, after all.

Just then, Rosemary's pager went off, but before she ran to attend to it, she reminded me that my turn to be in charge of the ICU would be coming up one day.

"It is an expectation of every nurse in the unit to take on this responsibility," she said. I could tell from her tone that this point was non-negotiable. "You have to know what's going on at the bedside, and beyond that, too."

"I don't think I could handle the responsibility of being in charge."

"When the time comes, you will be ready."

Okay, okay, I thought, but put it out of my mind for now.

I sat there for a few minutes after she left. On her desk was a journal article she had been reading. It was entitled "Hardiness: An Essential Attribute of the ICU Nurse."

I almost started to cry, but instead, I composed myself and returned to the ICU, where I could hear Laura busy expounding out loud at the nursing station, on her latest "theory" about the personality profiles of various medical specialists.

"Haven't you ever noticed that cardiologists are, by and large, musical and shy? They're slim and have long, narrow feet, and are very conservative lovers."

"How would *you* know that?" Nicole asked.

Laura ignored her. "Anesthesiologists are crass mercenaries, just in it for the money. They do lots of little procedures and make the big bucks. Patients get very attached to them because they put them to sleep or get rid of their pain. They're usually womanizers who drive fast red sports cars, and they're often drug addicts, too, because of their easy access to narcotics. Gastroenterologists are just grown-up kids who still like to dissect frogs and muck around with worms and mud pies. They love anything gooey or slimy. Surgeons are mechanics and technicians. All they care about is their little organ and only if they can fix it. If not, they move on. The patient could be having a heart attack, but the brain surgeon couldn't care less. Know what I mean? As for psychiatrists –" Here, she stopped for dramatic effect and rolled her eyes. "Need I say more? You get my drift. Endocrinologists are the only nice ones because they actually talk to patients. They listen to them, too. That's how they make their diagnosis. Neurologists are tight asses. So pedantic! They care way more about numbers and statistics than about people and pain. They care more about the diagnosis than the treatment. An exact identification of a rare, malignant astrocytoma in the subarachnoid space fascinates them so much that these nerds might just overlook the fact that there's no treatment for the poor patient who has that terrible tumour in their brain. Neurologists can't see the forest for the trees. In fact, they can't even see the trees for the leaves. Yeah, neurologists are leaf men," said Laura, ending her diatribe. "Strictly leaves."

"Aren't you generalizing, just a bit?" Nicole asked.

"No. I know what I'm talking about."

"Why don't you research all of this?" I asked Laura in mock seriousness to cajole her out of her crankiness. "You could do personality tests on the various groups of specialists, test out your hypothesis."

She walked away, but I could hear her going on about another of her theories. It was something to the effect that people peaked at different times in their lives. Let's say you were a rotten, miserable grown-up, she explained. You might have been a great baby. Maybe your peak was back then. Some people were great at being a teenager, but then went downhill in their twenties.

Perhaps my peak was yet to come?

By the time I had worked there almost a year – just two months short of my year-long commitment to the ICU – I finally felt competent. Of course, I wanted to be more than competent. I wanted to be a nurse like Laura, for her intuition and skills, Tracy for her calm helpfulness, Nicole for her kindness and fairness, Frances for her compassion, and Justine for her chutzpah. How Justine could make us howl with laughter! Was it that she saw everything as funny or was it that funny things always happened when she was around?

"Will you look at that?" she said just then. We were still standing outside of Rosemary's office. She pointed at Glenda, our housekeeper, who was just coming out of a patient's room, holding her rainbow-coloured feather duster up high across her chest, brandishing it like a drum majorette, hoisting her baton to the tune of some marching band that only she could hear.

"Oom-paa-paa, oom-paa-paa!" said Justine to her. "You go, girl!"

EARLY ONE MORNING, on a day that I wasn't scheduled to work, I got a phone call that woke me from a deep sleep.

"Could you come in for an overtime shift for us today, Tilda?" It was Cynthia, the night nurse in charge. "We've just had two sick calls – one of them Nell, of course, I should have predicted that – and we're really short-staffed."

The extra money would be great, but I was just coming off a stretch of nights and I was tired. I thought for a moment. It would be nice to help out, show them I was a team player. On the other hand, I didn't feel like going in and I wouldn't have the security of working with my gang. Cynthia needed my answer right away, so

I stilled my chattering mind and decided to offer whatever answer came out of my mouth. Let my unconscious decide for me.

"Okay, I'll come in," I heard myself say.

As I drove to work, I listened to the local news on the radio: a gang murder, an abducted child, and a devastating house fire, at least two people confirmed dead. There would likely be enough sadness and tragedy awaiting me during the day ahead, so I turned the dial to music – a peppy Blue Rodeo song.

When I arrived in the ICU, there was the usual bustle of activity. By then I knew all the other nurses because of our overlapping schedules. I easily joined the group gathered at the nursing station, the buzz of their conversation now comforting and familiar. It felt as much like a social gathering as part of the daily work routine.

"There's your assignment today, Tilda," said Cynthia. She pointed to a room outside of which a policeman stood watching the passing parade of the slower-moving night nurses leaving one by one, and the perky day nurses taking their place.

"Did you hear about the terrible fire in the West End overnight?" Cynthia asked me. "Well, the wife, she's one of the few survivors – she's your patient. They got her out in time and her husband's okay, too, but their baby died. Your patient has been in the hyperbaric chamber for decompression and just came out. She's doing well. You'll have a good day."

"Hello," I said to the policeman and stepped into the patient's room.

The smell hit me first. It was a smell I'd never encountered there before and it seemed out of place in the ICU. It was the wild, elemental scent of smoke. It was a natural smell of the outdoors that was so different from the chemicals and antiseptics or the human smells of infection and bodily fluids. It was the lingering aftermath of a bonfire on the beach, the fire tamped out, the embers dying down, but the ash smouldering, alive and still dangerous. It was also the smell of happy, carefree times – a campfire – but in this setting it seemed ominous.

"The patient is improving and her husband survived, too – he didn't even have to go in to the hyperbaric chamber, but – it's so sad – her mother, father, sister, and her eight-month-old baby all perished, burned to death in the fire this morning," said the night nurse. "No smoke detector, can you believe it? Anyway, so far only the husband, two brothers, and the wife have survived. The bodies of the parents, the sister, and the baby are still in the morgue, awaiting official identification."

"I haven't taken care of a smoke inhalation case before," I said. "What goes on in the hyperbaric chamber?"

"It looks like a submarine and it's based on the same concept. They put the patient in for a few hours. In the chamber they raise the atmospheric pressure so high that more hemoglobin and oxygen molecules bind together. Then they lower the pressure and decompress the patient slowly and gradually as they bring her out so that she doesn't get the bends."

"And what's with the cop outside the door?" I asked. I had noticed him peeking in the room from time to time, trying to get a glimpse of this unfolding drama.

"He's there to ensure that no one tampers with anything. He explained it to me, it's called continuity of evidence."

After she left, I proceeded to do my assessment. I could see the outline of a slight, still body under the yellow bedspread. Like all our patients, she was attached to the cardiac monitor. The breathing machine pumped oxygen into her lungs, and an assortment of other plastic, chrome, and wire attachments criss-crossed over and around her body. Her heartbeats moved across the black screen in green lines, and I noted that her rhythm was fast, but steady and regular. So far, so good.

I parted the tubings and made my way through the equipment and the stiff linen to get to her body and her hands. It still occasionally felt awkward to talk to intubated patients, but touching them was easier and more immediate. However, this time was different, because my patient opened her eyes a little and nodded her head in response to my voice.

Darryl Price, a visiting doctor from Ireland, specializing in critical care, came in to check on her. He reached under the covers for her hand, leaned down toward her and spoke softly, directly into her ear; his silk tie dragged across her chest. "You're going to be just fine, m'dear. Coming along nicely. We're hoping to get that breathing tube out, right away. You've got a great nurse taking care of ye." He winked at me.

He spoke like he was crooning a song and I loved listening to him. Even more, I was moved at the startling phenomenon of this doctor, speaking so personally and personably to a patient whose eyes were closed and who was just barely able to respond.

"Isabella," I said, afterwards, emboldened to show even more compassion by the example of this new doctor, "you're in the hospital, the intensive care unit. There was a fire in your house, but you are okay. I'm your nurse. Do you understand what I'm saying?" She squeezed my hand in reply.

As the morning wore on, I could see marked improvement from hour to hour. Isabella opened her eyes and began to look around. She began to breathe more on her own and I started to wean her off the ventilator. I gave her a warm bath and scrubbed the soot stains from her face, hands, and body. I explained everything I was doing, as I monitored her lungs, her heart, her stomach, and her mind.

"Isabella, you're doing really well," I kept telling her.

It was true. I could see she was getting better under my very eyes. What I suddenly realized was that she was getting better, in part, because of the care I was giving her.

Throughout the morning I spoke to her constantly, so that she would have a voice to move toward. I did not mention the loss of her child; she did not ask and I did not feel it was the time to tell her. She was pretty and looked so young, a lot younger than her thirty-one years. She had a long thick braid of black hair that I tried to keep neat and tidy. Someone from the family came to the door and pressed a tiny plastic Madonna and a gold cross into my hand and asked me to put them next to her pillow, and I did.

Rosemary came to tell me that the husband had recovered sufficiently from smoke inhalation to visit his wife.

"Why don't you go out to the waiting room to bring him in while I cover for you?" she asked.

The waiting room was full of visitors, but it was easy to spot which family was mine. Fernando Alvarez was the short, slight man, still greasy and grimy from the fire. He was covered in soot and looked like a shell-shocked soldier, just returned from battle. Aunts, uncles, and cousins accompanied him with me to the ICU to see Isabella for the first time since the fire.

"She's doing well," I reassured him, along the way. "She has been waking up slowly and is starting to move her limbs. Her blood pressure is very stable and soon we will have her off the ventilator. She's going to be just fine."

Once in the room, he approached the bed slowly. He could face her only in gradual increments, taking tentative, sideways glimpses, so his mind could catch up with his eyes. He looked at the bed, then at the floor, and then glanced back at the bed.

I guided him closer with my arm across his back, as I had seen Frances and Nicole do.

"She won't be able to talk to you right now. She's still not fully awake and she has a breathing tube in her mouth that goes down into her lungs. But she's alive."

I couldn't tell if it was too much information or, perhaps, not enough.

Mr. Alvarez approached the bed and forced himself to look at his wife. He took a long, straight-on look at her and then suddenly reared backwards in horror.

"*Jesus! Meu Deus! Ai, ai . . . não, não! Porque?*" he cried and collapsed in a heap on the floor. The other family members rushed to him where he lay.

"But she's improving!" I said. "She'll be just fine. Look, she's opening her eyes. There! Look. Isabella, look who's here. It's Fernando."

The other members took a look at her, then they too reeled back.

A cousin came forward to explain to me, in gasps. "This is not Isabella! This is not her. It's Isabella's little sister, Alva. And if it's Alva Machado in the bed . . . that means . . . that the body downstairs . . . oh, my God. Poor Fernando," he sobbed into his hands.

That meant that the charred remains of a human being that lay awaiting identification in the morgue must be his wife, Isabella.

His grief at the death of his baby was instantly doubled – if the laws of mathematics apply to such emotions. His anguish expanded to fill the room as he began to howl. He twisted and writhed on the floor. The cousins, aunts, and uncles surrounded him, and each one pulled up on his arms and legs to get him to his feet – even the policeman came in to help. But he fought against them; he did not want to be brought to his feet. He wanted to stay down there on the floor and die as his wife had. I saw what it meant to be beside oneself with grief. I thought fleetingly of joining him.

The ward clerk moved in swiftly. The patient's name band had to be changed, as well as the health insurance number and the information in the computer. She had to let Admitting know about this mix-up, right away.

I couldn't sit. I couldn't stand. I couldn't summarize the notes in the chart or tally the in's and the out's on the fluid balance sheet. I couldn't even find it in myself to be happy that at least we had saved someone and a young person, at that. I felt myself shutting down, until I felt nothing. I felt my heart closing off to save myself. It was too much for me.

Rosemary told me, "Tilda, go take a break in the lounge. Give yourself time to pull yourself together. Maybe you would like to leave early?"

I was a failure.

Leave early, Rosemary had said. Did she mean for the rest of the day or for the rest of the year? Leave the ICU altogether?

She came to check on me and then sent me home in a taxi, and another nurse took over for me.

6

SISTERS OF THE AIR

I took a few weeks off work, but moped around at home and thought of little else than work. How could I strengthen myself enough to do this work, keep enough of a separation that the sadness didn't affect me so much, yet stay emotionally connected to my patients and their suffering? I wanted to be efficient and empathetic, compassionate and capable. Competent was not enough. But more than these concerns, I missed the work – and my friends.

"You had fun at work," Ivan commented, one evening over dinner.

It wasn't meant as a criticism, but I took it that way. Enough to set down my fork and face the imagined attack.

"How could anyone do this work if they didn't have a few laughs now and again? It's perfectly harmless. We never do it in front of the patients. Laughing is our coping mechanism."

"You don't have to give it a fancy name. You're allowed to have a good time. There's nothing wrong with having fun." He chuckled at my indignation. "I was merely making an observation."

He knew what he was talking about. I considered him somewhat of an expert on fun, and I knew I had a lot to learn about the subject. In my family, when I was growing up, I never even thought about fun. Having fun was taboo. How inconsiderate it would have been to be light-hearted when there was my poor mother, lying on the couch, always sad and disappointed by life. How could I have *fun* when *she* could not?

It was Ivan who introduced me to the concept of fun, but it was the nurses of the ICU who taught me its practice. I was thinking about all this when the phone rang. It was Justine.

"Yo, Tilda! Listen, since you've gone incommunicado, I'm calling to tell you the latest news. The hospital has a new mascot. She's this huge woman who sits outside the front entrance every day in a wheelchair, calling out to everyone who walks by. I swear, she's the world's ugliest woman. Her legs are wrapped in drippy bandages and she's holding her IV pole with one hand like it's an umbrella and smoking a cigarette with the other. She gets people to collect cigarette butts off the lawn and then she stuffs them all into one butt and has a free smoke! Then she chatters away all day about how she used to be in show business, but the doctors took out her ribs and shocked her and now she can't shovel snow any more. She keeps calling out that they're using her as a guinea pig, a scapegoat, and a miner's canary – all because of the bomb that was dropped on Hiroshima. Get the picture? Then at the end of the day, the Wheel-Trans bus comes and – what that poor driver has to put up with – takes her away!"

Of course, I burst out laughing, but tried to stifle it. It wasn't right to laugh.

"Thanks for that information, Justine. I can hardly wait to meet her," I said.

"So, Til, when are you coming back to work?"

"Let me talk to her," I heard Laura say and could just picture her grabbing the phone from Justine. "Get your butt back in here, Oh Sensitive One. We need you. Do you know how short-staffed we are? We have two doubles and a sick call – one of them Nell Mason, of course – and I've been on the phone all morning calling for overtime. Some team player you are!"

Frances was next. "Howya doin', Tillie? Oh, we miss you so much. Come back already. You're not going to quit, are you? We're all going out for drinks this week, it's Justine's birthday. Can you join us? Work has been so interesting lately. We've done lots of transplants – lung and liver – and we even did something new – a combined kidney, pancreas, plus liver and intestinal transplant on a young boy who had a rare idiopathic coagulopathy. He's doing really well for a guy that was so sick when he came in, with clots throughout his abdomen and pelvis, one of them obstructing his –"

"Time's up, Jabber Jaws," I could hear Laura tell her. It sounded like Laura was trying to yank the phone away.

"Old Bossy Boots here won't let me talk any more. You come back, soon," Frances managed to call into the phone as Nicole got on the line to tell me she was dating someone new – a nephrology resident, Oliver, who had rotated through our ICU and was very well liked – and she was very happy. "This might be the one," she said.

Then Tracy came on the line to tell me quietly – she wasn't ready to tell the others – that she was pregnant. She was a few weeks along, but she and Ron had been trying for a long time and were ecstatic.

I called Rosemary the next morning and told her I was ready to return.

IT HAD TAKEN me only two weeks away from my work to recover from that disturbing mix-up with the smoke inhalation patient, plus the residue of sadness I couldn't seem to shake off after caring for the Sikh family and their son. During that time I came to the paradoxical realization that I loved being a critical care nurse and wouldn't want to work anywhere else. I had worked so hard to master the skills; I couldn't give up now. How could I ever have thought otherwise? In fact, at times I even felt a little sorry for people who didn't have work as fascinating as mine.

On the evening before I returned to work, the group of us, along with boyfriends and husbands, met at a pool hall in Little Italy to celebrate Justine's thirtieth birthday. She announced that she was going to university part-time to work on her degree and then mentioned in passing that she and her boyfriend of only a few months, Tom, were engaged and we toasted all of those things.

I noticed that everyone was calling her by a new nickname and I asked why.

"It's because of what happened the other night at work," said Nicole. "Tell Tilda about it."

Justine needed no prodding.

"Some lab technician calls to tell me that my patient's potassium is 3.1 mmols. This guy hardly speaks a word of English – 'verry creetee-cull reee-sult,' he's saying. I say to him, okay, it's 3.1, gotcha. Goodbye. But then he asks my name. What right does he have to ask my name? Why do you need my name? I ask. Some new policy about verification. Okey-dokey. I say, 'My name is Pippi. Pippi Longstocking.' A minute later his supervisor calls back to ask my real name. It's his job, he says. This is serious business and he has no time for games. I say, 'Pippi' – and slam the phone down."

"Did she ever!" said Nicole.

"So the guy calls back and I say, okay, you're right, I was kidding about Pippi. My name is Morticia. Morticia Addams. And he buys that!"

"We laughed about it all night," said Tracy.

The name stuck. She became Morty.

The next night there was a sequel.

Never one to leave a prank well enough alone, Justine rummaged around in the refrigerator, which was always cluttered with Tupperware containers of old food and plastic bags filled with abandoned lunches. She found a Thermos with some sort of slimy substance in it and slapped a big yellow sticker on it, labelled "Biohazardous Material: Handle With Caution" and sent it off to the Microbiology lab, along with a requisition to identify the contents!

WE STAYED OUT late that night and had a few drinks – I drank a watermelon wine cooler and endured incessant teasing for it – but we all had to leave by midnight, because we had to get up early the next morning for work.

It seemed like no time at all passed between the moment my head hit the pillow and the ringing of my alarm clock at 6:00. I jumped out of bed and hustled off to work.

By lunchtime, it felt like I'd never left. In fact, I was reminded it was lunchtime by Navreen, the travelling Roti Lady, whose real job was in the hospital laundry service. She stuck her head into the opening of the curtains in my patient's room to ask if I wanted to buy either a spicy chicken or vegetarian roti – that was all she had left.

I could hear Laura arguing with someone on the phone.

"The order is in the computer, you say? . . . It says I'm supposed to bring the patient down for an ultrasound at 1300 hours? I see. . . . Maybe, just maybe, I'll take an order from a doctor, but from a computer? Never!"

Frances had been tied up in the quiet room for over an hour with a distraught family, participating in a drawn-out family meeting conducted by the Irish doctor, Darryl Price. He did tend to go on and on.

Tracy and Nicole came to get me for lunch.

For some reason, Justine was patrolling the refrigerator, still looking for something.

"Who stole my can of Diet Pepsi?" she yelled into its depths as she rummaged around. "I was just getting ready to drink it."

I didn't think it belonged to anyone. It had been in there for weeks. I must have looked guilty, because she looked right at me.

She pointed her finger at me. "You?" She made the motions of chugging back a drink.

I nodded. "I was thirsty. Here, go get yourself another." I tossed her a loonie. "My treat," I added graciously.

"Thirsty? Thirsty, you say? I don't care if your mouth is as parched as the Sahara Desert. Don't steal my stuff," she grumbled.

"You don't scare me," I laughed and the others joined me.

Later that day, Rosemary came over to Justine, who was working beside me that day. She had a puzzled expression and held out a lab report to Justine. "Is this for you, by any chance?" she asked.

It was addressed to Morticia Addams, Staff Nurse, Medical-Surgical ICU.

Microbiology Report
Identification of Thermos contents: Ravioli.

MY PATIENT ON the day that I returned to work was a thirty-year-old Cree woman from a reserve near Manitoulin Island who had swallowed paint thinner and antifreeze. She had a history of drug and alcohol abuse, but whether she had gone on a desperate binge or made a deliberate suicide attempt was not clear. However, this time her actions had put her into a hepatic coma that had so badly disrupted her body's clotting mechanism that she was bleeding from both her mouth and rectum, as well as internally, because of her destroyed liver. She was in a deep stupor, but roused from time to time and uttered incomprehensible sounds. As the day wore on, we had to insert a huge tube into her stomach to stem the bleeding and a breathing tube into her lungs to protect her airway from aspiration. I knew that only a brand-new healthy liver could save her life, but these weren't so readily available.

"I hope she's a candidate for a liver transplant," I said during rounds.

"Of course she is. She's right at the top of the transplant list," said Dr. Bristol. "Is there any reason you can think of that she wouldn't be a suitable transplant candidate?"

I drew a blank at this test question and luckily he turned it over to the entire team to consider.

"I want to know if she's made a commitment to taking better care of herself, if she's going to abstain from drinking and taking drugs so that she doesn't ruin her new liver," one of the nurses said.

"Something as precious and rare as a liver isn't to be taken lightly," someone else commented.

"Isn't it her right to live her life as she chooses?" asked Dr. Bristol. "What if she isn't completely rational? Do you believe that receiving an organ transplant confers a moral obligation?"

Some of us nodded.

"What if this unfortunate woman is mentally ill and unable to keep such good intentions? Is living a healthy lifestyle something that can be legislated? Even if it could, should it? What if her home environment, social conditions, personality – whatever – predispose her to make decisions that might jeopardize her new liver? Let me put something else to all of you. Would you put a death-row prisoner on the transplant list to receive a new liver? Should our criteria be strictly medical need or do lifestyle choices figure into the mix? I want you all to think carefully about these things before you're so quick to pass judgment. Once we make medical decisions based on our emotional reactions, we set a very dangerous –"

Just then Justine – now known by all as Morty – sauntered over to the team, carrying a large metal basin filled with murky grey water that was sloshing from side to side.

"Here's a real ethical dilemma," she said. "Who volunteers to drink a medicine cup full of my patient's dirty bathwater for a million dollars?"

Just the thought made us scatter back to our patients' rooms.

Rounds were over.

"FLORA KNOWS EVERYTHING about living in the bush," the young woman at my patient's bedside said proudly. She wore a filthy plaid jacket and her hair was scraggly.

"Who is to be contacted in case of an emergency?" I asked.

I had to complete the form in the chart but I knew that the emergency had already arrived. This was it.

"That'd be me. Flora's my sister and I'm her sister. We're sisters of the air. She knows everything about me. I know everything about her, even though we don't live nowhere together no more." She took off her jacket and folded it at the foot of her sister's bed. "Flora's on the Rez and works in a factory, but we don't need to talk. If she's there, then she's there and if she's not there, she's still there. She's with me wherever I am, all the time. I call her my sister of the air. How's she doing, anyway?"

"She's . . ." I looked at this young woman before me and did my best to ignore her dishevelled appearance and unwashed smells of the back alleys of the city, where she likely lived. I looked over at Flora, stretched out in the bed, bleeding and unconscious, then back at her sister of the air. "She's very sick."

"But she'll make it, won't she? Isn't she going to get a new liver? That's what the doctor said. One of those trans*plane*tations?"

"We hope so," I said. "If she can hang in until a liver becomes available."

"I guess she can't eat nuthin' yet, huh?"

"No, not yet."

The sister shook her head and let out a sigh between her teeth.

FRANCES CALLED ME one day at home.

"Listen, I'm planning to pay a visit to Nell Mason. She told me not to come but she's been off sick for weeks and I'm worried about her."

For a number of years, it had been Nell's pattern to work a few days, then call in sick, just at the last moment before the shift started, often leaving us in the lurch. One year Nell had accumulated more sick days than days at work. However, she invariably offered a variety of creative excuses.

"Yeah, like the Ebola virus," Nicole recalled one day while we were shooting the breeze in the cafeteria. "Remember when Nell called in sick because she thought she had the Ebola virus?"

"Yeah, the only problem was that although we had that suspected Ebola patient in the unit, she hadn't had contact with him. She must be a hypochondriac," said Laura.

"How about when she called in with Chinese Food Syndrome?" said Nicole.

"What the hell is that?" asked Justine.

"You know that funny throbbing feeling you can get from eating MSG?"

"How 'bout when Nell called in to say she couldn't make it in to work because her best friend was dying and she had to help her plan her funeral, choose the music, and everything? Do you remember when she called to say she couldn't come to work because her mother was just diagnosed with a brain tumour and then Morty, without missing a beat, asked her, is this the same mother who died two years ago and last year was in a fatal car crash?" someone else recalled.

"How 'bout when she called to say she couldn't come to work because she had ringing in her ears?" Laura said. "I was in charge and when she told me that I said, perfect, then of course you can come to work. There are bells and whistles ringing here all the time!"

We knew Nell well, as we did most of the other nurses, but she was not part of our circle. Nell had no group. As it turned out, she was more alone than any of us realized.

After her call to me, Frances went alone to see Nell and in the cafeteria the next day she told us about the visit.

"Nell sat on a low window ledge in her empty apartment – she hardly had any furniture – and just stared at me. This was not the Nell we know. She was silent. Didn't say a word."

"Probably couldn't get a word in edgewise, with you there, Jabber Jaws," I heard Laura mutter.

Frances continued. "Her silence was the strangest thing. I tried to get her talking, but she didn't answer me. No adventures or tall tales. None." Frances ended the story sadly. "But she says she'll be back at work, soon."

"I loved her story about the night when she took care of Glenn Gould after he had a massive cerebral hemorrhage," I said. "I could just picture it when she told me how she propped up his arms and hands on pillows and his fingers began to play 'The Moonlight Sonata,' or so she claimed."

Nell had often spoken about a period of her life when she was a hockey mom to five orphan boys in Thunder Bay and how as a child she used to ride a camel to school. It had been given to her family by an itinerant circus troupe. We all remembered her recount the day the camel broke out of his pen and rampaged through the town. It crashed into a strawberry social the ladies of the local church were holding and soon whipped cream, shortcake, and berries were flying everywhere.

We all knew of times when we were working with her and she had to run out to the Eaton Centre on her lunch hour. If she was a little late getting back, she had a ready explanation for her delay.

"I had to do CPR on someone who had a cardiac arrest in a shoe store," she'd say. Or "I got stuck in an elevator and all of a sudden, it cut loose and started plummeting downward. I kept jumping up and down, figuring I'd have a 50 per cent chance of being in the air when it came to a crash landing, and that's exactly what happened. What luck!"

Sometimes, if work was slow, I was guilty of prompting her and goading her into recounting stories of her exotic vacations where she always had fantastic adventures and narrow escapes, just like Indiana Jones. There was the time she was walking along a secluded beach in the Galapagos Islands when she was chased and attacked by a pack of wild dogs. She swam far out into the ocean to escape them, but they tore into the water after her. Then one by one, as the dogs plunged in after her and set upon her, snarling and growling, brave Nell had the presence of mind to poke out their eyes and blind them, then drag them under the water, one by one, and drown them.

The funny thing was that when she did show up to work, Nell was a wonderful nurse. She had a wise, calm presence, vast knowledge, and expert skills. Patients adored Nell, always asked for her and gave her gifts of money, flowers, bottles of fine wine, and job offers for private nursing for astronomical wages.

We were grateful that Frances had gone to visit her. We were all so comfortable and experienced with diseases of the body – heart attacks, respiratory failure, liver disease – but the mind? No one knew anything about that! If a patient in the ICU ever showed signs of depression or anxiety, we'd call a "psych consult" and they would come in and talk to the patient for a few minutes and then order a cocktail of meds, such as Valium and Prozac, or Haldol and Ativan.

"I HATE NURSING. I can't wait to get out of this hell hole."

I was horrified to hear Laura saying this to a tall, slim, beautifully coiffed woman in a navy suit who was standing at the nursing station. She had come to visit our ICU to gather data on research she was doing about nurses' work lives. It also turned out she was one of the new vice-presidents of the hospital who was getting out to meet and greet the "frontline workers."

"I hate this job," Laura added, as if her first statement wasn't clear enough.

The woman looked a bit taken aback, but kept her cool. "Do you have any specific concerns?" she inquired, but Laura shrugged her shoulders and turned away.

"Gotta get back to my patient," she mumbled discourteously.

"What good is that?" I asked when I confronted Laura later. "Either articulate your complaints constructively or don't be such a bitch. It reflects badly on all of us. If you're not part of the solution, you're part of the –"

"Stop lecturing me! I'd like to see that fancy lady put on a pair of scrubs – she did mention she was a nurse, didn't she? – and pitch in here and give us a hand. She's probably one of the ones behind the move that's underfoot to oust us, lay us off – especially us old-fashioned, uneducated, diploma nurses – and hire the cafeteria sandwich makers and housekeeping staff to replace us. She's the one who wants to institute some new theory of nursing, but hasn't a clue what nurses really do in practice. I don't trust her for a minute. She's going to sell us up the river when the next swing of the pendulum comes around and the government decides there's too many of us."

Morty, freshly revved up from a union meeting and never one to miss out on a good argument, joined in.

"Laura's right, Tilda. Nurses make up the vast majority of the hospital workforce – over 95 per cent – and we're the only ones who are at patients' bedsides twenty-four hours a day. We're the ones out there risking our lives, exposing ourselves to infectious diseases – hepatitis, tuberculosis, HIV, and now these new super-bugs, these drug-resistant bacteria that every other patient seems to get these days. Not to mention the hazardous working conditions, the radiation exposure, the toxic chemotherapy spills on the countertops – I had a fingernail melt away from some of that stuff. There's Aspergillus fungus blowing in at us from the ceiling vents and Acinetobacter in the plumbing. And believe me, girls – and boys," she added with a nod to Bruno and Charles, who had come over to listen in, "it's way worse on the floors. You wouldn't believe their workload or the conditions they have to put up with. We've got it made here in the ICU, especially with a nurse manager like Rosemary – we couldn't have a better one – but I bet you they'll give her the axe one day, too."

"See what I mean, Tilda?" Laura felt vindicated. "You're incredibly naïve. So what's the point of talking to this new corporate nurse person? And what's the incentive to stay here – all these hassles, no respect, stressful work environment, fighting politics with the doctors, abusive patients, and angry families? Oh, yeah, and an extra fifteen cents an hour for the additional responsibility of being in charge. Your turn is coming up soon! You better get ready. You'll see, the additional $1.80 you make will just barely cover the cost of the extra coffee you'll need to keep you going."

"What's the incentive?" I stammered. "What's the incentive? What about all the reasons you went into nursing in the first place?"

"I do this job because I like to think that there will be someone there to care for me when I get sick one day," Laura said.

"How do you know –?"

"We're all going to get sick of one thing or another. Get real, Tilda. We're all going to need a nurse one day. We're all potential patients. I just hope there's a good nurse there for me when it happens. Maybe that's why I do this work. Superstition or hope or wishful thinking that if I do my part, someone else will do theirs."

"I'm not listening to you any more," I told Laura later that day. "I'm not listening to you complain all the time unless you can come up with some constructive plans to improve things. You say what's the incentive? I'll tell you – doing work that's interesting and challenging. Helping people. Having the opportunity every day to make a difference in people's lives. Having the skills to relieve pain, comfort an anxious family member, assess a wound and know exactly what's needed to heal it. I don't believe these things aren't satisfying to you, because you're one of the nurses around here who do those things best. I don't believe you, anyway. If you hated nursing that much you wouldn't be as good a nurse as you are. Besides, if you really hate nursing, as you claim you do, what are your plans to change careers? If you're really planning to leave this job, have you updated your resumé or taken any courses?"

"Booze and cheap drugs, that's my escape from this place . . . and chocolate," she said.

"Very good, keep it up. You'll be here forever."

I simply didn't believe her. I stood watching her warm her patient's cold hands in hers. I watched the steadiness in her arm that guided the crying family from the quiet room. I watched her titrate the dose of Levophed with the dips and surges of her patient's erratic blood pressure. She was brilliant. I would let her do open-heart surgery on me. Yet her bitterness was a poison I wanted to expunge from her heart – for her own sake and because I was afraid it would infect too many others.

"Tell me, what's the real reason you take the longest route to the cafeteria?" I asked her.

"There you go again," she said with a sigh. "I need the exercise, okay?"

"You claim I'm the one who's so sensitive . . . I'm not so sure."

"I have never, ever cried over a patient," she said, "and I never will."

NICOLE LONGED TO be married and have a houseful of kids. She wanted to have a boy and a girl and a Sharpei, named Liam, Sophie, and Chin-Chin, respectively. Things were going well with Oliver, but it was still too soon to say for sure. Nicole knew, as the others did, that she'd better start taking courses toward her degree, even if only part-time. The problem was, another world pulled her in a different direction. She was a scratch golfer and once had dreams of trying out for the professional circuit. She had taken a year off work and golf training in order to care for her dying mother. We knew she was still working toward paying off her student loan and was in no position to take on the cost of tuition. Apparently her game hadn't suffered too much from the time off, however. When Daniel Huizinga and David Bristol challenged her to a round of golf, she trounced them – to our delight.

According to David's sheepish report, "Nicky double bogied at the opening hole, then strung 17 pars in a row."

What a pleasure finally to see the personal side of him.

"She was amazing," he added, in awe. "We didn't even bother to add up our score!"

JUSTINE CLAIMED SHE wanted to get into politics or acting and keep nursing as a sideline. Nonetheless, she kept working hard toward her degree and had aspirations for further education. Her love of centre stage found opportunities in local theatre where she had played Bloody Mary in an amateur production of *South Pacific* in Scarborough and a role in the chorus line of *Grease*. She also claimed it was a good place to meet guys, something she was very successful at, anyway. In addition to these activities, Justine also took her duties as our union rep very seriously and spent a lot of her spare time attending meetings, rallies, and dealing with grievances, which was just as well, because she was the first to admit that her forte was not patient care.

FRANCES CLAIMED SHE was happy. It was strange to hear someone say that. I hadn't ever heard it said before.

"I love being a nurse," she said simply.

Even stranger.

"HAVE YOU THOUGHT about going back to school to get your Master's degree?" Rosemary asked me. She was working on one herself, taking evening courses.

"I'm not ready to go back to school," I said. "I still have a lot to learn about patient care. I want to continue doing what I'm doing."

It was late afternoon on that first day back at work, after my brief leave of absence. I sat with Rosemary in her messy office. The exuberant Trout Symphony played softly from her computer and I caught a whiff of her vanilla-scented cologne from the Body Shop:

she smelled like cookies. She wanted to know how work was going and did I plan to stay on after my year was up, in a month's time? She didn't mean to pressure me, she explained, but she needed to know, as full-time positions were becoming scarce once again.

"The trend keeps repeating itself," she said. "The need for nurses stays the same. What changes is each government's willingness to pay for them. Now the pressure is on us to move our staff toward part-time and casual positions and bring in agency nurses as needed." The tense expression on her face made me realize she wasn't pleased about these changes. She explained the administration's position. "It's a cost-saving measure so the hospital can avoid paying nurses benefits or offer any assurance of job stability. Ultimately, we're trying to avoid layoffs." She smiled at me. "As for your work, Tilda, it's quite satisfactory," she said. "You give safe care."

My heart sank. I wanted to do much more than that.

"You are competent, but very emotional. I worry about you. There might be other departments in the hospital where –"

"No, I want to stay here, Rosemary. I want to get over my emotions."

"I understand," she said and paused, to consider her reply. "It's like this. Certain patient emotions, for example, anxiety, can be contagious. Patients' emotions belong to them. Your ability to be helpful to patients and families will be impaired if you share their feelings – fear, anxiety, anger, despair – whatever. The nursing literature on this subject calls it 'emotional contagion' and it's like an infectious disease itself. It's hard to stay immune to it. It's very easily spread and difficult to treat. Some nurses vaccinate themselves with emotional disconnection and apathy, both of which lead to burnout and attrition. However, on the other hand, over-identifying with the patient can prevent a nurse from functioning as a professional. The course of action I suggest is this: prevention. Take good care of yourself so that you are in a position to take care of others. Eat properly, get exercise, do yoga or meditation, whatever it takes to be healthy. Take mental health breaks from this work, as you wisely did. Make sure you have good support systems outside of work, develop hobbies – I love gourmet cooking, for example, and my husband and I breed Jack Russell terriers. Find a balance between your work and your personal life. It's important to ensure that your own life is healthy, especially when you're in the profession of taking care of others. All those who wish to serve others have these same challenges."

"Sometimes, when I'm not at work, I think a lot about the patients and wonder how they're doing. Certain cases really get me down," I said glumly. "Sometimes the situations we deal with are really –"

"Hopeless?"

I nodded.

"It is hopeless only if you see death as a failure, if you see death as the worst possible outcome. Many doctors see death as a personal failure, but nurses have the chance to make a valuable contribution in these cases. We can do everything we are able to do to save a patient, but then we have to let go and recognize our limitations. Besides, not everyone here dies, but it's human nature to dwell on the catastrophic cases. However, I believe that there is always something to hope for, even if a full recovery isn't possible. These are the things that are at the heart of nursing's domain. I've heard you say it yourself. It's all that you learned at school and from the examples of your colleagues. I must say, you have chosen to make friends with quite a wild bunch, but I have a lot of respect for each of them. If you focus on those things that are at the heart of nursing – comfort, dignity, nourishment, promoting well-being – you'll find that you'll alleviate some of the suffering, and you'll always have hope."

After I left Rosemary's office, I thought about what she had said and also about a conversation I'd had that very morning with Tracy. She was telling me about the liver transplant patient she'd taken care of last week who had done so well. Within twenty-four hours of his surgery, new liver intact and working, he was transferred out of the ICU to a general floor, smiling, talking, and rejoicing with his family. She told me about him, because the patient had suddenly deteriorated that morning and needed to return first to the operating room and then to our ICU. He was in shock, still bleeding internally, and his room was swarming with people.

"It's a zoo in there," said Tracy, standing just outside the door, looking in.

"Why didn't you ask to be his nurse so you could follow up with him? You knew him and his family so well."

"I got pretty close to them," she admitted. "They were so glad to see me the other day on the elevator and told me how well he was doing on the floor. Even so, I think it's better if someone else takes care of him today."

It's probably better for you, too, I realized in that moment.

To do this work properly, I was going to have to keep something back. I would have to learn to create and nurture that peaceful harbour within myself that Rosemary described. Otherwise, how could I go on opening my heart and having it broken again and again? But if I closed it altogether, what kind of nurse would I become?

ANOTHER FRIENDLY FACE on staff in the ICU was that of Father Vincent Szigetti. Because he wore casual blazers and no clerical collar, I didn't realize at first that he was a priest. He had the rotund belly of a sensual man who enjoyed his food and drink a little too much, and because he confided in me, I knew those things to be true. He visited us often, both the nurses as well as the patients and families, and regaled us with hysterical jokes and fascinating stories about his missionary work in Africa and his travels through war-torn Bosnia.

"When you went to Nigeria, did you take the wife and kids?" I once asked him.

"Oh no, my dear, I'm a priest. I'm married to the church." He looked at me with mock seriousness and twinkling eyes. "Many of us don't wear the collar any more. Not us modern ones, anyway. But we follow the tenets of the Vatican, just the same. Now, don't forget, I'm the R.C. chaplain."

"Oh," I said and giggled. "Now, don't *you* forget, I'm the J. nurse!"

"I thought so, my dear."

"Would you ever take confession from a Jew?"

"From you, anytime, my dear! But surely you don't have anything to confess!"

"You'd be surprised," I said and left it at that.

I often helped him figure out from the patients' names whether they were Roman Catholic and therefore might be in need of his services – confession or communion, the sacrament of the sick or last rites. Sometimes, when things were going badly and I asked the family if I should call the priest, it sounded like a line from a movie.

"Is it that bad?" they would ask. "Is he that far gone?"

"You deserve a commission from all the referrals you've made to me," Father Szigetti joked.

"I'd be rich," I said. "But everyone could use your services, not just Catholics."

"You'd be surprised!" he said. "Now, dear, if you ever need to speak with me about anything that's troubling you, please come by my office or have me paged."

I often shared with him things that troubled me, as well as many hearty laughs about silly things. For example, if he wanted to know about a patient who had been discharged from the ICU, he would ask, "Discharged upward?" with a heavenward glance.

"Going up?" I would say if I saw him waiting for an elevator.

"I hope so and I will see you there, too!"

We also had serious discussions about many things, such as the assassination of Yitzchak Rabin, the prime minister of Israel, budget cuts to health care, the choice of soups that day in the cafeteria, and our sweet-tooth indulgences.

"I realize I should eat less, swim more. My joints are getting creaky. That's the problem, we realize these things, but we don't do them, God, please forgive us."

Once I called him during the night to administer the last rites for a patient.

"I'll be right there, my dear."

Within fifteen minutes, he was.

"Is he conscious? Is he still able to hear me?" Father Szigetti asked me as he took the patient's hand in his and bent down close to his face.

"He's not conscious, but he may very well hear you. We have no way of knowing for sure. We always talk to patients anyway, just in case. You never know what they take in."

"Well, my dear, I will pray for his soul and sit with the family, but I can't administer the sacrament of the sick or the last rites to an unconscious man. There has to be a conscious will in order to accept the blessing. It can't be done without the patient's participation."

I wondered if I should hold back the morphine that was keeping the patient comfortable, but drowsy, in order that he might be more awake to participate in these rituals. Which need took priority, the body or the soul?

"But isn't prayer supposed to be a consolation?" I asked, annoyed with him that he was being such a stickler, withholding something that might comfort the family. Why did a prayer come with conditions? I pressed further. "I don't understand, Father. A man is dying. Wouldn't he want it said? Besides, maybe he *can* hear you. Why don't you take that chance?"

"I'm sorry, my dear, but if this unfortunate gentleman can't participate in acceptance of the sacrament, it cannot be administered. I can bless him with the holy water. That I can do. The edicts of the Padre must prevail." He dipped his pinky finger into a little silver vessel that he carried with him and made the sign of the cross on the patient's forehead. He closed his eyes, and whatever the prayers were that he was saying, I stood there and joined him.

"How do you deal with all the suffering that you see in the hospital, especially in the ICU?" I asked him sometime shortly after that meeting with Rosemary in her office.

"Death and sickness are a part of life," he said quietly. "None of it surprises me, nor does it sadden me. I accept it as God gives it to us. Sometimes I wonder what will happen if modern medicine and science manage to eradicate illness altogether. How will we learn the important lessons of humility, faith, hope, gratitude, and compassion, that these mortal conditions teach us?" Father Szigetti gave a nod toward Mrs. Zaiken's room. "By the way, she's one of yours, I think," he said with mock solemnity.

"That's true. I'll look after her," I said and smiled.

"Speaking of which," said Rosemary, tapping me on the shoulder, "Tilda, could you give us a hand with Mrs. Zaiken? Bruno is her nurse, but there's a problem you might be able to help us sort out. I'll stay here with your patient and cover for you."

The family were Orthodox Jews and didn't want their mother taken care of by a male nurse.

"Bruno is an outstanding nurse," I said and put my arm lightly around him. He was looking a bit crushed. "He's a complete gentleman and will respect your mother's modesty. Not only that, but Bruno is a *mensch*."

"Isn't there a female nurse available who could look after our mother instead?" a black-suited, black-hatted man inquired, keeping his gaze on the clock on the wall beside the door where I stood. I recalled that even eye contact with a woman was prohibited.

"We'll try to keep your request in mind from now on," I said.

A man was sitting in the corner of the room, rocking backwards and forwards vigorously and loudly chanting Hebrew psalms.

"By the way," I asked, my curiosity, as usual, getting the best of me, "what are you praying for?" I glanced down at Mrs. Zaiken's chart: Alzheimer's disease. Ovarian cancer. Kidney failure and coronary artery disease. Seventy-four years old, living in a nursing home.

"That the Lord might see fit to grant her more days," the spokesman answered.

"I see," I said.

WE MADE A point of meeting once a month, our group, Laura's Line. We went out for lunch or dinner and a movie or just drinks, but wherever we went, we stipulated that we would not talk about work.

"But who else can we talk to about work? Sometimes I need to go over this stuff to get it settled in my mind," I wailed. "I can't tell Ivan or any of my friends. They tell me it's depressing to hear about my work. It upsets them so I never can talk about it."

"Go see a shrink," said Laura.

"I can't tell anyone, either," said Nicole.

Perhaps Tracy was the wisest. She kept quiet, listening to us and keeping her own counsel. How I envied her self-containment.

"I tell people what I do, but no one believes me. Can you imagine if people knew what we *really* do?" asked Morty. "I mean the truth? No one would believe it. Hey, Tilda, no drinky-poo for you tonight. You're still feeling the effects from that silly Kool-Aid drink you had last time."

"No one could even describe some of the things we do," said Laura with an involuntary shudder. "No one has seen what we've seen. Did you see that cavity in Mrs. Claggett's chest after they removed her lung? You could get lost in there. I had to shove my arm in up to my elbow to pack the wound and they hadn't even ordered any pain medication for her, 'cause it dropped her blood pressure. I feel like a member of Hitler's army when I do that dressing."

"Enough!" we yelled out in a group mutiny.

"There's more to life than work!" Nicole said.

"I agree," said Tracy, who was sipping ginger ale. She still wasn't ready to tell them her news.

Frances also wanted to change the subject. "Let's talk about something else, shall we? How are the Leafs doing in the playoffs? Nicole, what about that new guy, Tiger Woods, do you think he'll win the Masters? Not only that, but there's a war going on in the Middle East. Bosnia, Ireland, and Zimbabwe, too. What about all of that?"

Of course.

"I wonder if my patient got a liver transplant in the end," I murmured. I was thinking about the Cree women, those two sisters of the air.

"Tilda!"

7

GIFTS AND DONATIONS

'Twas the day before the night before Christmas, and all through the hospital lobby joyful music rang out!

I made sure of that.

My loathsome childhood piano lessons turned out to be worth it, after all: I approached the hospital administration with the proposition that the flagging morale (the place had been abuzz lately with ominous rumours about layoffs and cutbacks) of the staff and patients could be lifted by an infusion of Christmas spirit. How better to do this than with the glorious music of the season? However, certain objections were raised. We live in a city of multicultural diversity. We have to be sensitive to the needs of all groups. If Christmas is celebrated, others will feel marginalized. They will not feel that their voices are heard; they will feel excluded. Why not embrace them all, I asked. Have an African group come in and sing the melodies of Kwanzaa, a choir of children from a synagogue, and so on. They would look into it, they said. Maybe call a meeting, form a committee, strike a task force . . .

Meanwhile, I managed to convince them that this year at least, Christmas wouldn't be Christmas without carols! I opened the keyboard and started off the morning by launching straight into

Joy to the World!

It was in a high-pitched key and I didn't know how to transpose it down a notch, but luckily, some soprano cleaning staff showed up by 0730 hours and helped me carry the tune.

With all my heart and soul I

Let Heaven and Nature Sing!

The lobby did look festive, in a restrained sort of way. A few tired-looking green and red tinsel streamers had been draped here and there. The electric lights on a forlorn artificial Christmas tree that was a permanent fixture, all year round, were turned on for the week. "Seasons Greetings to All" announced the banner that was strung across the entrance to the lobby.

I sat at the piano, which was positioned near the information booth at the main entrance, under a sign written in the green and black colours of the hospital that read, "Taking Care of You is a Corporate Priority."

Even at that early hour, the hospital was already bustling. A trolley with an industrial-sized urn of hot apple cider was set out and people helped themselves. The secretaries from radiology and the kitchen staff, a staff pathologist, a few social workers, and the chief librarian were all there, clustered around the piano. The lady who gave out the uniforms (known throughout the hospital for her surly manner and her habit of handing out lab coats with buttons missing) was positively *ebullient*. Even she joined me in song.

On the twelfth day of Christmas
My true love sent to me . . .

My heart was about to burst with jubilation – how I loved this music! My fingers flew recklessly over the keys. I flubbed a few sharps or flats here and there, but I didn't let that stop me. I'm the kind of pianist who can't play "Mary Had a Little Lamb" without a full score of sheet music in front of me, yet with notes up there, I can play anything.

Then, after playing "Rudolph, the Red-Nosed Reindeer," I had to take a brief pause to dry my eyes and blow my nose. I was such a sentimental fool! The part when the other reindeers make fun of him and don't let him in on their reindeer games really got to me.

Dr. Bristol rushed by with a wave, but didn't stop. "I don't sing," he said by way of greeting.

At mid-morning, I took a break and came up to the ICU to visit my friends. The unit looked magical. Laura and Nicole had taken charge of the decorations and had chosen a Disney theme. They plastered photographs of each of the staff doctors, plus a few senior residents, onto the faces of each of the seven dwarves. Rosemary was Snow White.

"No nativity scenes allowed. Nix on that," Laura said in mock admonition, making an x with her index fingers. "Christmas isn't politically correct. I'm surprised you got away with playing Christmas carols, Tilda. Soon even that will be outlawed. Everything has to be watered down to accommodate Chanukah." She bowed in my direction. "And Kwanzaa, thank you, Althea and Belinda," she said and nodded at two of our Jamaican nurses. "When the hell are Diwali and Ramadan, with all due respect to any of us around here that celebrate those holidays?"

Morty harrumphed in agreement and shook her head, making her little dangling mistletoe earrings swing vigorously. "I want to know why there was never any mention of Kwanzaa when we were kids. I think it's a made-up holiday, invented by Toys R Us. There's a conspiracy going on against Christmas."

Althea and Belinda looked bemused. No one could be offended by Laura, who was mad at the world, nor by Morty, who insulted us all equally.

The red, white, and gold lights on the tree twinkled on and off as we sat around the nursing station admiring Laura and Nicole's hard work. Nicole was waiting for the arrival of her patient, who was coming in from her home on a farm near the town of St.

Jacobs. She was to be admitted to the ICU for only a few hours in order for us to perform specialized tests of her lung and heart function, something that could be done safely only in the ICU. Dr. Bristol had told us about her in rounds that morning.

Alice Heidebrecht was a twenty-five-year-old woman with no previous medical history. She'd been symptomatic for a few weeks with an as yet undiagnosed problem – shortness of breath upon exertion and even sometimes at rest. It was "idiopathic," meaning no known cause – but the slightest bit of activity made her weak and dizzy. She had even fainted a few times at home.

"They're Mennonites," said Nicole, who had reviewed the patient's chart, which had been sent ahead. "She can't do any of her farm chores or take care of her three children, who are all under the age of four."

"Check out if they're bringing in any pies," said Morty, "or quilts."

"Where will they park the horse and buggy? Special rate for livestock, don't you know," said Laura, in a mock Maritime accent to poke fun at Frances, who prided herself on her familiarity with rural customs.

Rosemary had kept me as extra in case of a new admission, which left me free for my carol-playing duties, as well as floating around the unit and helping the others.

Nicole admitted Mrs. Heidebrecht in a room at the end of the hall, partly because we thought she might prefer the privacy, and also because it was farthest away from the TV lounge where *The Grinch Who Stole Christmas* was playing at top volume to the delight of some children we'd put in there while their parents were visiting a sick relative.

"That's my favourite movie," said Nicole, one of the most un-Grinch-like people I'd ever met.

"Go take a break, Nicky, watch it with them," I said, "I'll admit her for you."

ALICE HEIDEBRECHT LOOKED up from where she lay in the bed and gave me a wide smile when I came into the room and introduced myself. Her broad, round, sturdy face was wan, and she was breathing heavily from the effort of having got up onto the bed. Her pale skin was exactly the colour and texture of one of those pies, still raw and unbaked, that Morty had mentioned. Wire-rimmed glasses magnified her eyes, making her look startled, which she probably was. Her husband, Jakob, was at her side, holding her hand.

She had draped her long dark dress, black bonnet, and under-garments over the chair beside her bed, and I noticed the handmade stitches in the garments, the buttons fashioned from wood chips.

Under the sheet, which she'd pulled up to her chin, I could see that she was naked, as if in total submission. Perhaps that was what she thought a hospital in a big city expected of her.

The room had become suffused with their combined earthy smells, smells that I was unused to but that were not unpleasant. It was the natural smell of bodies accustomed to a life of manual labour, the smells we usually wash away.

I placed an oxygen mask on her face to ease her breathing and helped her into a blue hospital gown. I took her vital signs, started an IV in her arm, and then sat down with both of them and explained the complicated tests for pulmonary hypertension, the disease that Dr. Bristol suspected she suffered from. A nurse would be with her, I assured her, during every moment. The tests were not painful, but were definitely uncomfortable. There would be times during the testing when she would be adminis-tered different drugs, and we would be monitoring her closely for side effects.

She listened to me, but was more focused on her husband's watchful gaze, as if she heard what I was saying only when it was filtered first through his ears.

The moment I stepped away from them to record my notes in the chart, they instantly became oblivious both of me and the hospital around them. He turned to her and spoke in hushed tones in the German dialect that they shared. Then he bent down low over her body and drew back the sheet. He lifted the blue hospital gown and placed his ruddy, chapped lips on her pale pink ones. He cupped her

small breasts in his large, rough farmer's hands – hands that bulged
with the circulation of the hard physical life that he lived.

I watched them for a few minutes. I wanted to keep on
watching them and not disturb those intimate moments, but David
Bristol arrived and wanted to begin. I made some rustling noises
with the curtain to let them know we were ready. With that, Jakob
Heidebrecht stood up beside his wife, pulled up the covers, picked
up his wide-brimmed black hat that he had laid on the bed, and
went out the door.

With Mrs. Heidebrecht under mild sedation, we inserted a
deep catheter into the right internal jugular vein in her neck
and threaded it down into her superior vena cava, right atrium, and
into her right ventricle. Then we floated a tiny, air-filled balloon
until it reached the pulmonary artery. With that balloon, I
measured pressures in the chambers of her heart at the same time
that I was administering various potent drugs – pure oxygen, a beta
blocker, nitroglycerin, nifedipine, and nitric oxide – and then
new experimental drugs that hadn't yet been proven to be useful
in this condition. We were hoping to see if any of them would alleviate her symptoms. If they didn't, there was only one option: a
lung transplant.

Throughout the day, the carols stayed with me, coming and
going in my mind, both the stirring words and the glorious music,
both when I was at the piano and when I was away.

Angels we have heard on high, sweetly singing over the plains

Each one, as I played it or sang it to myself, was my favourite
at that moment.

NICOLE JOINED ME and together with the doctor, we reviewed the
patient's numbers and trends and tried to find helpful correlations
between the drugs given and the patient's reactions.

We called Mr. Heidebrecht back in and immediately understood the conclusion that Dr. Bristol had drawn when he handed

Mr. Heidebrecht a beeper. He explained that either he or Mrs. Heidebrecht would have to carry it with them at all times so that they could be reached if lungs became available. This was the only option, he explained. A social worker would be in touch with them to go over the details, but in the meanwhile, they must carry this beeper and remain within an hour's drive of Toronto.

Mr. Heidebrecht looked at it and shook his head.

I imagined it was how an Orthodox Jew might regard a pork chop: not as much with distaste, but rather, with disinterest. Anyway, he explained, with a shrug of his shoulders, they didn't have a telephone in their farmhouse.

Dr. Bristol tried to impress on them the importance of being available every day, twenty-four hours a day. Only a lung transplant could possibly save her life.

On a cold winter's night that was so deep.
Noel, Noel, Noel, Noel.
Born is the King of Israel.

I was back at my Christmas gig for the lunchtime crowd.

God rest ye merry, gentleman,
Let nothing you dismay . . .
O tidings of comfort and joy.

I was building up to my personal musical Everest: "Jingle Bells." To do it properly, it's gotta fly! I could barely keep up the tempo. The tune kept getting ahead of my fingers.

"That's funny," said Dr. Huizinga, stopping by for a sip of apple cider. "You, Tilda, of all people, playing Christmas carols. You, being, er, you know, celebrating Chanukah, and all. It's very ecumenical of you."

"I'm nothing if not ecumenical," I said. (Usually I could play the piano and keep up a more intelligent conversation, but "Jingle Bells" required my full concentration.)

"Merry – er – Happy Holidays to you," he said and placed his paper cup full of cider on the piano top. "They should spike this stuff. It's vile." He rushed off.

Next, the stirring "O Holy Night."

Who could not be moved by the supplication: "Fall on your knees"? I thought about the devotion of Christians or true believers of any religion. I admired how they lived by their principles, especially the moral ones. The rules about food and clothing seemed much less important to me. But sometimes I did feel a longing to belong to a church, temple, mosque, or synagogue in order to experience prayer and faith within a community.

The synagogue services I had attended as a child with my father had been cerebral, intellectual exercises. The prayers were about ancient, archaic laws and the pursuit of justice. They didn't speak to my soul like the exhortation "Fall on your knees!"

I recalled that when the Sikh family had prayed in Manjit's room, I'd become aware of a certain phrase they kept repeating. I asked the father what it meant.

He broke off his chanting to tell me: "God is one. God is one."

That was exactly the same as the central prayer of the Jewish faith, the Shema, I had thought at the time. The Shema says, "Hear oh Israel, the Lord is our God, the Lord is One." What, really, was the difference? Weren't there more similarities than differences and weren't the differences primarily cosmetic, or involving costume, custom, and cuisine?

O bring us figgy pudding
And a cup of good cheer.

From which I slid smoothly into

Go, tell it on the mountain
Over the hills and everywhere

There was a tap on my shoulder. It was Rosemary.

"We need you to come back to the ICU, Tilda. You're getting a new admission."

A stretcher was being wheeled down the hall as I arrived back in the ICU. Since I could see that it was the body of a young man, I assumed that the two people who were trailing close behind him were the mother and father, still in their snowy boots and coats, their scarves flapping open. They looked like any frantic parents facing life's worst nightmare.

"No spontaneous movement, no eye opening, no gag or cough reflex, no response to deep pain." The doctor who had accompanied the patient on the flight from North Bay was reporting to Dr. Bristol, standing at the foot of the patient's bed. I joined them there and listened in. "An eighteen-year-old boy, sudden collapse . . . likely cerebral aneurysm. Normal medical history. Blood pressure and heart rate stable, but no spontaneous breaths. Unresponsive."

Even the paramedics, who prided themselves on their cool demeanour and emotional control under all circumstances, seemed shaken.

Early that morning, when I was sipping cider and playing carols in the lobby, far away in North Bay this young boy was busy being the team's star forward, playing in a regional hockey tournament. He scored a first-period goal, then had a breakaway with another shot on goal, and then a blood vessel burst in his brain and he collapsed on the ice, face down. A CT scan showed a massive intracerebral bleed and global oxygen deprivation. His brain was swelling up rapidly inside the vault of his skull.

"Can't something be done?" the mother asked Dr. Bristol in the hallway.

"The neurosurgeons have examined him. They had hoped to be able to insert a drain to release the pressure in his brain, but have decided it would be of no benefit. The damage is too extensive."

"Is he in a coma?" the father asked, clearly hoping for a coma, rather than what he must have begun to suspect.

"After we examine him thoroughly, we will have more to tell you." Dr. Bristol pulled the curtains around the patient's bed and directed the parents to the door. I accompanied them to the waiting room and returned to the patient, who was being examined by the doctors.

This was not the first patient like this that I had taken care of, so I was familiar with the methods used to sustain a body until a final determination of the situation could take place. I knew there would be a period of limbo, a time of ambiguity between this hovering life and the slamming down of one of the two most likely pronouncements: persistent vegetative state or irreversible brain death. These seemed to be the only two possible outcomes for this young hockey player.

As I went about my work, I thought about the parents in the waiting room. They were probably imagining the worst – which in this case would be accurate – and I hoped for their sake that the testing period would not be too prolonged. Waiting was torture for families. However, I also knew how thorough and exhaustive the testing had to be in order to avoid a pre-emptory or mistaken declaration of death.

Perhaps this waiting period was a good thing. Perhaps it gave the family the time they needed to register the shock, say their goodbyes, and consider some important decisions. There was no doubt in my mind that if this young boy was declared brain dead, the family would be approached regarding organ donation.

I TURNED TO my patient. He had a beautiful, young man's body – veiny arms, defined muscles in his legs and arms, a taut flat stomach. The other nurses came to admire him and to give me moral support.

"Gosh, what a hunk. Look at that six-pack," Justine said.

Frances shook her head sadly as she came closer to look at the young man's handsome face and his athletic physique. "I had a brain-dead patient like this last week. She ended up being a donor. Can you imagine – she'd just been to the hairdresser. Her hair was perfect." She sighed.

"I know," I said. "It seems unreal, as if he's playing a trick on us and will pop up any minute. C'mon, the joke's over, I feel like saying to him. Enough is enough, I keep thinking."

Tracy shook her head. "It looks like he's just sleeping. He looks a lot better than all the other patients here. He looks just like a real person. I can't believe it." She walked away.

"How're you doing, Tillie?" Frances stayed back to check on me. She peered at me and saw at once that I was fine. "I have to run off. There was a big car crash on the Don Valley Parkway. Another possible donor is on the way in from the Trauma Centre at Sunnybrook. Can you believe it? This always seems to happens during the holiday season."

DR. BRISTOL AND the senior fellow, Jessica Leung, came back to perform the tests that were done only under these dire circumstances.

"Keith, Keith!" we all called out. "Open your eyes!"

"Keith!" Dr. Bristol shouted in his ear.

Jessica made a fist and pressed her knuckles deeply into the boy's sternum, which was already rubbed raw from other, previous attempts to elicit some response. There was no flinching, grimacing, or withdrawing to that sternal rub, nor to a ballpoint pen rolled along his nail beds, nor to sharp squeezes to his nipples or presses on his eyebrows. There was no reaction to anything at all.

The reflexes were tested with a slender hammer. There was nothing.

Jessica rubbed the end of the hammer along the soles of his bare feet. We all noted the abnormal upward curl of the toes, and we glanced at one another with a grim understanding of where this all was likely headed.

Dr. Bristol observed the patient closely. He set his teeth hard after each test and then nodded to the resident and me to proceed to the next test.

I held open the eyelids and shone a flashlight in them. There was no constriction of the pupils.

The corneas did not flinch and there was no protective blink, even when Jessica flicked the eyeball with the rolled-up tip of a cotton tissue.

We moved his head from side to side to check for eye movement, but like a porcelain doll with immobile glass eyes, the
patient's eyeballs stayed motionless in his head. In fact, that was
the name of the test.

"Positive doll's eyes," Jessica said.

With each test, a shift was taking place within me. I was moving
from thinking of him as a young man, a star hockey player, a son
and a brother (I began to try to put all that out of my mind) to a
patient in the bed, to a body, to a potential organ donor, to what
he really was – a corpse.

For the next test, I brought over two basins, one filled with ice
water, the other with warm water, and a large syringe that the
doctor would use to inject water into the outer ear canal.

"cows," I reminded myself. "Cold, Opposite. Warm, Same."

In a normal person, the cold water in the ear should make the
eyes move in the opposite direction, toward the other ear. With
instillation of warm water, the eyes should move in the same direction, toward the ear. This was the normal response, but this
patient's eyes deviated neither to the opposite, nor to the same side,
with either test. His eyes did not move at all.

Finally, we removed him from the ventilator and waited for an
independent breath – even a single one of his own breaths would
rule out the diagnosis of brain death.

We had a strong instinct about this case, and all our tests and
knowledge were leading us in the direction of one clear-cut,
definitive diagnosis. Yet, at the same time, the search was conducted in order to prove ourselves wrong.

We waited and waited. The patient remained disconnected from
the ventilator. His chest was still. His oxygen saturations began to
fall and his heart rate began to block down, slower and slower. Dr.
Bristol waited a little longer, and then looked at his watch. For a
full ten minutes we waited for any sign of respiration from this
boy's body. Any rise or fall of the chest? There was nothing. The
doctor looked again at his watch and said quietly, 1430 hours,
December 24.

None of us could say for sure if that was truly the time of
death. Was *this* the time of death or had that time occurred this

morning, out there on the hockey rink when the hidden bubble burst in his brain? Was *this* the time of death, now, or would it occur when we finally turned off the ventilator and stopped the flow of powerful intravenous drugs, and allowed his body to die, as his brain already had?

As horrific as brain death is, as devastating as such a loss of a previously healthy person is, I had come to believe that in these circumstances, it was preferable to another, closely related diagnosis: persistent vegetative state. But some people preferred that latter diagnosis over death. I was never around to find out if any of those families ever regretted the decision they made on behalf of their loved one.

Until the declaration of brain death was made, during all those exhaustive neurological tests, we were on the alert for any sign of life: a slight twitch, a blink, or a minute constriction of the pupil in response to a source of light, a minuscule movement of a finger, an effort to make even one breath, or a primitive reflex. Any of those signs would mean there was still some brain activity. Families often interpreted these things in the most hopeful way possible and chose to believe that it was the start of a process – albeit a long and arduous one – toward a full and meaningful recovery. I had seen only a few of these cases diagnosed in the ICU. However, from what I had seen and learned, these patients were transferred out to the wards and soon became contracted into a fetal position and bedridden. Their days consisted of being turned from side to side, breathing shallow breaths through a hole in the neck (a tracheostomy) and being fed through a tube. Pneumonia and other infections were likely to develop, as well.

As for Keith, the tests confirmed what we had suspected: he was dead. We were keeping blood and oxygen flowing to his organs to give us time to explain all this to the family and then to give them time to make some important decisions. I went over it again in my mind as I prepared myself to bring in the parents. By now a sister and brother had joined them. First I stepped back and gave them privacy to grieve and to come to their own conclusions.

"Keith, Keith, wake up!" I heard them call out.

"Time for hockey practice!"

"Come on, the Leafs are going to make the playoffs this year!"
They sobbed.

Then we led the family back out to the quiet room, where Dr.
Bristol explained the situation.

"We have performed exhaustive tests on your son's brain
functioning. Those findings, coupled with the CT scan that shows
massive global infarction, led us to the conclusion that, unfortunately, your son is brain dead. I am very sorry."

"Dead? What do you mean?" the father cried into his hands.

"Dead means a total and irreversible cessation of brain functioning, even in the presence of a beating heart," the doctor said,
reciting from the textbook of his mind.

"How can he be dead?" the father cried. "He was fine this
morning. He's perfectly healthy. He's never been sick a day in his life."

"Keith has no brain function. He is in an irreversible coma. I'm
very sorry. There is nothing we can do."

"Is he dead or just brain dead?" the father asked.

*If it's just a technicality, we'll overlook it. If it's just his brain
that is dead, we'll take the rest of him.*

"He is not alive." The doctor tried other words to help explain.
"He is dead. He is not just brain dead. The machines and the drugs
are keeping the blood flowing and the oxygen circulating. We are
perfusing his organs and keeping the cells alive."

"But what about the life-support machines? Aren't they doing
any good?"

"The ventilator is maintaining oxygenation, but it is not
keeping him alive. It is purely biological life. It is life at the cellular
level, only," Dr. Bristol said.

"Have you ever seen a case like this get better?"

"No."

"How long could he live like this?" the mother asked.

It was too much for anyone to grasp, much less a mother or a
father. However, more time with their son, even if he was in this
condition, must have seemed preferable to . . . that. The other. The
alternative to life.

"Not very long," said Dr. Bristol. "A few hours, a day, perhaps.
His brain is not working and already complications are setting

in. His brain cannot control his temperature and he is becoming hypothermic. His kidneys are not functioning properly and are producing large amounts of watery urine. His blood pressure is very erratic, high then low. These are commonly the things we see that happen to the body in these situations. He cannot continue like this much longer."

"But his heart is beating. Surely given time, he'll recover?" the mother reasoned. "Keith will wake up from this coma, I know it. We've all heard of cases where –"

"Recovery is impossible in the presence of brain stem damage," said Dr. Bristol. "Your son suffered a massive subarachnoid hemorrhage. A blood vessel burst in his brain. Likely it was an anomaly present since birth, but undetectable, asymptomatic."

"The family doctor never told us anything about it."

"He couldn't possibly have known, and it could not have been prevented."

"What's to be done? You're going to pull the plug on him?"

"We won't do anything until you are ready, but there is something very important for you to consider. You have the opportunity to donate Keith's organs. His heart, lung, liver, and kidneys could all go to help other people who are terribly ill."

The mother sobbed as she asked her next question. "What if you took his organs and he was still partially alive?"

"There is no such thing as partially alive, and we do not harvest organs from living people," Dr. Bristol stated. "Now, should you wish to donate Keith's organs, you will have to decide soon, as we are under time constraints. In these situations, we have to preserve organ perfusion to maintain the viability . . ."

He droned on but they couldn't bear to hear any more.

If only he could show a little emotion, I thought. In some situations, I had the feeling that families cared more that we cared than they cared about what we knew. When Dr. Bristol said he was sorry, he said it as if he meant it and I knew that he did. Of course he did. He was not heartless; he was not made of stone. After all, he had children of his own. He had shown me pictures of them and of his beloved horses that he kept at his country home. Perhaps he simply did not know how to show his caring to the family, other than by being the superb doctor that he was, without losing the image of who he was. Perhaps it would disturb him too much if he showed his emotions and it might render him unable to do this work, day in and day out. Perhaps it would exact too high a price. Perhaps it was too much to ask of anyone. But I believed that if he could show them his feelings, share even a tiny portion of their sorrow, it would help them and be remembered always.

I tried to make up for his detached manner with my sorrowful eyes and my arms across their shoulders, but my gestures also seemed inadequate. I decided instead to sit there and simply be still. I would bear witness to their grief in the hope that my presence alone might offer some comfort.

After a few minutes, to no one in particular, I said into the suffocating room, "Perhaps the family would like some time alone, to think about all this?"

They looked at me, stunned, but grateful.

They gave consent to donate Keith's organs and then came to the bedside to spend some time with their son and say goodbye.

The mother sobbed into her son's bare chest and the father stood on the other side of the bed, holding his son's hand. He looked at it in sheer amazement. That hand that had gripped a hockey stick hours before, now was lifeless.

As I went about my work, I made a point of not talking to my patient as I always did. If I spoke, whom would I be addressing? It would be without purpose and confusing for the family. He was dead, after all, despite the apparently normal activity on the monitor, despite his composed, youthful face and good colour, despite the rise and fall of his chest.

I was the caretaker of their son's body. The guardian of his vital organs.

In just a matter of hours, he had gone from a young healthy boy to a critically ill patient, to a dead body, to a treasure trove containing precious gifts. Waiting inside this body were the spoils of an untimely, tragic death. But were we pirates, pillaging and plundering the human body for its booty? Our haste and efficiency made me feel at times as if we were treating a person as a means to

an end, but in order for the organs to be viable for transplantation, we had to act fast. Organs did not live long inside cadavers,
even less in buckets of preservative fluid. How can we make this
experience more respectful and honourable, yet do our work
quickly and effectively? I wholeheartedly believed in what we were
doing. The boy was dead; he was a body. A casing, a container, a
jewellery box containing sapphire lungs, a ruby heart, an emerald
liver. To others, now, it might mean a chance at life: as precious as
gold, frankincense, and myrrh.

> We three kings of Orient are
> Bearing gifts we traverse afar.
> Field and fountain, moor and mountain following yonder star
> O star of wonder, star of light
> Star with royal beauty bright
> Westward leading, still proceeding, Guide us to thy perfect light.

The parents' backs, as they turned and walked out the door,
moving farther and farther away from the body of their son,
leaving it behind to us, entrusted in our care, was the saddest sight
I had ever seen.

"Their Christmas is fucked, for sure," said Morty, standing just
outside the door.

> Silent Night.
> Holy Night.
> Shepherds quake, at the sight.

Hell, I was quaking too, but there was no time for that. There
was so much work to do.

Prep the body for the OR. X-ray, echocardiogram, and
bronchoscopy – all to verify that the organs were in good condition for transplant. Treat the complications of brain death: the
buckets of colourless urine spilling out from his bladder, caused by
a type of diabetes due to a hormone disruption from the brain
damage. Cooling his body when it suddenly heated up, warming

it when his temperature erratically dropped. Levophed up, Levophed down with each swoop and dive of his blood pressure. I thought of Laura's oft-repeated quip: Levophed? Leave 'em Dead!

The brain was no longer in control – we are, or so I was trained to believe. I administered medications for no other reason than to maintain good organ perfusion. *Stop, isn't this too bizarre, too macabre?* No, I answered myself back. He's dead and now his family has given the ultimate gift. Their son's organs and tissues may save other people's lives. Focus on that, I told myself. Isn't it good that something positive might come of this tragedy? Two voices – there were at least two – kept up a dialogue in my mind.

> *And all the bells on earth shall ring,*
> *On Christmas Day in the morning.*

The room was quickly becoming crowded.

"Have we reached a consensus?" the surgeons asked about each organ. "Are we ready to roll?"

The thoracic surgeons who wanted the lungs arrived, already in their OR scrubs and rubber clogs, hopeful for an expedient retrieval. The liver team was there, asking me to draw more blood tests.

The harvest would soon begin. Then a long winter of recovery, then hopefully, new life would spring forth.

WHAT HAPPENED LATER that Christmas evening, just as we were finishing up that shift and getting ready to leave, makes me tremble to think of it still. And when I do, I reach out to touch my loved one's hand to make sure he is safe. It makes me pause before I get into my car. It makes me say a prayer – even though it's not really my way or habit to do so.

"Everything has already been decided, no matter what you do or don't do . . . whether you will arrive safely or make it to your next birthday," my husband, the cheery existential fatalist, says. "It's all been decided, but you still have to do the right thing."

"Who shall live and who shall die?" the rabbi said each year during the solemn Yom Kippur service, the prayers for the Day of

Atonement. "Yet, whether it has been decided or not does not absolve you of the responsibility to do the righteous thing," he made sure to add.

Frances told me just a few of the details that she knew as she admitted her patient and rushed around trying to get as much done as she could before the end of her shift. My "donor" patient had gone to the OR for organ retrieval. I could have gone home a few minutes early, but I stayed to help her.

From the little she told me, from what I heard from the paramedics, and from what I knew about these situations, I could easily imagine the details.

There must have been a patch of black ice, undetectable, unavoidable to the driver of a car that was on the way to visit grandparents for the holidays. Margot Heinz, a twenty-seven-year-old woman was sitting beside Steve, her husband, their two children in the back seat. Steve swerved to avoid an oncoming driver who had wandered crazily into their lane.

"That guy must have had a few too –" he must have started to say, when suddenly, the tires couldn't find purchase on the road and the car went into a skid. Steve slammed on the brakes, the car spun around, flipped over into the ditch. They were found, a few moments later, the horn blowing, the children crying, and Steve, sitting, motionless, his eyes glazed. Margot, slumped forward; not a sound from her.

Ambulances raced to the scene and paramedics began resuscitation efforts. They called ahead to the hospital to let them know what they'd found. Two small children in shock, but VSS – vital signs stable. One thirty-something white male, multiple fractures, contusions, possible concussion. Young white female, appears to be pregnant, VSA – vital signs absent. Letters are faster than words. The driver races to the hospital with the siren screaming, but takes the time to put in another call, this one to the provincial trauma centre, to alert them about a possibly brain-dead victim, a potential organ donor.

A pager goes off in the jeans pocket of a young woman working late at the hospital. It's Christmas Eve, but she's on call for the entire province, ready for just this sort of eventuality, which

unfortunately, with drinking and festive merry-making, is statisti-
cally speaking more likely to happen at this time of year than at any
other. She is responsible for all the lungs, hearts, livers, and kidneys
that become available for distribution to transplant centres. It will
be a long night ahead, and as tired as she is, and as disappointed as
she is to be missing Christmas with her family, she hopes that some
good may come of each tragedy. She loves her work.

The ICU is dangerously short-staffed. Casey is in charge on the
night shift.

"Belinda," she'll say as she enacts an impromptu skit of how
she'll call one of our nurses who managed to get Christmas off,
at home: "We interrupt this Midnight Mass and the ho, ho, ho,
opening of your presents. Don't bother taking down your
stocking! Dump your eggnog down the sink and turn off the oven
with the undercooked turkey – who cares about salmonella? – and
come to work in the ICU. We're working with a skeleton staff, but
we can't afford to lose an organ!"

I could see the grandparents, the stricken look on their faces as
they waited for their children and grandchildren to arrive. It is late
and dinner is getting cold.

"Where are they?" I can hear them saying.

"Now, don't fret, dear. They're on their way. There must be
traffic or they got delayed somewhere."

"It's not like them to be late." She stands at the window, waiting
for a sign.

I picture the police car pulling up to the front of the house and
see the grandmother falling in a faint to the floor. Two officers get
out and begin their slow solemn walk up the driveway. Margot's
father knows without being told. One of the police officers,
perhaps a young woman, near Margot's age, will hold his hand
and sit with him. She may also be wishing she were home with her
family for Christmas dinner, but it was her turn to work.

"WHEW!" SAYS CASEY, glancing at me. "We could use more Jewish
nurses. We can always count on them to work on Christmas."

Rosemary is getting ready to go home, but comes to tell us

that if we are desperately short-staffed, she will come in and help out if necessary.

Margot is declared brain dead. Steve, who has stabilized in ER, is notified, and although he is beside himself with grief, he believes that even though Margot hadn't signed the donor card attached to her driver's licence, she would have wanted to donate her organs. Her life was lost, but maybe others will be given the opportunity for life. That is the kind of person – that *was* the kind of person, he corrects himself (how cruel the rules of grammar can be) – that Margot was.

The surgeons on call are paged. The ophthalmologist will want those clear, young corneas. Someone will harvest the kidneys and the pancreas together, along with a few metres of bowel. A thoracic surgeon will procure the lungs and a cardiovascular surgeon, the heart. One hopes the organs are in good condition, but they may be used anyway, even if there are deficiencies. The potential recipients for these organs are desperate and will take any chance at life. Even imperfect or iffy organs – a bruised liver or smoker's lungs (after one transplant, the nurses swore they got a whiff of smoker's stale cigarette smoke every time they came near the patient) – may be put to use.

Margot's liver was severely lacerated in the accident, but her other organs are in excellent shape and will go to those whose need is greatest and who mostly closely match the donor. However, the most pressing question still needs to be addressed. What about the twenty-two-week fetus inside Margot? Is it still viable and if not, who should be saved? Whose life takes precedence? Should the body of the mother be sustained on life support until the fetus can be safely delivered, even though such a delay puts her precious organs in jeopardy? Or should one life, a precarious one at best, be discontinued so that others might be given a chance? Are we doing the right thing, this tampering with life, this tinkering with death? Pretending to play with the stars, as if we even could? Have we gone too far? Perhaps it all has been decided already, but that does not exempt us from trying to do the right thing.

God and sinners reconciled.

It was time to go home. It was already late, and Ivan and I were invited to friends' to share in their Christmas Eve celebration. It was also Chanukah, so I would bring the menorah and light the candles and we would have carols and songs together, plum pudding and latkes.

I lingered for a few more minutes in the lobby and because the piano was still there, the open keyboard was an invitation I couldn't resist.

Bearing gifts we've traversed afar
Field and fountain, moor and mountain,
Following yonder star

It was the most Jewish of all the carols. It was as sombre as any of the Hebrew songs I knew, even the so-called cheerful ones. Its minor key echoed with the melancholy in my heart. How can such joy and such sadness co-exist simultaneously within me and in the world around me? Yet they always have.

Westward leading, still proceeding
Guide us to thy perfect light

But I couldn't bear to end the day on such a mournful tone.

Hark the Herald Angels Sing!
Glory to the Newborn King!
Joyful, all ye nations rise,
Join the triumph of the skies

I sang along with a few other people who gathered, just as they were leaving the hospital. My hands stretched out vigorously past the octaves, using more muscle than was really required and let my heart soar along with the words and music. Yes, that's it, we have to give glory. Glory to our good health, to our friends, family, and yes – I'll dare to say it, though quietly to myself – to God.

8

GRATITUDE

As I was transferring a patient to the floor, she asked me to make a stop by the pay phone. She was an elderly woman who had suffered a severe bout of pneumonia related to her chronic lung disease, but now had improved and would likely be sent home in a few days. She asked me to put the quarter she had saved for this purpose into the phone and called out the phone number from a little folded piece of paper. It was the number of a local funeral home. She took the receiver from me and proceeded to make arrangements to purchase a burial plot. She held up her credit card for me to read off the numbers, which she then repeated into the phone.

"No, I'm not dead yet," she explained to the person at the other end, "but I may be shortly."

ON ANOTHER OCCASION, we admitted a Mr. Tom Kettle, and as I was inputting his name in the computer chart, he said, "That's T. Kettle, for short."

I looked up and met Laura's eyes, then Frances's eyes. Such tiny jokes didn't warrant the uproarious laughter with which we all erupted, but it seemed to, at the time.

"Mr. T. Kettle." I paused to wipe tears from my eyes when we were still laughing about it later, in the lounge. "That reminds me. Remember that British patient whose first words when we extubated her were 'May I please have a cuppa tea, luv?'"

"Wasn't that when Morty brought a pot of tea to her room wearing the tea cozy on her head? When the patient saw her coming in with that, she lost her dentures in the bed from laughing so hard!" said Nicole.

Of course, all this silliness set us off again.

PEOPLE WHO ASKED about my work always raised the same questions. How did I manage to keep my emotional distance? Why was I so drawn to such catastrophic illness? Wasn't it depressing? Why didn't I choose a happier place to work, where more people got better? Whatever I answered did not satisfy them.

I began to suspect that people asked these questions because hearing about my work raised uncomfortable feelings and new questions in them. It disturbed them and made them feel squeamish. It provoked them to think about their own safety and their mortality. It made them wonder if such devastating things could ever happen to them or their family. It made them feel unsafe.

Frances told me how she dealt with this reaction from her friends and family.

"I tell them that I love being a nurse, especially here in the ICU. You get to solve problems and know that it's all up to you. You have your patient's life in your trust for these hours and you can really help people. Sometimes you get to bring people back from the brink. I wouldn't work anywhere else."

Nicole explained her position. "Taking care of people who may or may not make it is not depressing when it's not your own family member in the bed. Even if you get very involved with them and care a lot for them, at the end of your shift, you leave." But then something occurred to her. "But if it happens to be your own family member, then that's different."

I didn't ask Laura, but she overheard and told me anyway.

"It's not the work that depresses me, it's the doctors. We do all the work and the doctors get all the credit. We're the ones who really know what's going on with the patient, but the family rushes in and asks, where's the doctor? What does the doctor say? People don't realize that it's nurses who make people better."

Sometimes I responded to inquiries about my work by giving the example of the Cresswell family. I accompanied them into the ICU when they arrived for the first time, explained everything to them, helped them get used to the scary machines, demystified the alarms, encouraged them to ask all the questions that were on their minds, allowed them to visit their father whenever they wished, and, in the end, ensured that he was pain-free and comfortable.

"But how did he do? Did he get better?" my friends asked. Of course, everyone wants a happy ending.

"Well, no. The treatment was unsuccessful. He had serious illness and a lot of complications. But he had a good death."

Even we nurses could sometimes get fixated on death and dying and forget about the success stories that we'd had a part in. There were many lives we saved and people we fixed and cured and sent on their merry way. If they came back to visit us, what a bonus! But we never expected it. In fact, we were a little surprised whenever former patients walked in the door. Why would they want to revisit the scene of such horrors? Even with the most compassionate and gentlest of nursing care, so many ICU experiences were unpleasant: the IVs, the drugs, the intubation, the ventilator, and the noise. Surely they wanted to forget about us and put the whole experience out of their minds? Nevertheless, from time to time, a patient would walk in the door and want to shake the hands of those who cared for him. They made a point of thanking us one by one and often placed a box of doughnuts or a big green plant on the nursing station counter. We waved them off and did all we could to limit or relieve them altogether of any sense of obligation. We *did* want to be appreciated, but we didn't want gratitude.

We wanted acknowledgement, but not indebtedness. There's a big difference.

Those cases – those success stories – were the reasons that we went in to nursing in the first place. But even when our patients didn't get better, if we believed we were helping in some way, we could do our work with a clear conscience. So long as we believed that the pain of the treatments was worth enduring for a reasonable chance of improvement, we loved our work in the ICU and did it wholeheartedly. Most of us wouldn't have worked anywhere else. Those nurses who left often ended up coming back. Occasionally, we received a card or letter of thanks.

> We would like to acknowledge with grateful hearts the care you provided to a woman who was very special to all of us. Although we gave her up to God, we are so appreciative of the skilful and loving care you gave her during her time with you. Thank you to all of you.

Our work was stressful, but I believed that many of us thrived on the stress. It energized and exhilarated us. We craved the stress of challenging cases, of solving complicated problems, and putting our knowledge and expertise to good use. Stress was the price of doing work that was fascinating, challenging, and invigorating.

Often, if I stopped a nurse in the middle of a busy day or night, when he or she was caring for a sick or "crashing" patient, and asked how it was going, the answer would be something like "I'm having a great day. Gosh, look what time it is! The day is flying by so fast."

The work made us feel vital, needed, and alive, alive, oh!

I remember coming into Nicole's room one day to give her a hand. I knew she was busy. The crash cart was in there, off to the side, most likely put there because she believed she would need it soon. She had even gone ahead and attached external pacemaker pads to her patient's chest, just in case, because she had noted an occasional ominous heartbeat on the monitor that sometimes foreshadowed a lethal arrhythmia. I drew her blood work for her, looked up lab results, prepared and hung an antibiotic while she gave me an update on her patient.

"Pressure's in his boots," she said, nodding at the monitor. She was mixing up more dopamine, the powerful vasoconstrictor drug to elevate the blood pressure. The problem was that her patient needed that drug, but it could also dangerously speed up his heart rate. Nicole narrowed the high and low alarm parameters so that she would be warned even sooner in the event of a problem.

"He's just had a seizure and has been going in and out of a tachy rhythm with lots of irregular beats. He's pretty sick, but thanks for the help, Til, I'm cool now."

I looked at her. Nicole was flushed with excitement. She was doing five different things at the same time, planning ahead for another five. She was totally focused, in her element, in control, completely at home with the chaos. There was a huge smile on her face.

Nurses like to fix things. If they can.

I COULD ONLY hear one side of the telephone conversation, but it stopped me in my tracks.

The organ transplant coordinator was sitting at the nursing station making phone calls. A cup of cold coffee sat on the counter beside her and at her feet was an oversized red plastic picnic cooler that I knew contained some newly dead person's body parts. She leaned forward as she spoke into the phone.

"How soon can you get him to the hospital? . . . Yes, a pair of lungs . . . it's a very good match. . . ." She smiled, sharing the excitement with the person at the other end. "He's waited a long time for this call . . . over a year, I know . . . yes, it's for real! Now, I don't want you to rush, but we do need you here as soon as possible . . . don't forget that there's always a chance that once we're in the OR, the lungs might not be satisfactory. Sometimes there is some reason that we cannot go through with the transplant. If that happens, we'll have to wake him up and he'll go back on to the list. . . . We're here waiting for you. Drive safely."

We smiled at each other as she hung up the phone. I clicked my pen at her. It was one of the ones she had given out to all of us – key chains, too – that bore the slogan "Don't take your organs to heaven. Heaven knows we need them here."

We weren't supposed to know which organs went to which recipients, but often we had a pretty good idea. It had happened to all of us more than once that we would care for the brain-dead donor, send the body off to the OR for organ retrieval, and then come in the next shift and take care of the recipient. At first it seemed ghoulish, but I got used to it and soon it became what it still seems to me now: incredible. Awesome in the true meaning of the word: I was full of awe.

WE TRIED TO keep Margot's body going until the fetus was at least twenty-four weeks' gestation. That was the decision the husband made, to try to save the baby. The mother would not live, but maybe the baby could have a chance if the mother was kept alive for as long as possible. All the nurses cared for her, some of us with nagging qualms.

A small group of nurses spent extra time in the room, playing soothing music to the fetus, talking to it, and holding gatherings in the med room to pray for divine intervention on its behalf.

I hung back, along with the other secular or merely skeptical nurses who didn't believe such disproportionate efforts should be made for a fetus. All our efforts and resources, both human and financial, should be directed toward the living, we believed. Margot was dead, merely hatching a life that was tenuous at best. With each day that passed, her organs become more vulnerable, more exposed to deterioration and infection and therefore less suitable for transplantation to someone else. After a few days, the matter was decided for us when Margot's body became too unstable and the doctors had to deliver the baby at twenty-two weeks and disconnect Margot from life support. The baby was stillborn.

"First I'll read a psalm," said Father Szigetti as he laid out the doll-sized body on a sterile green towel on the countertop in Margot's room. It looked like a strawberry jelly-baby candy spit out from a child's mouth, still glistening and wet. "Then we will pray for the soul of this baby."

"Can you offer the last rites to the mother or the baby?" requested one of the Catholic nurses.

"We do not anoint the dead," Father Szigetti reminded her firmly and gave her a look that told her she should know better. He did offer what comfort he could to the nurses.

Margot's lungs were still usable, but unfortunately not soon enough for Alice Heidebrecht, the Mennonite farmer's wife with pulmonary hypertension. Her condition had deteriorated rapidly, and she became too unstable to undergo a transplant. She was cared for at home and died there.

I didn't know for sure, but I suspected that Margot's lungs went to my patient, the one I cared for a few days later. Jeremy was an eighteen-year-old boy who had cystic fibrosis. He hadn't had a day of his life when breathing hadn't been an effort. In order to replace missing enzymes in his body, he had to swallow over two hundred capsules a day.

"I realize a lung transplant won't cure his CF," said his mother, "but whatever help it can give his breathing, we would be so grateful. He's struggled all his young life."

Clearly, she had too, along with him.

Jeremy did well. Within a few hours after the surgery, he was awake and weaning off the ventilator. His vital signs were stable and by the end of the day, we removed the breathing tube. The look of astonishment on his face, his expression of pure amazement that he could breathe with ease, probably for the first time in his life, moved me to tears.

Jeremy looked around and simply breathed. In and out, and we watched.

"It's so quiet," his mother said, sobbing in my arms. "I never heard him not coughing. I can't believe it!"

"Ma, I'll need an alarm clock, now," he said with a grin.

"He had never needed one before," she explained. "His coughing woke him up every morning."

SYLVIE HAD BEEN waiting for lungs for almost two years. She also had CF, but had never been as sick as Jeremy. Now she was. Only seventeen years old, her lungs were shot through with holes, from mucous plugs and recurring infections.

I came over to help Tracy, who was her nurse, and we stood on either side of her bed and watched Sylvie gasping for breath. We had her on an oxygen mask at 100 per cent and even though each breath was a struggle, she used what little energy she had to mouth words.

"Mommy, help me. . . . I can't breathe."

Her mother was holding her hand. "Do something, please," she pleaded with us, standing by.

There was nothing we could do. We couldn't give her any sedation because that would make it likely she might not breathe enough to meet her oxygen requirements. That, in turn, would make it more likely that she would need to have an endotracheal tube inserted and then a ventilator to take over her work of breathing. All these events would be a setback and would cause Sylvie to be removed from the transplant list.

It was a heartbreaking situation. None of us could bear to watch, so we stepped outside the room and kept an eye on her from there.

"What's going on in there?" asked Laura, from across the hall.

"Sylvie needs sedation and intubation," Tracy explained, "but if we do that, they'll take her off the transplant list."

"If she gets intubated, it will be a one-way ticket out of here," said a medical resident passing by. "They'll downgrade her or take her off the list, for sure, and right now, she's at the top of the list in Ontario."

"I think she would tolerate a smidgen of sedation," said Tracy. "I think she could handle it. It would lessen her anxiety and would help her to breathe." I watched Tracy thinking it through. She was calculating Sylvie's height and weight, deciding which drug would be best and at what dosage. She was taking into account all the other drugs that Sylvie was on and the various effects and inter-acting effects they might have on Sylvie's rate of breathing, blood pressure, heart rhythm, and emotional state. She was thinking back to previous times when she had taken care of Sylvie and recalling her reaction to sedation, to analgesic, to anti-anxiety medications. She was putting the whole picture together and adding in her instinct and kindness to come up with her plan of action.

A resident came over and took a look at Sylvie from the door of the room. "If you snow her, she won't breathe, and we'll have to tube her and that'll end her chance for a transplant. She's small, and even a pediatric dose of sedation might be too powerful for her. I wouldn't take the chance."

"But you're not in there with her," Tracy said. You haven't stood watching the terror in Sylvie's eyes, her struggle, the mother's helplessness, I thought. Overall, it was a small thing, but it was a big thing to Sylvie and her mother. It had the potential to be a big thing, in the long run. I could see in her eyes that Tracy was going to take a chance.

"I've had asthma all my life," Tracy said, revealing something that none of us knew. "I know how terrifying it is when you can't breathe. There's nothing scarier. I know it's a fine line, but I think a touch of morphine would ease her anxiety and open up her airways. I can't bear to see her like this."

The resident shook his head. "I disagree. It's not worth the risk."

"I'm going to page Dr. Bristol," Tracy said, knowing the repercussions that might ensue by trumping the resident and going over his head, and more importantly, by possibly jeopardizing Sylvie's chance for a lung transplant.

"He's not going to like it," the resident called out.

Tracy came back in tears. "He said, 'Do what you have to do. You know I don't approve,' and slammed down the phone. I'm going to give it anyway."

She knew he wouldn't back her up if the plan backfired. But we would.

Tracy went back into the room to talk to Sylvie and her mother. Bruno joined them and offered Sylvie a soothing massage until the drug arrived. I retrieved the narcotic keys and went to the locked cupboard to get the morphine. I think I saw Tracy's hands trembling as she injected the drug.

"Just the tiniest dose," Tracy assured the mother.

All those things – the nurses' words, touch, and positive intentions, along with the morphine – helped ease Sylvie's breathing. It was something only a nurse could know. You had to be right there to judge that delicate balance. Tracy had a finely tuned intuition and a tough analytical mind. She knew a lot, but didn't even know she knew it or how she knew it.

Sylvie's mother smoothed her daughter's hair. "You look better, dear, don't worry about anything. Your brother is back home taking caring of the cats. I'll call Papa and tell him you're doing better. Now, don't try to talk. Just rest."

AS FRANCES AND I got on the elevator the next morning, Sylvie's mother was just getting off.

"I'm goin' out for a quick smoke. I've gotta get right back 'cause Sylvie's going to the OR. They found lungs for her last night!"

We smiled automatically in response to the mother's smile and tried not to show the trepidation we felt. We couldn't bring ourselves to rejoice as she did. We knew that in Sylvie's case the recovery would be long and difficult and likely complicated, if she even made it off the operating room table. She had deteriorated so quickly over the past day before going into the OR; she would be a high-risk case.

> Thank you not only for your expertise, but also your generous and caring hearts.

Most of the nurses were comfortable with the idea of organ transplants. For the most part, we believed in what we were doing. We knew that many people were out there in the community, living each day by the phone, praying for that call that might save their lives. Even when families refused organ donation, everyone respected their decision. We understood that either grief or certain moral or religious beliefs might preclude a family from agreeing to organ donation. However, sometimes there were occasions when a person had signed the donor card on their driver's licence, but the family overrode that decision at the time of death. Those occasions made many of us feel disappointed, even affronted, on behalf of the dead person. Their wishes had not been carried out.

"We don't own our bodies – or anything for that matter – once we are dead," explained Dr. Bristol. "The law is very clear about this point," he added.

But there was one case that wasn't so clear-cut. It left us all flummoxed. I still wonder about it, now, from time to time. That night I learned a new word.

"I put you in with the donorcycle," said Casey, the nurse in charge on days.

"The what?"

"A daredevil. He was in a motorcycle club doing a stunt. Anyway, he's brain dead and a potential donor, but there's a catch." She smiled and said, "I thought you'd have the tact to handle it, Tilda. That's why I put you in there."

Dr. Bristol and the hospital's lawyer were already in the room. I tried to listen in, but Morty kept talking loudly over them.

"It's like *The People's Court*," Morty said, referring to the afternoon TV show. "*The case you are about to witness is real. The participants are not actors. They are actual litigants with a case pending in the California Supreme Court.*"

"Hush," I said. "I want to hear what's going on."

"The victim did in fact sign his organ donor card on his driver's licence, but the common-law girlfriend – she's the next of kin, there's no one else – states she'll overrule if we don't allow for retrieval of sperm for posthumous fatherhood," the lawyer was saying.

"Sperm retrieval would be impossible in the conventional manner," explained Dr. Bristol to the lawyer, "technological advancements notwithstanding." The two exchanged boyish grins. "The patient is brain dead and sperm retrieval would be possible only by way of an invasive procedure. At any rate, more importantly, does the next of kin agree to organ donation?"

"Yes, but only on condition of receiving . . . the other. In hand, so to speak. It has been explained to her that sperm retrieval is not allowed in this case. There must be clear, prior intent on the part of the deceased to put his post-mortem sperm toward such a purpose."

What other purpose is there for the stuff, I wondered.

"He's my fiancé," a distraught and pretty woman standing at the bedside said. "We've already set the date, Valentine's Day!"

"You can understand why this matter must be sorted out most expeditiously," said Dr. Bristol to the lawyer. "If there is any chance he is still to be an organ donor, that is."

"I won't agree to anything if I can't have his sperm," she said.

"It gives new meaning to the term dead-beat dad," said Morty, who was trying to whisper, but was probably incapable of it.

"Shhh," I hushed her.

Dr. Bristol came up with a creative suggestion.

"Could the sperm be obtained, then quarantined in a cryogenic storage facility? That would allow the proxy – and the courts – the time to make a more considered decision."

"I want his baby!" The woman began to wail and threw herself across the husky, extensively tattooed body in the bed and sobbed into his broad chest. "He wanted me to have his baby," she said, amending herself.

Dr. Bristol addressed her. "It is doubtful, or at best uncertain, if Raoul would have wanted to be a father after his death." He spoke slowly and carefully.

"If you call that being a father!" said Morty under her breath, but just barely under.

"At any rate, we will never know his wishes in this regard. Did you ever talk with him about having a child?"

"Of course. We talked about it many times."

"Did you ever talk about having a child, even in the event of death?"

"Of course not," she cried in exasperation. "He never thought he was going to die! Why would he? He's only twenty-five. He doesn't even have a will."

The lawyer drew Dr. Bristol and me to the side of the room and Morty included herself.

"Her motive must be determined. Is it truly her desire to have his child, or is there possibly a financial incentive, for example, inheritance of his estate? What if in the ensuing year, she finds a new partner, what is to be done with the, er, sample?"

"That's going too far! I'm not prepared to probe into her psyche or her love life," exclaimed Dr. Bristol. "I doubt whether she is even in a rational state of mind at this moment to discuss any of this."

"She doesn't seem to have even registered the loss," I noted.

A surgeon walked by and beckoned me to join him out in the hall.

"What's the holdup?" he asked with a glance at his watch. "We've been ready and waiting for him in the OR for over an hour."

"There's a bit of a hitch . . . I mean a glitch." I stifled a giggle.

He was tired and wanted to know if he could grab a nap before the long night ahead, or if there was even going to be a long night ahead. I understood all of that but sometimes in their eagerness for the "harvest," the surgeons acted more like hunters than farmers.

When I went back into the patient's room, the doctor and the lawyer had left and the girlfriend grabbed my arm. The intensity of her gaze frightened me. Would she attack me? How would I manage to call security for a Code White – a violent patient? Where was Morty now?

"I need his sperm," she said. "I want you to help me."

Did she want me to somehow procure it for her?

"It is impossible and against the law," I said sternly, in imitation of both the doctor and the lawyer. She softened and slumped again over the body in the bed.

What a conundrum: if something is impossible, did it even matter that it was against the law? If it is against the law, did it even matter if it was possible? There was a surgical procedure available, but it would be against the law to perform it, so what did it matter that it was possible?

"What about the old-fashioned way? Would it work?" she asked with a weak smile.

At that moment, Morty turned up again and handed me an urgent report she'd scribbled on a piece of paper.

"Necrophilia!"

"I doubt if ejaculation is still possible when there is brain death," I said, temporizing after glancing at the note and glaring at Morty to stop. "But I can't say for sure." There were certainly a number of questions that were coming up in my practice that had not been covered in the nursing curriculum. "But you heard what the lawyer said. Raoul gave consent to donate his organs, but he didn't give consent to father children after his death."

I rejoined Dr. Bristol and the lawyer, who were continuing their discussion just outside the patient's room. They were talking about electro-ejaculation techniques (I noticed both men wince imperceptibly at the mention of that) and the feasibility of procuring viable sperm after a period of oxygen deprivation. It will certainly make an interesting case study to write up for publication, Dr. Bristol must have been thinking.

After a few minutes, the girlfriend came out of the room. She had a beatific expression on her face. "I got what I wanted," she said, patting her purse and licking her lips. "You can take what you want."

We looked at each other in disbelief. Was she bluffing?

We would never know for sure.

IN MOST CASES the organ procurement phase went smoothly, causing little distress or confusion, at least among the nurses. Once the declaration of brain death was made, our work was straightforward and mostly technical, although it was done under the intense pressure of time constraints. However, when it came to allocating those precious and few organs to recipients, it became harder to suppress judgment. Sometimes our reactions were explosive.

"I can't believe this!" exclaimed Morty one morning on team rounds. "I took care of this patient a few months ago and I had to give him whiskey down his nasogastric tube so he wouldn't go into the DTs. I remember how the psychiatrist said this is not a detox centre and that we'll have to address his alcohol abuse in another setting. Now, it's a mere few months later, and he's in a hepatic coma and his liver enzymes are sky high, but he promised to stay sober, so they put him at the top of the transplant list. They found him a liver right away and guess whose liver matched? A victim of a drunk driver who ploughed into another car on the 401, a mother of two kids, on New Year's Day! What guarantee do we have that he won't go back to drinking and ruin this new liver?" she demanded to know. "Couldn't they have found a more deserving candidate?"

Silently, we were grateful to her for having the courage to ask the question that was on all our minds.

"Do you believe that a patient suffering from alcoholism warrants different treatment than a patient with a congenital disorder of the liver?" Dr. Bristol challenged her back. "All things being equal, why should there be a bias?"

"But all things aren't equal and you know it," Morty said. "The reality is there is an imbalance in supply and demand. There aren't enough organs for everyone who needs one."

"What about the overdoses? I sometimes have a problem with them, too," admitted Tracy. "I realize these patients must be mentally ill to do something so irrational, but what if they go on to a second attempt and destroy their new liver? It's such a waste."

"Surely we mustn't create a hierarchy of diseases so that mental illness or alcoholic cirrhosis have inferior status and fewer rights than a congenital disease such as, say, a biliary tract atresia, or even a contracted disease such as hepatitis. We aren't here to apportion blame or pass judgment. We're here to treat patients impartially, based on their medical needs. Why should transplantation be treated any different than any other treatment we offer? Don't we treat overweight diabetics without compunction? We treat smokers with respiratory diseases, don't we?" His eyes twinkled with the love of these questions.

"Even if we do regard alcoholism as a disease, why can't we expect someone to exert some control over themselves, especially if their behaviour is ruining their health and harming their family life?" I asked. "Organs are scarce. Is it too much to ask?"

"What about the cost of all of this in dollars and cents?" asked Morty. "We can't ignore that any longer."

"David, you'd offer Osama bin Laden a kidney transplant," said Laura.

"You'll have to find him first," said Morty.

"Well, we would certainly put him on the list. That's the beauty of Canadian medicine," said Dr. Bristol, content that questions were being raised and not the least bit perturbed that no answers were found. We all knew there weren't any, anyway. Although we always argued with great zeal, we all knew that resolution of these perennial questions was never really possible and we just had to live with the uneasiness these situations created.

"Okay, I'll give you an ethical dilemma," said Morty. "Let's just say that Princess Diana had been wearing her seat belt and her organs had been intact after that car crash. Do you think for one minute the Royal Family would have offered them up for donation? I can just see some homeless low-life rubby staggering around the London Underground drinking away his new royal liver! Or even some poor deserving commoner getting her lungs? The blue blood in his veins would be a dead giveaway!"

IT SHOULDN'T HAVE been easier or more pleasant to take care of the grateful, "nice" patients, but for most nurses, it was. We tried to be above such bias and never let it affect our care, but a card we received from a woman we'd cared for following serious complications after abdominal surgery did make us feel very appreciated.

> Even though the odds were stacked against me, the care and dedication of the staff and God's hand have saved me. I have been given the opportunity to once again enjoy the love of my children and grandchildren. I thank you with all of my heart for being so aggressive in my treatment. My memory of my ICU stay is limited, which may be a good thing, but everyone filled me in on just how incredibly relentless and compassionate all the doctors and nurses were and I thank you.
>
> With love and gratitude.

"I prefer a card like that to the chocolate bunny with the bitten-off ears that we got last Easter from some family. Do you remember that?" said Laura with a snort. "Some gratitude!"

"How about the bottle of rotten cherry kirsch?" I added.

Then a letter came that put us all in our place:

I know I was difficult during my stay with you, and I want to apologize to those to whom I may have lashed out at in my frustration. Being in the ICU was the most harrowing, terrifying experience of my life and I am still plagued with nightmares from my ordeal. However, my thanks go out to all of you. You saved my life.

THERE WASN'T ALWAYS the luxury on days to socialize or to discuss the cases that troubled us, but during the long night shifts that we worked together, there was time to talk about everything, and we did. It was cold in the hospital late at night, or maybe it just felt that way because our bodies were slowed down. If all was quiet with the patients, we sat out in the hall, flannel blankets draped over our shoulders, at various, odd distances from one another, so that we could keep an eye on our patients and the machines, and spring into action if necessary. We propped our feet up on little stools that we normally used for standing on at the bedside of patients while doing CPR chest compressions.

Of all of us, Morty found night shifts the hardest, for she slept poorly on days. "When I work nights," she moaned dramatically, "I feel sick. It runs my metabolism down to a slug's or maybe a two-day-old cadaver's."

Nights were a hardship for most nurses, but some nurses chose to work nights exclusively.

"I don't like working days," said Pamela. "I used to do them, but no way. I'd never go back to days."

"Is it because of your kids?" I asked.

"Hell, no," she said. "My kids are little and I sleep when they nap. No, I can't stand the politics and all those doctors hanging around on days. And there's so much commotion with the families. Nights are usually quieter, and you're more in control of your work at night."

"I don't like when you tell people you're going to night shift they give you such a pitying look, like what a loser you are, especially if it's a weekend and everyone's out having fun and you're going off to work," said Tracy, getting up slowly to do her vital signs and then do mine for me, while she was at it.

I must have looked like I was about to nod off because she asked, "How're ya doing, Tillie? Hangin' in there?" She gave me a little shove.

"Just barely," I muttered.

When Tracy came back, she added, "I don't like when people call it the graveyard shift. It's so demeaning. We do this for a living. We're professionals around the clock."

I sat up to make myself be more awake and to add a complaint of my own. "I can't stand going to bed when the sun is up and going to work when it's dark. Whole days can go by when you don't see any sunlight because you have to waste the day sleeping. It makes me feel out of kilter with the rest of the world." I yawned just thinking about it. "It feels abnormal and unhealthy."

From time to time we worried about the effect on our health of working the night shift. Someone would bring in a newspaper or magazine article that reported on research that showed that shift work could take years off our lives, make us more prone to depression, diabetes, and heart disease.

"At this rate, I'll be a hundred before I'm thirty," said Laura.

Sometime, during every night shift, a wave of exhaustion came over me, so powerfully that I felt like I would collapse. There were moments when I envied – even slightly begrudged – the patients their beds. There came a time, a moment I could pinpoint every night shift I worked, when I ran out of energy. I was afraid I couldn't go on. I temporarily lost faith that I would be able to carry on. It was usually between 3:00 and 4:00, sometimes 4:30. Sometimes my eyelids closed and opened again like a blink. I had to glance at my watch to be sure that it wasn't more than a blink. A few more of those micro sleeps somehow helped me make my passage on to the reliable gift of the second wind. Luckily, almost always, at some point, the second-wind phenomenon kicked in.

Occasionally, and only when it was quiet and safe to do so, we took turns covering for one another during breaks and took short naps. The doctors certainly did, and we knew we would be able to function better and more safely if we could lie down for even a few minutes. A storage room with mattresses piled high worked well for our purposes or an empty patient bed would do in a pinch, if we were desperate. (There was some disagreement among the nurses about the minimum "cooling-off period" required between a patient's death and subsequent removal to the morgue, and the bed's use for napping. How much time was enough for the bed to slough off its residue of death in order for a nurse to feel comfortable to curl up on its clean sheets? For me, as soon as the hard gurney rolled down the hall, away from the unit, with its load under a white sheet, the bed was immediately fresh once again, its karma newly minted.)

But one night I walked past a locked room and noticed a note taped to the door.

"Do not disturb. Nurse sleeping."

Now *that* was going too far.

ONE NIGHT I was working beside Bruno. We loved working together and joked that we were like brother and sister. We moved our tables out into the hall because we kept the patients' room dark and we needed the hall lights for charting, conversing, and sharing a bag of microwave popcorn. It was just around that desperate time of waiting for the arrival of the second wind, praying it would come – sleep would be so easy, it was so close – when I looked up to see five men in dark three-piece suits enter the heavy double door of the ICU, stride toward us down the hall, in a tight formation like a phalanx of troops. Visitors at this hour? Who was so sick that visitors showed up in the middle of the night? I looked at Bruno and he mouthed the answer to me.

"It's the mob."

He got up to meet them and then ushered them to the room of the patient they had come to visit. "Come right this way, gentlemen," he said graciously, like the maître d' of a fine dining establishment, leading customers to their reserved table. I wondered what would happen next because it was Pamela's patient and she didn't tolerate unannounced visitors at the best of times.

"Should I warn her, so she doesn't throw them out?" He chuckled. "There may be repercussions. They may give her an offer –"

"– she can't refuse! Yes, you better," I advised.

But it was too late by the time he got down the hall to Pamela's room.

"Sorry sirs, visiting hours are long over," I heard her say. "Come back in the morning. Our patients need to sleep. Next time, call in first on the intercom in the waiting room, to see if it's a good time for you to visit."

I couldn't hear their response, but Bruno was standing outside the door, out of their line of vision, motioning "pow, pow," with his fingers as a gun, but Pamela wasn't getting the hint. Fleetingly, I wondered how he might pantomime a bloody horse in a bed.

"Are you people family or friends? Are your names in the chart? I only give out information about patients to family members. Oh, you're family? Ahhh . . . I see." She must have noticed Bruno's signals. "Oh. In that case, here are some chairs. Have a seat. Stay as long as you like."

It took the Mafia to keep Pamela in line.

IT MUST HAVE been a month or two later when a tall young man carrying an artist's portfolio and a petite woman wearing black bicycle shorts arrived at the ward clerk's desk. I heard my name called over the loudspeaker, requesting me to come to the nursing station. There was someone to see me.

"Remember me?" The young man smiled. I didn't recognize him, but knew I should.

"It's Jeremy," he said.

"Jeremy!"

"Yes, it's me!" He beamed and stood tall to show off our shared accomplishment, his health. "Look, I can breathe!" He took in a deep breath to demonstrate. "Sylvie's here too, of course." He put his arm around her waist.

Here they were, the two of them, yet I sensed the eerie presence of four. The two lives that were lost and the supreme gifts they had given, so that these two young people could breathe. Here they were that day, members of this exclusive club. They had joint membership in a lung fraternity, their friendship cemented by the rare experience they shared.

Jeremy had returned to graphic arts school and Sylvie to living her life however she chose.

"What do you remember of your stay in the ICU, Jeremy?"

"To be honest, I try to block it out. I look around at all these other cyborgs stretched out in the beds and attached to machines and I think, I was just like you, man, but I made it. It doesn't make me feel great though, 'cause I know that some of these dudes won't make it out of here."

"But do you remember anything specific?" I asked. "Did you have pain? Did we manage to keep you comfortable?"

"I didn't have any pain, but I had nightmares. Stuff about the doctors and nurses being Nazis, doing experiments on me. I know it's not true, but the mind plays tricks on you. Oh, I know. I dreamt some hockey players came to visit me."

"That actually happened, Jeremy. Mats Sundin and Tie Domi from the Leafs came to visit you. You must have been too sedated to take it in."

"Wow. Now that I know about it, it makes my day. Nah, I don't remember too much about those guys coming in – I think my mom told me about it – but I remember you."

"How do you remember me? There were so many nurses who took care of you."

"You took care of me right after my transplant when I got back from the OR and you seemed to know just what I was thinking. It seemed like you were right inside my head all the time. You knew I wanted to see my parents right away and then the next big thing on my mind was getting that damn tube out. You were with me every step of the way. You were me until I could be me, again."

"That's better than a Timbit," said Laura, passing by and helping herself to one from the box on the nursing station counter.

"I'll say."

Jeremy grinned and I watched him breathe.

Mostly unconscious while in your tender loving care, but I remember well the soft, reassuring voices of comfort in the surrounding space.

With gratitude.

9

CELESTIAL HOUSEKEEPING

Rosemary, our nurse manager, had a firm policy. She insisted that every nurse take a turn at being in charge of the ICU. At the end of my first year of working there, my turn came. Although I had resisted taking on the role, I came to enjoy the challenges it offered. That slight remove from the bedside helped me understand some of the bigger issues in the hospital and in the health-care system.

"Busy day?" I asked Casey, who had been in charge on the day shift, as I came on to the night shift to take on the role for the first time.

"Not busy or slow. Just steady, but I'm exhausted. Pull up a chair, darling, and I'll give you report. First off, there's a possible brain-dead donor. It's Stuart Bradshaw, a twenty-seven-year-old man who was thrown and trampled by his horse in a show-jumping competition and suffered massive head injuries. The docs are in there now, doing the brain-death testing. Next to him there's Nadia Kholodenko, a twenty-five-year-old with psychogenic polydypsia. You remember what that is." She glanced at my face. I must have had a "systems failure" kind of blank expression. "It's water poisoning. She's a psych patient and voices of Satan told her to drink about six litres of water all at once. She's managed to screw up her electrolytes, but good. Her sodium is only 115! I thought of sprinkling table salt all over her! Next is Mrs. Derczanski, who had carotid surgery today for removal of calcifications but there are complications and she's not doing well. You need to arrange for her to be transferred out for a neurosurgical consult. In the next room is Mr. Joe Binder, a thirty-five-year-old, four-hundred-pound man with a history of alcohol and IV drug abuse, admitted with diabetic ketoacidosis and abdo pain. Came to us from jail – assaulted his mother. He is also in acute renal failure and on dialysis. Had a bowel obstruction that ruptured and was in the OR for eight hours today and now has a colostomy. Peter Hollander, forty-six-year-old, four days post-op for repair of an aortic aneurysm. I don't have a good feeling about him. His numbers are great, but he looks terrible. Ha! They'll put that on his gravestone: 'This man had great numbers.' Sarah Mitchell, thirty-three years old, previously healthy, went into acute liver failure after a week of flu-like symptoms, now decreased level of consciousness, liver enzymes rising, waiting for a liver to become available. Hey, if we can't cure a previously healthy young person like that, who can we save? Then there's a tourist from Greece, a fifty-two-year-old Elias Roussos, here in Canada visiting his lover, when he had a massive MI[*]. Came in with symptoms of SOB, but no CP, N. or V. Came in with HIV, HIT positive, and CMV. Oh, and PCP, to boot. No OHIP, of course. This is a freebie! We're paying for it!"

"He's got most of the letters of the alphabet," I noted.

"And how! Anyway, we had to put him in isolation today for MRSA[†] – you know, it's one of those new super-infections that are resistant to most antibiotics – plus he's growing a new little bug,

---

[*] Myocardial infarction. Definitions of remaining acronyms: shortness of breath, chest pain, nausea, vomiting, human immunodeficiency virus, heparin-induced thrombocytopenia, cytomegalovirus, Pneumocystis carinii pneumonia, and Ontario Health Insurance Plan.

[†] Methicillin-resistant *Staphylococcus aureus*.

Cryptococcus malformans! Let's see how the rest of the passengers – I mean *patients* – are doing here . . ."

Casey had once worked as a flight attendant for Air Canada, back in the days when she was young, thin, and beautiful, as she described herself, and I wondered if that slip was a joke or not.

"Okay, who else have we got on board tonight? Mr. Dwayne Pickup – yup, that's really his name, believe it or not – who's got necrotizing fasciitis, climbing up both legs. Started with an ingrown toenail that got infected. It crawled right up his legs and into his scrotum and buttocks within twenty-four hours. He was in the OR all day for debridement. You should take a look at it – it's a complete anatomy lesson. My husband once worked in a fur barn and this patient's leg looks like one of those skinned animals. It's right down to the bone. Anyway, he's got huge dressings. It takes two nurses over an hour to do it and he's in septic shock and very unstable. Then there's –"

A tall and imposing woman stared down at us through large glasses with shiny mother-of-pearl frames. "My husband, Dr. Laurence, needs to see the doctor right away."

Casey sighed. "Is it urgent, Mrs. Laurence?"

"He's coughing."

She looked from one of us to the other, trying to decide which would be of more use to her. It was a toss-up: I was coming on and Casey was signing off.

"Yes, it's urgent," she said to Casey, whom she had seen all day, rather than me, who was unfamiliar.

"That is something his nurse at the bedside can take care of," Casey said. "I'm in the middle of giving report to Tilda. She's in charge tonight."

"I need to speak with the doctor. A staff doctor."

"Have you ever noticed how it never helps to tell families that there are nineteen other patients, most of them in a lot worse shape than their loved one?" Casey said quietly to me. "They only care about their loved one, of course, but neglect can be a good thing in this place."

She turned back to the patient's wife. "Mrs. Laurence, believe me, if it was an emergency, the doctor would be there, *tout de suite*."

Mrs. Laurence stalked off, unsatisfied.

"Aren't doctors and their families the worst patients? Always expecting special treatment. She tore a strip off Belinda, who was his nurse today, about something trivial and reduced her to tears. I was sweating bullets, but I went in there and told her off. I threatened to call Security and have her escorted out of the hospital if she ever talked to one of our nurses like that again! Imagine! Anyway, where were we? – Mrs. Wei Chong, seventy-nine years old, with end-stage everything, you name it – renal disease, coronary artery disease, and dementia. She doesn't speak a word of English. Come to think of it, doesn't speak a word of anything, since she's unconscious. Family is gathered at her bedside. It's going to be an all-night vigil, I can tell. Someone needs to have a chinwag with them and tell them the score."

"Which is what?"

"That she's dying. You know how the Chinese families have difficulty letting go. Pang-Mei was on today and she explained it to me. Chinese people are terrified of their ancestors, and they don't want the ghosts to come back from the grave and accuse them of sending them off too soon. Anyway, Mrs. Chong came in with failure-to-thrive syndrome. Was living at home, stopped eating and drinking, and the family brought her in. She's been tapped, scoped, scanned, prodded, and cultured and they still can't find anything wrong with her. The daughter was force-feeding her some soup and she aspirated, then arrested, and was brought down from the floor. First thing she did was pull out her endotracheal tube and her IVs. We had to put them back in and tie down her arms. Did they ever stop to think that maybe she's trying to tell us something? Oh, and last but not least – you met the wife – I think she's the ex-wife – of Mr. Laurence – excuse me, *Dr.* Laurence. She insisted I put 'Dr.' on the patient name board. Geez, some people!"

"What's he got?"

"Chronic lung disease. Congestive heart failure and cancer of the prostate, but doing well, for now, anyway. Blood gases are acidotic, so he's here for monitoring. He's a repeat offender."

"What?"

"You know, he's had multiple previous admissions here. Take a look at his mile-high chart. Anyway, he's doing well, for now. If you need the bed for an admission, Dr. Laurence is the one who will have to be transferred out because, believe it or not, he's the most stable one here tonight. But I'm sure the family will raise a stink if you do. Good luck. Just remember what Rosemary says: 'You're not here to win any popularity contests. You're here to do what's right for the patients.' Oh, there were two Code Blues from the floors. The cardiac arrest didn't make it – I don't know where we would have put him if he did. We simply don't have a bed or a nurse to spare – the other Code Blue, a respiratory arrest, did make it and belongs to us, but we didn't have any beds, so he's being bed spaced in the Cardiovascular ICU. Be prepared in the morning for the chief of CV surgery to come roaring through here like a lion because he needs that bed for his own heart surgery patients. Well, as you can see, it's been a pretty busy day, but hopefully you've got a horseshoe up your butt and you'll have a quiet night. Oh, by the way, see if you can find out who's been leaving these religious quotations all over the place." She pointed at one stuck on the refrigerator door of the med room.

Those who hope in the Lord will renew their strength.
They will soar on wings like eagles
They will run and not grow weary.
They will walk and not be faint.

— Isaiah 40:31

"Probably one of the bible thumper nurses," Casey said. "Well, good luck. See ya in the morning. Tootle-loo. Ciao, baby."

Mrs. Laurence peered down over the counter at me and she pressed her fingers into her temples. "Could you please give me two Tylenol."

"Is it for your husband?"

"No, it's for me. I have a headache, but my husband – in 618 – is a doctor."

"I'm sorry, but I can't give you medication. There is a drug-store –"

"I'll pay for it, if you'll just give it to me," she said angrily.

"I can't. I don't know you or your medical history," I said.

"I don't like that nurse," I heard her complain to another visitor. "She's going to be trouble."

ONE OF THE main differences of being in charge of the ICU is that you're listening for phone calls, pagers, faxes, and call bells, instead of alarms, beeps, and the ringing of machines. All the while, you're playing a big chess game, moving all the pieces around – and you have to know which way they each go – and at the same time, you're planning your upcoming moves and preparing in your mind for various contingencies and likely scenarios. To play it well, it's all in the strategy. Intuition helps a lot, too. There are twenty patients, twenty beds and, maybe, enough nurses to go around.

As it stood, there was enough staff for tomorrow, unless someone called in sick. But it was only a few minutes into the shift when the ward clerk came to tell me that Nell Mason had just called in sick for the next day.

"*Quelle surprise*!" said Laura, whose room was right next to the nursing station. She rolled her eyes. "What's the excuse this time? Scurvy? The bubonic plague? Did she tell you that her mother died? If so, make sure you ask her if it's the same mother who died last year!"

"Laura," I said in a tone meant to remind her we knew that Nell had a serious problem.

IT WAS LESS than an hour into that shift when there was an announcement over the hospital public address system and we all paused to listen: "Code Blue, Code Blue."

"It's called change-of-shift syndrome," said Laura. "Some nurse doing evening rounds came across a cold body in the bed."

I went right away to prepare the room that had just been vacated by the organ donor, who had gone to the operating room. Everything had to be ready in case the arrest patient needed to come to the ICU.

"Please call housekeeping to come and clean this room," I asked the ward clerk.

"Laura already called them for you," she said and returned to her private phone call.

"Yup, let's go up there," said Mike, the resident on that night. "It may be business for us. We'll have a look-see."

It was our last empty bed and none of us nurses dared say it, of course, but it was our only napping bed, too.

THE ROOM ON the floor was chaotic with doctors, nurses, and respiratory therapists trying to save a life. A nurse was perched up high on the bed doing athletic-looking compressions on a patient's chest, and I could hear the unavoidable crunching of ribs with each thrust. A large plastic tube had been inserted into the patient's mouth and I noted by the rise and fall of the chest that it was in the lungs, where it should be. One nurse was starting a large needle IV in one arm and another nurse was injecting medication into the IV that was already in place in a vein in the arm that was flopped over the side of the bed. Yet another nurse was recording everything that was happening. She had filled the allotted page and was now scribbling on a long, torn piece of paper towel.

A nurse stepped forward out of the crowd to give me report. "Mr. Lilly is a 104-year-old gentleman, previously well, living independently at home. Came in with pneumonia. He had a respiratory arrest and then cardiac –"

"Did I hear you correctly?"

"I know." She smiled. "But he looks good, doesn't he? Just turned 104."

Mike came to talk to me. "They've got him stabilized, but he obviously needs to come down to the ICU. Do we have a nurse and a bed?"

"Did you know that this patient is 104?" I asked.

"That's his heart rate?" He peered at the portable cardiac monitor, attached to the bed.

"No, his age."

"Wow," he whistled. "He's in pretty good shape for 104."

"Not any more, he isn't. Do you think it's a wise idea to bring him to the ICU?"

"What do you suggest we do with him?"

"Well, get rid of all this equipment, give him morphine if he looks in distress, gather around, and hold his hand. Common sense dictates that this event signals the end of his life. He's lived to a ripe old age with dignity and you know what we're going to subject him to in the ICU. Do you really think we can buy him more time? And at what price to him?"

"But he was well before. Living on his own. You think we should just write him off 'cause he's old? That's called ageism."

"All I'm asking is should we be doing all of this? Does he have any advance directives? We can't just resuscitate by default, can we? Don't forget, Mike, it's our last bed. Anyone else who needs an ICU bed will have to go elsewhere."

"Let's not start playing God, here," he said. "These are choices that are way out of our control."

"But every choice has an impact on other choices and every choice we make affects people's lives. Even no choice is a choice."

Surely this was not the time to have such a conversation, regarding the life of a complete stranger, but that's exactly what we were doing.

Mike flipped through the chart and went off to consult with the staff physician. When he came back he said, "Nothing is known about his wishes. We have to take him. Besides, we've started everything already, we can't stop it all now."

"You're going to take him?"

People had cleared out of the room, and I was able to get closer now. The old man's face was in a grimace and his papery, wrinkled skin strained against the breathing tube, like a horse bucking against the sharp bit of a bridle. "Can he have some sedation at least?" I asked.

"It would drop his blood pressure and it's already too low."

I took a reading myself and barely heard the systolic, hovering around 80.

"We have to take him," Mike said. "You have a point, but we don't have a choice."

"What about his family? Where are they?" I suddenly felt desperate to spare this man the indignity of the ICU.

"There is none. He's outlived them all. He had a son who died and there's a seventy-year-old daughter who's in a nursing home with Alzheimer's. There's a niece in England, but she hasn't seen him in years. I spoke with the family doc, but he said he never spoke with him about it. You'd think the topic might have come up when he hit ninety, wouldn't you? There was a girlfriend, but unfortunately –"

"A girlfriend?"

"It's possible. Male sexuality can extend well into –"

"I'm not saying –"

"Anyway, the girlfriend died a few weeks ago."

"Oh." I gritted my teeth and pressed on with my campaign. "What if he arrests in the unit, what are we going to do then?"

"Do what you think is right. Tell me about it afterwards."

I hated the cowardice and the artifice of that charade. I'd done it a number of times before.

"Then this exercise is nothing more than protecting your –" I stopped myself as a nurse handed me a plastic bag containing Mr. Lilly's belongings, and Mike and I began to push the heavy bed down the hall.

It never failed to touch me when I saw the personal items that patients brought to the hospital. So hopeful they must have been when they packed them that they would use them once again. They seemed to me like souvenirs from a country to which they might, or might not, return. Over the years I had seen pink furry slippers, a knock-off Nascar racing jacket, a package of condoms, subway tokens, a three-hundred-page word-search book in which only the first few pages had been completed, a nibbled chocolate bar, rolled-up children's crayoned pictures: "Gamps, Get beter soon, Love Meagan."

Inside Mr. Lilly's No Frills shopping bag were the following items: a plastic container of false teeth knocking about in blue liquid, a pair of reading glasses, a rosary, a plaid flannel robe, yesterday's *Globe and Mail* and a Happy 100th Birthday! card signed, "Your Sweetie."

"I thought you said he was 104," said the resident as we got on the elevator.

"I imagine the demand for Happy 104th cards is rather limited," I said dryly.

When we got back to the unit, I assigned Nicole, who was freed up from the brain-dead donor patient, to now take over Mr. Lilly's care. When I told her the story, her face registered the same dismay that I had felt.

"I know we're not supposed to have opinions about these situations," she said, "but this is wrong." She took his hand in hers. "It's so cold and thin. It feels like it will break right off."

Mike came over to where I sat at the nursing station, going over the staffing for the next day.

"I'm starving," he said. "Is there anything around here to eat?"

"There's a tuna sandwich in the pantry. It was Mrs. Daley's."

"Maybe she'll want it?"

"She was the one who died this afternoon."

He raked his hand through his hair. "Man, I'm beat. My girlfriend – she's a resident too – says our jobs are a form of birth control." He was catching up on his notes in the patients' charts. "Hey, what's the usual dose of cefotaxime? Is it one gram four times a day or three times?"

What if I tell him and I'm wrong?

"I don't remember," I said.

"Whatever," he mumbled and scribbled something in the chart.

"What have you decided to specialize in?"

"Radiology or pathology most probably. Something without too much patient contact and a fairly decent lifestyle. Isn't it funny how it's the patient contact you think you want in the beginning and how that changes as you go through it?"

I looked at him and he could tell he'd gone down in my estimation.

"I know it sounds strange, like you're wondering, like, what's the reason he went into medicine in the first place? It's just that's the part I find the hardest, dealing with patients. I like everything else about medicine."

He means the science, the puzzles, the problems, and the math. The things that can be controlled, measured, understood, or fixed.

"I'm sure," I murmured. "Listen, Mike, the young woman in liver failure – her amylase is rising."

"I'm too tired to think of a differential diagnosis." He put his head down on the desk.

"She could be developing pancreatitis. Do you think we should do an ultrasound? Some blood work?"

"Maybe."

IT WAS 2300 hours and as it stood, there was enough staff for the morning, if we didn't get any more admissions and if no one else called in sick. As I made my rounds from room to room, I kept finding strips of masking tape on the wall or countertops upon which were written messages. There was one stuck on the ice machine that read,

> Bear with each other and forgive whatever grievances you may have against one another. Forgive as the Lord forgave you.
>
> – Colossians 3:13

Who was leaving these things? Oh well, they can't do any harm, can they?

"WHERE'S THE HOSPITAL assistant?" I asked the ward clerk, who was slumped over the phone at the nursing station, talking in hushed tones to her boyfriend. (Laura claimed she once overheard them having phone sex.) "Please call the hospital assistant. We need help to turn a four-hundred-pound patient."

"She's taking a nap in the lounge." She gestured to me to wait, then cupped the phone and whispered, "Hey, Trev, I'll call you right back."

"The hospital assistant is sleeping? She just came on duty!"

"She had a late night last night. She's still recovering. It was heavy, man. She told me to tell you to wake her in about an hour."

"What do you recommend I use to accomplish that? Dynamite?"

The ward clerk giggled. "She is a pretty sound sleeper, that girl."

"Where's Rodney?" I asked reluctantly. Rodney, the other hospital assistant, was a frightening sight, especially at night, with his shaved head, Doc Marten boots, and the dirty, frayed red string tied around his neck. But he had strong and useful arm muscles and without them, Emily, the nurse taking care of the heavy patient, wouldn't be able to reposition him in bed and make him comfortable.

"How ya doin', big guy?" I heard Emily ask her patient, Mr. Binder.

He couldn't speak because of the tube in his throat, but nodded at her words.

"We're goin' t'chill tonight, dude, is that okay?" she asked and smoothed back his shaggy hair and smiled at him. "Rod's here now and we're goin' t'turn you and I'll give you a nice back rub. You jiggy with that? How 'bout some tunes?" She found a heavy-metal rock station on the radio and snapped her fingers to the blast of sound.

How soothing her slangy speech and dropped-off verb endings sounded!

Her patient nodded. His eyes were wide. He must have been taken aback by the respect Emily showed him. How much kindness had this abused and violent, heroin-addicted, paranoid schizophrenic, homeless man ever been exposed to in his life?

GEORGINA, A NURSING supervisor, came by and mentioned to me in passing that the hospital had just received a bomb threat.

"Gosh, do we have to evacuate?" I asked. It would be my first Code Black!

"No, no, not to worry," she said. "Just look out for any suspicious packages."

I saw Morty suddenly busy with cardboard, scissors, and string.

"Georgina, I don't have time to go around looking for bombs," I told her. "What's a bomb look like, anyway? Doesn't Security take care of these things?"

She giggled. Georgina was an older woman, originally from Bombay, who had been put out to pasture years ago and had risen to the role of nursing supervisor. (We often wondered why she didn't bother to pluck her single, dark eyebrow to demarcate the hairy furrow above her eyes into two separate arches, but that was neither here nor there.)

Morty rolled her eyes. "We're busy taking care of patients. How do you expect us to look for a bomb?"

"I have no idea, girl!" she said with a jolly bounce of her head from side to side.

"Well, you've cooked your goose, Georgina," said Morty. "If you admit *you* don't know, how can you expect us to know?"

"Yes, indeed," she echoed. "Cooked my goose. Indeed. I cook it well done!"

"Everything else okay, Georgina?" I asked.

"Thanks for reminding me, girl. There's a family that keeps calling the hospital. Their father died in this unit and they're missing his glasses, his teeth, and his wallet. Have you seen them around anywhere?"

"Can't say I have. His wallet I can understand, but what do they need his glasses or teeth for? He's dead, didn't you say?"

"Yes, I know, hon, but they want him buried with his glasses and teeth."

"You know what my grandmother would say about that?" Laura asked and then told us. "Shrouds don't have pockets."

We couldn't find the items, but just as she was leaving, Morty called her over.

"Georgina. I found this. I think it's for you."

She handed her the little box she'd fashioned out of cardboard. Inside was a little piece of paper that read: "KA-BOOM!"

"Oh, you girls! So funny!"

I informed the resident about the bomb scare. "I'm not going to lose any sleep over it," he said, peevishly, "probably because I'm not going to get any sleep in the first place."

"Listen, we need to transfer Mrs. Melissa Derczanski."

"Remind me again who –"

"She's Laura's patient. She's the sixty-eight-year-old who needs neurosurgery, which is done only at the other branch of our hospital 'corporation.'" I couldn't help using the term with a tone of distaste. "She came here for vascular surgery and developed complications. Now she needs neurosurgery, which is only done over there now."

"Someone should inform patients that they aren't allowed to have two things wrong with them," said Laura, listening in.

"The surgeons are ready for her, but the paramedics haven't shown up to transfer her over there," I explained.

Laura had a new observation. "Here's proof that we baby boomers are aging. My sixty-three-year-old patient's first name is Melissa. One day elderly patients will have names like Grandma Tiffany, Grandpa Jason. Listen, Mrs. Derczanski is deteriorating fast. She needs a brain surgeon."

"I've spoken to the transfer team and they say it's going to be at least another hour," I told the two of them. "They were en route to us when they had to divert to another call – teenagers who took an overdose of Ecstasy. I'm going to call the dispatcher and tell them Mrs. Derczanski has been upgraded to urgent."

I returned to Mr. Lilly in Nicole's room.

"What can we do?" we asked each other with our eyes.

"It's so sad," said Nicole, "what we do to the elders of our society." She shook her head. "Look how groomed his hair and nails are, how well-used his rosary is."

I knew that hers was, too. She had placed it in his hand; into a blue vein on this hand a needle had been inserted to deliver a saline solution. I stood and watched the drops, one by one, falling like sand through an hourglass.

"I gave him just 2 milligrams of morphine because he was struggling so much against the tube. Mike is going to put in an arterial line." She shrugged, trying not to care as much as she did. Nicole filled a basin with warm soapy water and gave her patient a sponge bath, inch by inch, keeping him covered with lots of towels. I helped her for a few minutes.

Everyone else seemed to be doing okay.

Pamela was reading a magazine outside her room. Her sedated, unconscious patient was stable and undemanding. She had called in before her shift to request this particular patient. She said she was tired, had a migraine, was getting over the flu and PMS, too.

"That girl's a lazy bum. She hasn't moved off her chair all night," Laura came over to the nursing station to tell me. "I'm going to draw a chalk outline around her patient and prove to her in the morning that she didn't move him all night."

"Look," Laura cornered Mike and continued her rampage, "you better pull some strings, call David Bristol at home, do whatever you have to, but get my patient over to the neurosurgeon at the Western. Her neurological weakness is getting worse from hour to hour. She's barely moving her left side. If they don't get here within an hour, there'll be no need to come at all. She'll have totally stroked out by then and be paralyzed. Short of carrying her over there on my back or putting her in a taxi . . ."

"Okay, okay, I get the message," said the resident.

"I'm going to call Dr. Bristol at home," I said.

"Wow, you're brave," said Nicole, joining me at the nursing station to dip into the crumpled bag of sour-cream-and-onion-flavoured potato chips that we were sharing throughout the night. "He'll tell you to figure it out yourself."

"He should be informed about what's going on."

"You're a pistol, Tilda," said Frances, smiling at me, watching all of this from her room.

"Can you believe we raised her from a pup?" asked Laura.

"Yes, and now look at the monster we've created," said Frances proudly.

"A viper," said Laura, which was high praise, coming from her.

"CORINNE'S PATIENT IS dying." Laura came over to tell me. It could have been Laura in charge; she knew everything that was going on. "Corinne's fairly new, so I'll go help her out a bit. Once her patient dies, make sure you call housekeeping right away to come and clean the room, so you'll be ready in case you get a new admission."

"Don't listen to Bossy Boots," Frances called over to me. "You do your own thing."

"You've got to have the bed ready in case someone needs it," Laura said. "They're *dying* to get in here tonight!" She pointed to the single, hermetically sealed window and howled at it like a werewolf. "See, it's a full moon."

"I know," I said, thinking out loud. "As it stands now, the ICU is full. We'd have to send someone out if there's an arrest or an Emerg patient elsewhere. It will have to be Dr. Laurence because he's the most stable. I'd better go warn Valerie to be ready." Valerie was Dr. Laurence's nurse.

"The Laurence family won't be too happy about it," warned Valerie, "especially if we move him out in the middle of the night."

"I know, I know. I'm only telling you in case we have another admission such as an in-house arrest or an admission from the Emerg. Just so you know."

"If Dr. Laurence does have to transfer out tonight, make sure you tell someone to catch the family quick before they come in the morning and see the empty bed and freak before we have a chance to explain."

Her "nag list" of issues to be discussed with the resident was long tonight. She had written it on a strip of surgical tape on her table on wheels in the same embellished handwriting in which she wrote her long manuscripts, novels of mystery and romance.

1. Excessive adventitious sounds in all lung fields. A new finding. Temperature elevated to 37.5. Chest sounds crackly. Please check X-ray. Infiltrates noted bilaterally. Blood cultures drawn. Please order chest physiotherapy and change antibiotic for more gram-negative coverage?
2. No bowel movement in three days. Needs a laxative.
3. Patient needs subcutaneous Heparin for deep vein thrombosis prophylaxis.

There was another note, this one stuck to the door of the Greek patient with HIV.

> If a man has sexual relations with another man, they have
> done an abominable thing and both shall be put to death.
>   – Leviticus 20:13

Who would post such a notice there? Surely not Suman, who
was the nurse taking care of that patient. I looked around. A few
of the religious nurses were on, but they wouldn't be imposing
their beliefs on others in this way, would they? Probably the work
of someone on a mission to save heathen souls. Surely it couldn't
be Father Szigetti. The priest had probably been in the ICU this
afternoon when Mrs. Daley died, so maybe he knew something
about it. Corinne came to me and I saw she had been crying.

"This is going to go on all night," she said. "My patient is practically dead, but the family keeps pressuring me to keep her going.
They're sitting around her bed staring at the monitor. I swear,
those green lines on the screen make them keep hoping she'll
recover. Every time her blood pressure takes a dive, they tell me
to go up on the inotropes, increase the oxygen, but I'm now at
maximum doses of everything. They've got a little granddaughter
in there, who keeps singing 'Jesus Loves Me' in Chinese. It's
breaking my heart."

I felt for Corinne, who was caught in the middle of this situation. I felt for the patient, whom I hoped was too far gone by now
to be aware of what was going on. I felt for the family; I knew their
grief would soon engulf them. But that night, as the nurse in charge
of the ICU, the main thing on my mind was what would I do if I
needed that bed.

"I'M GOING TO put a pulmonary artery catheter in," Mike said
wearily.

"In whom?" I asked.

"Mr. Lilly. I've got to do it."

"You're not," I said, incredulously.

"He may still be salvageable. I need to know what's going on in
the guy's left ventricle. Was this a pure respiratory event, or is there
a cardiac component, too, like congestive heart failure?"

"Can't someone just die any more?" I asked. "I mean without an IV? I mean the natural way?"

"That's the point," said Mike. "We can now do things better than natural. In the old days, people used to die. Now, we can buy them more time. In the old days, dying was a painful process. Now we have ways of making it more pleasant for people. If we can do that, why shouldn't we?"

I thought about it. "Oh," was all I could come up with. "I always assumed natural was best."

"But we can improve on what's natural."

"Listen," I said. "Why don't we wait and see? Maybe he'll become conscious and then he can tell us himself if he wants all this done or not."

"Technically speaking, informed consent isn't required for this procedure. It's medically indicated. We'd be negligent if we didn't offer it."

"Just because we can do something doesn't mean we should."

"It wouldn't be right not to give him a chance."

"How is it going to change your treatment, or is this merely an academic exercise?"

At that, he looked sheepish. "In the morning, Bristol will ask if I've done it and –"

"Say no more." I put up my hand like a traffic cop to halt the flow of words.

Now when people ask me if my work makes me sad, I'll have a new answer, I thought as I stewed over this conversation: "No, not sad. Angry."

Corinne came to tell me that her patient had died. There was no blood pressure, no pulse, no cardiac output, no breathing. "The only problem is," she said, "she has an internal pacemaker and it keeps on firing and I don't know how to turn it off. The family are confused, because they see these occasional blips on the screen and they can't compute that she's dead."

"Where's Mike?" His on-call room was dark. "Wake him up, will you, Laura? Hey, do you have any idea who's been leaving these notes all over the place?" I pulled at another strip of tape, this one on the frame around a computer screen:

Professing themselves to be wise, they became fools.

– Romans 1:22

"Some religious psycho," Laura said with a yawn. "By the way, the paramedics just called. They say they're on their way to pick up my patient. I hope it's not too late. Mike? He got called down to Emerg to see a patient. Call the Coronary ICU. Ask them if their cardiologist can come over and turn off the pacemaker," she suggested. "Hey, you can tell him to prepare to meet thy pacemaker."

"You have to deactivate the pacemaker," the cardiologist said to me over the phone in a slurred, sleepy voice. "Move the magnetic doughnut ring around the anterior chest wall until you knock out the pacemaker and get a flat line."

"What magnetic doughnut? Could you please come and do it? I've never done it before," I said, glaring into the phone at him.

It's your job. I woke you up. Admit it. You don't want to get out of bed. That's what's going on here.

"I can't come," he said. "Someone's arresting. Get the magnetic ring, it's probably on the fridge door. Move it around the chest, up and then down and then all around."

"Up, down, and move it all around," I repeated, jiving a little to a disco beat in my head. I was giddy. The place was getting to me. I looked at my watch: 0400 hours.

The patient was dead but the pacemaker continued to make the heart beat purposelessly. After several tries, I finally found the exact location on her chest that made her heartbeats stop. Then and only then was the family convinced that she was dead. That was the signal for the wailing and keening to commence. They clasped their hands together and shook their clasped hands up and down in the direction of their wizened old matriarch. She had been a midwife back in rural China, delivering all the babies of the village. She had laboured on her hands and knees in upscale Toronto homes, scrubbing floors for years as an immigrant worker who never spoke a word of English.

A grandson sobbed loudly and shoved his wire-rimmed gold glasses up to his forehead and pressed his fingers against his eyelids to stem the flow of tears. The room was full of people now, chanting in Chinese, sobbing and kneeling on the floor beside the old woman's bed, bowing deeply. All the mourners were equal in their grief: the teenager and her uncle, the little singing toddler and the old cousin, the patient's elderly husband and the deaf, mute nephew.

Sad, grieving, angry, exhausted – I accepted it all. Corinne and I hugged them one by one and expressed our sympathy. I saw such disbelief in their eyes. Their shock was so innocent. It seemed as if it had never occurred to them that this old lady's life would one day come to an end.

I went into the med room, brewed a pot of strong coffee, and poured myself a cup. Caffeine would have very little stimulating effect on this degree of fatigue. Frances had brought in a home-baked pound cake, but it tasted weird – she had probably substituted salt for sugar, or maybe talcum powder for baking powder – and I spit out the dough as I walked past the garbage can. It was 0500 hours. I had read somewhere that this was the "witching hour." Soon it would be sunrise. My cozy bed at home called out to me. In the morning the house would be quiet. Soon, I would be there. I would pour myself a bowl of cereal with milk, take the phone off the hook; my little dog, Rambo, would curl around my feet . . . me, there, burrowing underneath my fluffy down duvet . . .

The phone rang. I looked at it. Taped to the receiver of the phone was a message:

> Write the things that thou hast seen, and the things that are, and the things which shall be hereafter.
> – Revelations 1:19

I picked up the phone.

It was Mike. "Tilda, is that you? I've examined this patient here in Emerg. He needs to come to the ICU. He's a twenty-year-old who drank antifreeze at a bush party. What's the situation? Do we have a nurse for him? Is there a bed?"

I took a sip of coffee. Held the cup for warmth in my hands. Stared down into it to await the answer to be revealed from within its milky depths.

IO

REDECORATING

Within a few years, sweeping changes were underway. The administration was "restructuring" and creating a new vision of the type of institution a hospital should be. Cutbacks, bed closures, and nursing layoffs were the new realities. The first shock was announced at a staff meeting. Rosemary, our beloved nurse manager, had been dismissed. She told us the news herself.

"No one's job is safe," she said. "They even told me that anyone who thinks they can fall back on their seniority is going to get a big shock. They joked that bringing your lunch to work is being overly optimistic."

We were stunned, except for Morty, who calmly explained the situation.

"Rosemary's right. Staff nurses may be laid off, too. There are plans underway to replace nurses with cheaper, unskilled workers, to save money. They figure that the cafeteria pastry chefs can be trained to do bed baths, vitals, and so on. They call it 'deskilling.'"

"Sounds like a frying pan," said Tracy.

"That's a skillet," I said.

Morty explained further. "They want to get rid of us and hire new nurses with less seniority at a lower salary. They think they can get by with fewer RNs. Oh, it's part of the Conservative government's new plan of health-care reform. It's only when the patients start dropping like flies that they'll realize the value of nursing care. Didn't you hear the premier of Ontario compare nurses to Hula Hoop makers? So much for the wage freeze and Rae Days of the NDP's Social Contract, welcome to the Common Sense Revolution. We're feeling it now – the patients will be next."

"I don't get it," said Nicole, who was the first to recover from the shock. "It's not as if business is down. Patient acuity is higher than ever. Everyone knows the trend is that the population is aging. We're going to need more nurses, not fewer. The ICU is always full with patients needing to come here and we're always scrambling for nurses, especially with all the transplants we're doing now."

Frances nodded. "Remember what happened when that pair of lungs had to be sent somewhere else because we didn't have enough nurses to care for the recipient?"

"Right now, all they care about is cutting costs. Slash and burn." Morty shook her head in disgust. Even her curly red hair looked inflamed in reaction to this news. "Hospitals are going to merge with other hospitals to streamline services and eliminate duplication. They're now public corporations and patients are now the 'clients.' Didn't any of you read the results of the patient satisfaction survey? 'Service is poor. I didn't see a nurse all night.' Or 'The mattresses are too soft and my sheets weren't changed for two days.' Sure, there's room for improvement, but the next thing you know, we're moving toward privatized medicine, a two-tier health-care system, and there'll be one standard for the rich and another for all the rest of us. We'll be like the States where people will have to mortgage their house to have their gall bladders removed. A lung transplant would bankrupt most people," said Morty angrily.

Sure, we were worried about the patients and the health-care system, but what about our jobs? one of the other nurses asked.

"After they get rid of some of us," continued Morty, "they're going to require all nurses to have a university degree. We all better get back to school if we want to stay marketable."

Everyone looked crestfallen and preoccupied as we took all this in, except for Laura, who didn't have a degree and had no intention of obtaining one. She knew what she was worth to the hospital and didn't care if they realized it or not. But it was worrisome news to me, even with my degree. Our jobs weren't secure, yet we all knew we were needed. Once a month the doctors met to review the cases of the patients we had treated in the ICU, along with the reasons that some patients had been turned away. Invariably, it was due to a shortage of nurses. Other than that, we didn't have much proof that nursing care made a difference. Yet we all knew that it did.

I looked at Rosemary, who looked more sad than worried. "But how can they get rid of you?" My voice squeaked in indignation.

I heard other rumblings and outcries from all the other nurses around me in the meeting.

"They can't get rid of you," Morty said. "It's not as if there's any problem with your performance. Your work is impeccable. They're obliged by law to offer you something else, another position within the hospital."

"They don't owe me anything." She gave us a weary smile. "It's called retrenchment. They say my job is redundant. They need someone with more management experience who could be responsible for all the ICUs. But they did offer me something." She spoke to us as a group in the same personal, intimate way that she spoke to each of us individually. "It's a desk job in the education department. No patients or families or nurses there, just computers and paperwork. Most of the people who work there haven't seen or touched a patient in years." She sighed and looked defeated. "It's sad because at the heart of it is the inability of administrators to appreciate what nurses do. They're figuring out how long each nursing task takes so they can then justify paying for nursing hours. Like a bed bath, how long does it take and how many personnel are involved? They want to know how many minutes nurses spend giving patients emotional support. Five or ten minutes, they figure? That kind of thing."

"How many points do we get for cleaning poo?" asked Morty. "We'll be in the money if they count that!"

"That's part of the problem," said Rosemary, ruefully. "That's probably all these administrators think nurses do. That's why they believe they can bring in less-skilled people to replace you."

Frances was in a huff. "It's not as if when you're doing vital signs or a bed bath it's a task like hammering in a nail. While you're doing that you're talking to the patient, explaining their meds to them, taking a good look at the condition of their skin. You're assessing if they need more pain medication. Planning when you'll do their wound dressing and what supplies you'll need."

"Well, anyway, I turned down that job they were offering," Rosemary told us. "I'm sure it's very important work, but what nurses *do* and what nurses *know* will never completely find its way into the record books or e-charts. Maybe some of the *doing*, but not the knowing, and certainly not the *being*. How can you apportion a number value to caring in minutes or in dollars and cents? They say we have to be more accountable, that nurses are a commodity and must be used efficiently like any other hospital resource, but nursing by definition is an unlimited commodity. You can never have too much caring. There is no limit to how much one can give as a nurse and the need from the patient's end is surely endless. Anyway, it's just not in me to do that job. I'll leave with the severance package they're offering."

We left to tell the news to the other nurses who were covering for us and get back to our patients.

"LET'S START A petition or write a letter to somebody," Nicole said to the group of us at lunch later that day. "There must be something we can do to save Rosemary."

"This place will never be the same without her," Frances said.

"Now, I love Rosemary as much as the next nurse," said Morty. She took an energetic bite out of her sandwich, as if to fortify herself for the fight ahead. "But she's not exactly a whiz with the budget. She's become a dinosaur. I'm warning you guys, you better get more involved in the union or we're all going to be the losers."

"Rosemary was always on our side," said Frances with a sigh.

"Yeah, remember when that family's son threatened us like a gangster – 'If Mama dies in this joint, I got a gun and I gonna come here and kill youse nurses.'" Laura made a slicing motion across her neck to show how the guy had meant business. It *had* been scary. When his mother did die, Rosemary took the threat seriously enough to have a security guard posted in the ICU for a few weeks to protect us.

"Remember how she baked a cake for the residents on the final day of their ICU rotation?" said Frances, who had already decided that she would carry on that tradition with Rosemary's departure. "Who else but Rosemary would attend all the nurses' weddings and baby showers and send flowers if we were sick? Remember that Christmas, when it was so busy with all of those donors and transplants, and she came in and took care of a patient herself?" recalled Frances.

"She could soothe the angriest family," I recalled.

"Rosemary knew all of the patients and their families by name," Tracy said. "She actually went out to the waiting room and sat and talked to upset families."

"She'd talk to families before they got around to blowing a gasket," added Nicole. "Remember how she would take them into that cramped little office of hers and she'd sit them down and ask them, what's *really* bothering you?"

"I liked that poster on the wall in her office that said, 'Go out on a limb. That's where the fruit is,'" I said.

We remembered it all.

A NURSING ADMINISTRATOR came to the ICU to quell the rising discontent among the nurses. We were heartbroken that Rosemary had been ousted and indignant that the hospital didn't appreciate her as we did. But a new nurse manager will be chosen who will raise the level of professionalism of the nurses, the administrator explained. Things were really slipping, she said, for example, the dress code. The appearance of some of the nurses was rather "inappropriate." ("Sloppy" was the word she probably meant but was too tactful to say.) She also noted on a previous visit to the ICU that many nurses were drinking coffee in patients' rooms and that some nurses had covered over the picture on their hospital identification badge with photographs of actresses and celebrities.

As she spoke, I looked down at my loose green scrubs. I always wore them about two sizes too large, for comfort and ease of movement, but truthfully, it looked like I was wearing pyjamas. There were a few drips of ketchup on my lab coat sleeve. I tried to hide my smile as I discreetly turned my hospital badge around so she wouldn't see the picture of a young Elizabeth Taylor where my face should have been. (One distracted family member had inadvertently called me "Liz" one day and later we both had a good laugh together when she realized the joke.) There had been a quiet night at work and Laura cut up *Maclean's* and *People* magazines and taped new faces on all our badges. Laura was Michelle Pfeiffer – a striking resemblance, I told her, give or take a few pounds; Nicole was Don Cherry's dog, Blue; Tracy was the Pokémon called Pikachu; Frances was Madonna; and Morty was Bart Simpson.

The administrative executive was clear about our priorities: the hospital was millions of dollars in deficit. We needed managers who could bring the budget in line. Reduce employee sick time. Cut costs. Streamline services to avoid duplication. Replace nurses with less-skilled workers and pay them less. Change the skill mix, which was too rich, by making use of unregulated workers to replace more expensive professionals. Lay off nurses if necessary.

WITHIN A FEW weeks, Rosemary's replacement had been chosen. Pencil-thin and statuesque, expertly made up and with a dark, sleek haircut, Sydney Hamilton was our new nurse manager. She strode into the ICU carrying a slim leather briefcase in her hand, a hand that was beautifully manicured and flashed a brilliant diamond ring. She could have been applying for the position of chief executive officer at a bank on Bay Street. Equally, she could have been pictured in a women's magazine cover story with the headline "Having It All: Superwomen Reveal Their Secrets."

At the staff meeting of the nurses and doctors, she brought out an easel, which she had set up ahead of time, upon which she had written her mission statement for the ICU. She stood before us and reviewed a series of graphs, charts, and diagrams to demonstrate the cost-saving measures and long-range planning she had in mind for the unit, based on her thesis for a Master's in business administration, which was on implementing cost-containment measures in critical care. Then she sat down and opened a leather folder to a prepared typed speech.

"These are challenging times in health care," she stated, turning to face each of us in turn. "But where there is challenge, there is also opportunity. It is a time of re-evaluating our vision of health care. Unfortunately, for many of our hospital workers, layoffs will be the new reality. . . . We need to look at ways to serve the customer better . . . increase hospitals' revenues . . . become more fiscally responsible. . . . We need to make effective use of our health services through judicious allocation of our precious medical resources."

"I think we are looking at real nursing leadership here," said the nursing administrator when she returned to the unit to pay us another visit. "Sydney Hamilton has the polish and professionalism to make a strong nursing presence at the corporate table. She will be a force to be reckoned with if the topic of nursing comes up."

I hoped that the topic of nursing *would* come up from time to time when the directors of the hospital corporation met for their annual general meeting.

"WE'LL WEAR THAT Barbie doll down until she has a nervous breakdown," vowed Laura. We were sitting in the lounge for our break. "I'll fill that briefcase of hers with laxative beads. When she opens it at some meeting, they'll fly all over the place. I'll make fake poo with K-Exelate and cascara and leave it in a box on her desk. I'll make a Sydney voodoo doll and we can put IVs into it with 16 gauge needles." She rubbed her hands together. "Once she spends time with us, she'll be running screaming to get out of this place. We'll have a mutiny until they give us Rosemary back."

"What are you guys plotting? Something I should know about?" asked Morty, joining us.

"Yeah, we're cooking up schemes to get rid of Sydney Hamilton and bring back Rosemary," said Nicole. "Even David Bristol said there's no one like Rosemary. He said to know her is to love her and that she has a sterling character and a heart of gold."

"Yeah, she's a real gem," said Morty, chuckling at the precious joke. "I think Daniel Huizinga already has the hots for Sydney, though. 'Impressive credentials, a stellar performance,' he said after that meeting, but I think he was referring to her legs. Listen, guys, get over it. I liked Rosemary as much as any one else, but it's time to move on. Come on, if a head nurse is supposed to be a manager and not everyone's friend, Sydney might be right for the job. Anyway, let's give her a chance. Don't worry, the union will keep her in line."

Laura narrowed her eyes and spoke like a demon from *The X-Files*. "Satanic nurse manager rises to power, but there's still no evidence of widespread devil worship."

WE THREW A going away party for Rosemary. She had taken a job as an old-fashioned head nurse in the orthopedic ward of a small community hospital in Arnprior, Ontario, a country town where she and her husband, Bill, intended to retire. She promised to keep in touch.

IT WAS IMPORTANT to Sydney that the unit look attractive and she set about sprucing up the place. All the ward clerks were given brand-new office supplies, a pine green blotter for their desks, and colour-coordinated vests. New curtains were chosen for the patients' room: Pepto-Bismol pink with matching vinyl swivel chairs for each room.

"When she gets done, this place is going to look as charming as a Victorian bed and breakfast," said Laura. "Who's been advising her – Martha Stewart? More importantly, why doesn't she sort out the room number in this place? We've been merged, reorganized, moved, decentralized so many times that you can read the whole history of this place in the room numbers. Why is room 670 next to 605 and 616 next to 620 and why are none of these rooms on the sixth floor? They put one plan in place and by the time that's carried out, a new one is already in the works. Not a day goes by when I don't come upon some poor lost soul, stranded somewhere in this labyrinth, holding a pathetic piece of paper, looking for a room, or an office, or a department."

Sydney beefed up the activities for Nursing Week. She helped make it more than just a roving cart of coffee and doughnuts for all staff. She made it more than just a free visit to the stethoscope clinic to get your instrument cleaned and oiled. She brought in guest speakers and provided workshops on stress management and career counselling, and offered gift certificates for massages for all the nurses.

But there were a few things she did that irked us. For one, she disbanded the lines that we had worked in for so many years.

"Nurses are not factory workers on an assembly line, punching in a time clock. You are professionals who can determine how and when you work. You have power over your work life, within the union agreement, of course," she added with a nod to Morty.

She instituted flexible scheduling to enable nurses to go back to school, to take courses, to arrange their schedules to accommodate child care needs.

Another thing she did that felt strange to us was to put price tags on the equipment. Barrier cream to prevent pressure sores, $12 a tube. Ceftazidime, $88 a vial. Chest tube suction bottle, $23 each.

"Think twice before opening that pulmonary artery catheter tubing," she wrote in the communication book. "Make sure you understand the rationale for its use and remember that each one costs $75!"

She wanted us to fight for frugality with the supplies, help rein in any profligate use of hospital resources, and eliminate wastefulness.

She tracked everything carefully so she could report the extent of the money she had saved the unit after six months.

"Maybe Sydney could get a good deal for medical supplies on the Shopping Channel," said Laura.

We eventually got used to Sydney's ways and learned to respect her, but it was also around that time that a number of other disturbing things happened.

One evening at home I got a telephone call and I could hear only sobbing at the other end.

"Tilda, it's me. Father Szigetti. Vince Szigetti."

"What's wrong?" We were friendly at work – he was with everyone – but he'd never called me at home before.

"They've fired me, my dear."

"Why you? Surely you don't cost the hospital any money!"

"I've been called before the parish and they've taken away my hospital duties. They've sent me on a silent meditation retreat for penitence. They say I've been too familiar with the nurses. They say I hug the nurses too much and touch them inappropriately."

"I can't . . . I can't believe it." Some things made me speechless.

"That's not all, my dear. They've accused me of telling homophobic jokes. I've always known there's a Lavender Mafia out there and it's been going on for years. Some of us call it 'Notre Flame.' I may have told a joke or two, in fun of course, but no harm was ever intended."

"You know how sensitive people are these days, Father. One has to be so politically correct."

I couldn't help but remember the joke he'd told in the med room one day about the gay church where only half the congregation was kneeling. Didn't we *all* laugh at that one?

"But I've always said that homosexuals can make good priests. Of course they can. As long as they remain celibate. The teachings of the Bible must be upheld. We need to bring more discipline back in the church. And there's another crime I'm wanted for, my dear. They accuse me of proselytizing. They say I've been putting graffiti around the hospital, just to offer a bit of inspiration to the nurses and the patients."

"But is it true, Father? Was it you who did that?"

Was I taking confession from a priest?

"It's perfectly harmless. In these trying times, my dear, all the more is the need for people to hear the word of God. A man is a priest forever, either to his greater glory in Heaven or to his damnation in hell. Please write a letter on my behalf to vouch for my character."

"Of course I will," I said.

"I will need your prayers, my dear, to get me through this crisis."

I assured him that he had them and vowed to start praying.

But another call I received a few days later informed me that even more urgent prayers were needed.

"Tilda, it's Tracy."

"Hey, Trace, how are you feeling?" She was ten weeks pregnant with their second child – Jake was already three years old – and was having a rough first trimester.

"I was feeling better until I heard this news. I've got bad news and bad news. Which do you want to hear first?"

"Let's go with the badder one."

"The first one is badder for me and the second one is badder for you."

"Okay, shoot." I was feeling great. We had just bought a house. I was pregnant too, feeling fine. Nothing could bother me.

"You remember that patient I took care of a week ago? He was a travelling businessman who had gone to Singapore and has had a respiratory infection ever since he returned? Well, he's really sick and the test results just came back showing that he's got tuberculosis! I took care of him and that exposed me to an active case of TB. They want me to have a chest X-ray and are recommending I take a course of rifampin and isoniazid and all those other TB drugs."

"Did you tell them you're pregnant?"

"They say it's safe to take the drugs during pregnancy. I don't know whether to believe them or not. What choice do I have? They say my risk of getting tuberculosis is greater than the risk of the drugs harming the baby. Now, are you ready for your bad news? I'm sure Sydney will call you later, but a bunch of us at work just discovered that pink slips really are pink. Five hundred nurses have been laid off at the hospital, twenty of them from our ICU, and I'm sorry to tell you, Tilda, but you're one of them."

II

TRANSFIGURED WORDS

As it turned out, I didn't have to mourn the loss of my job for very long. Two weeks after we received our lay-off notices, the hospital was scrambling for nurses. The human resources department invited all the laid-off nurses to submit applications to be re-hired at the hospital. Only now they were offering us part-time or casual positions.

"What's this all about?" I called Morty at home to ask.

"Union-busting. They wanted to get rid of as many of us as they could. The hospital is under pressure from the provincial government to cut costs. They figure they can save on us by having a flexible, transient workforce of nurses and bolster it with agency nurses if they have to. This way also, they don't have to guarantee you any shifts or pay you sick time or benefits."

Sydney Hamilton called us individually at home to encourage us to re-apply for our jobs. But many nurses were fed up and had already left or were planning to leave – either the profession of nursing altogether, or else the province of Ontario – to seek employment elsewhere. Many nurses started going to the job fairs that were being held to recruit nurses to work in the United States.

Indeed, many were lured away by offers of relocation bonuses, education opportunities that included tuition reimbursement, a significant night shift and weekend differential, and a range of career choices in every specialty of the hospital.

"I'm thinking of taking a job in Florida," said Suman, a nurse originally from Iran who had worked in the ICU with me. "I know I'll love the weather, but I really don't want to go."

We met over coffee to commiserate with each other.

"In Tallahassee they're offering me free housing and full-time hours, but I don't want to leave my family and my fiancé. We just got engaged. So I'm taking a casual position here."

"Back in the ICU?"

"No, I got bumped out. They offered me a job on one of the medical floors, but I'm not getting enough hours. Last paycheque, I only clocked four hours of work in one pay period. I'll manage somehow, but if I wasn't living at home I wouldn't be able to stay here. I'd be forced to go to the States."

I knew of many nurses who did leave.

I returned to the ICU, on a part-time basis. I was lucky because I was pregnant and would soon be off on maternity leave, anyway. In the meanwhile, following in Rosemary's tradition, Sydney did everything she could to help us further our nursing education. She sponsored me to attend a critical care conference and there I made a new friend.

It was in the Delta Chelsea Inn, amid a throng of critical care specialists from Washington, Paris, and Helsinki, that a strong hand reached out to grip mine and shake it warmly. It was connected to a tall elegant man with a shaved head and an earring. It was Darryl Price, who had done a fellowship in our unit in critical care. He had recently joined the staff of the ICU as an intensivist. I had always admired the way he talked to patients and I wanted to learn from him. Besides, there was something about him that made me think he would make a good friend.

"I've noticed you at work, Tilda, and you're a very good nurse."

His voice was soft so I had to move closer to hear him better. He sounded just like the voice I heard in my imagination while I was reading *Angela's Ashes*, the book I was obsessed with at the time.

"Have you read *Angela's Ashes*?" I asked.

"I can't bear to read that book," he said with a sigh. "I knew too many families back home who lived like that in such wretched poverty."

One morning, a few weeks after that encounter, I was kneeling on the floor emptying my patient's urine bag when I heard Nicole speaking to someone.

"You want to hear the nurse's head-to-toe assessment? Tilda is the nurse taking care of this patient. I guess she must have just stepped out for a moment."

They couldn't see me, but I could see she was talking to Dr. Darryl Price, who had just entered the room. The entire entourage of ICU residents and the rest of the team were converging *en masse* around him. I stayed down there beside the bags of urine and stool and thought of hiding out for a while, not coming up until after rounds. Would they miss me? I was holding a graduated cylinder, a large metal calibrated cup that we used to measure urine.

"Do you know Tilda? She's going to be a famous writer one day," I heard Nicole say. I cringed.

"So you're a writer too, as well as a nurse, are you?" asked Darryl, coming around to my side of the bed and peering down at me. I looked up from where I was kneeling on the floor, holding my jug of urine under the steady stream of fluid. I almost made a joke about the pint of ale I had on tap, but stopped myself in time.

"Yes, she is. She's the editor of the hospital's nursing news-letter," said Nicole on my behalf. "It's called *Vital Link*."

"Yes, but we all call it *Vital Stink*," said Morty in her booming voice. "Or sometimes *Vicious Link*."

Nicole glared at her and pulled me up off the floor.

The pitcher of urine was full to the brim and I couldn't just leave it there on the floor. I bent down to retrieve it as gracefully as I could and carried it carefully to the bathroom, where I dumped it into the toilet.

"And *that's* one of the more glamorous parts of our job," I said as I emerged from the bathroom, grateful for the laughter of the assembled team.

As the resident launched into my patient's past medical history, his referring complaint, and a complete review of the biochemistry and microbiology workups, Darryl leaned toward me and whispered, "If I was that bloke in the bed with a bag of urine, I would want a nurse as intelligent and respectful as you to wipe my ass."

I blushed. I kept my head down and pretended to be Princess Diana, once a commoner, but singled out of the crowd by royalty.

Then it was my turn. I proceeded to give my detailed assessment of the patient's condition, while everyone listened intently. Darryl made sure of that by commanding silence and attention. The resident continued his report, and Darryl interrupted him frequently to make a correction or to challenge him, or to refer to a new research finding.

"It's incorrect to say that multifocal atrial tachycardia is always indicative of an underlying respiratory –" Darryl broke off suddenly, lifting his head as if he had heard a far-off cry or as if he were a bloodhound, sniffing a scent. In a few quick leaps, he dashed across the room to Nicole's patient, a young man who was suddenly gasping and struggling to breathe. His oxygen saturation was dropping, 90 . . . 84 . . . 79 . . . 71 . . .

How had Darryl sensed this even before the alarm sounded?

Nicole raced to her patient's side and quickly turned up the oxygen concentration on the ventilator so that it would deliver 100 per cent and then drew up a syringe of emergency medication.

Darryl took the young man's hand and said, "Lad, you're just fine. We're going to fix you up right away." He cleared the patient's airway, the passageway into his lungs, then adjusted the breathing tube, and in a few minutes, colour returned to the young man's face.

All the time he was doing these things, it seemed as if Darryl kept holding on to the patient's hand, but I couldn't figure out how he could manage that. I had seen all these actions and interventions many times before, but the way Darryl did them made the machines, equipment, and medicines he was using seem incidental, almost imperceptible. Darryl's focus was solely on rescuing the patient and reassuring that frightened person in the bed.

Later, when everything settled down, Darryl came back to my room to speak with me about my writing aspirations, about music, and about the literature we both loved.

"Are you nuts about the Irish writers? Seems like everyone else is these days."

"I'm just discovering them," I admitted. "I've tried to read *Ulysses*, and *The Dubliners*, but it's difficult. I love William Trevor's short stories. Roddy Doyle is funny, but there's a lot of jargon that I don't get."

"About Joyce," he said. "Forget about everything else but *Portrait of an Artist*. That's brilliant. The rest is rubbish."

"Oh, and I like Edna O'Brien a lot."

"She's rather . . . earthy, isn't she?"

"Very sensual. She writes a lot of sex scenes."

"Oh, you always gotta have that, don't you?"

"Absolutely."

"The book you're writing, does it have sex scenes in it?"

"Lots," I said, and silently vowed when I went home that evening to write some.

"IT'S A GOOD thing Darryl Price isn't from India. You'd be reeking of curry," Morty said to me at one of our monthly nights out. "You'd be making us meditate and listen to whining sitar concerts."

This time we were at The Rebel House, on Yonge Street, an Irish pub where they played Celtic music. We had just seen the movie *The Commitments* in a review theatre and were having drinks and were trying, as usual unsuccessfully, not to talk about anything related to work.

They had taken notice that I was deep into Leon Uris's *Trinity* and had developed a sudden collection of Chieftains' CDs. I guess the tipoff was when I kept asking them to join me to see Riverdance. There was no point trying to keep anything from my friends.

"Does your husband know about your infatuation?" they asked.

"I'm going to call Ivan and tell him," threatened Morty.

"There's nothing to tell. I like Darryl as a friend, and because there's something I want to learn from him."

"What about Daniel Huizinga? David Bristol? Jessica Leung – she's probably going to be staff soon. They're no slouches."

"They're superb doctors. All I'm saying is that there's something different about the way Darryl talks to families and patients and I want to learn more about it. I like the words he uses."

"Why *do* you like him so much?" Tracy asked, joining us late. She was feeling better after that terrible TB scare, and as far as we knew, her pregnancy was progressing normally.

"Have you ever heard how he talks to patients? Have you ever been in a family meeting with him?" I asked.

"He has a great accent," said Nicole. "It reminds me of that soap commercial for Irish Spring: '*Manly, yes, boot aye loik it too!*' "

"So, what's so great about the Bald Leprechaun, anyway?" Morty asked. "He's a control freak, don't you think? He came down hard that time when I turned off the alarms on the cardiac monitor. They were going off all the time because the patient was moving around in the bed and creating artifact. I told him I couldn't hear the hockey game on the radio with the alarms going off all the time, but he didn't look too impressed with that. Let's face it, the guy has no sense of humour." She grinned to show that at least she did.

"He's no better than any of the jerks," said Laura. "I tell them what needs to be done for the patient, they argue with me, and when I come in the next day, what do I see? They've gone ahead and done exactly what I told them to do in the first place. Anyway, he's an anesthesiologist, as well as an intensivist, isn't he? I can't stand anesthesiologists. Of all the specialists, they're the worst." Laura was off on one of her favourite rants. "All they care about is money, money, money and doing procedures, everything is just another billable procedure to them. All they do is give a few drugs, put the patient to sleep, and then monitor them. They're no better than a nurse. They're the most boring of all the specialists."

"I disagree," I said. "Anesthesia is the one specialty concerned with the whole body. They're not like cardiologists, just focused on one organ and forget about the rest of the body. They're the doctors who really understand pain and how it works and care about how to relieve it. You'll sure want an anesthesiologist pretty fast if you're delivering a baby. Do you know how important it is to patients to feel confident in their anesthesiologist? For many people that's the scariest part of an operation, going to sleep, worrying that they might not ever wake up. What about that phenomenon of being awake under anesthetic?"

"What's that?" asked Nicole.

"I've been reading about it. Some post-op patients have reported that they were actually awake during their surgery. They remembered everything, felt everything, and could even recall accurately what the surgeons and nurses said during their operation. It's very rare and can usually be detected, but it's a scary thought for people undergoing surgery. That's why I'm telling Laura that anesthesiologists are underappreciated. Besides," I turned to her as she was draining the last drop of beer from her glass, "is there anyone you actually *do* like? Do you have a good word to say about anyone?"

"Can't think of anybody, offhand," she said. "Yeah, Liam Neeson. Now *that's* an Irish hunk!"

"Yeah, Darryl is an excellent doctor. He's very smart," said Frances, "but he's too touchy-feely. And his rounds go on all day. I can't get my work done because he drones on and on. I know if I go into a family meeting with him, it'll be hours until I get out. I feel like saying, get to the point!"

"Yeah, just like you do, Jabber Jaws," said Laura.

And as usual, we ended the evening in high spirits from the pleasure of one another's company.

ONE DAY I was taking care of a post-op lung transplant patient who was crashing. His blood pressure was falling and his blood gases showed a dangerously low level of oxygen. Quickly, the room filled with people – the surgeon and his residents who had just performed the surgery; other nurses who'd come in to help me; the respiratory therapists; and Dr. Jessica Leung, the senior medical fellow. Darryl Price stood at the foot of the patient's bed, quietly surveying the scene before him.

"We've increased his oxygen," I told him. "I've already called X-ray for a stat chest. I drew a set of 'lytes and a troponin and I have a chest tube all ready in case he's blown a pneumo. I just did an electrocardiogram. Here it is."

Darryl's gaze didn't leave the patient before him, and he pursed his lips in consternation. Clearly, he was seeing something that none of us were seeing.

"Have I forgotten something?" I asked.

He cleared his throat. "The family. We have to speak with the family."

The family? I hadn't given them a thought. Who was out there, even? I looked at the chart. A wife, some kids, two, I thought.

"But what can we tell them? He's crashing and we don't know what's going to happen."

"That's exactly what we have to tell them. Look, there are enough people here to take care of this situation now. I have a feeling it's just a mucous plug or fluid overload and they'll be able to fix it. Tilda, I want you to come with me."

Together we walked through the long corridor toward the elevators that would take us to the waiting room. Massive renovations were being undertaken throughout the hospital to merge units and consolidate departments, and the waiting room had been permanently relocated far away from the ICU to another floor altogether. The nurses had written a letter of protest, explaining the necessity for families to be in close physical proximity to their loved one and the difficulty many elderly visitors had in walking so far to the ICU, but to no avail.

In the elevator, Darryl and I exchanged a few words. He was reading Robertson Davies and listening to Emmylou Harris's melancholy *Wrecking Ball*; I was reading whatever Oprah had chosen that month and rediscovering the Chopin nocturnes of my youth.

"You must read Thomas Mann's *The Magic Mountain*," he said. "If you haven't read it already. That's the best book to help you understand the experience of illness from the patient's point of view."

I took it like a prescription.

In the waiting room, Darryl introduced us to the family. They were easy to spot. It could be no one else but the huddled group sitting around the Thermos of coffee, some still slumped on couches that had taken on the shapes of many other haggard bodies before theirs. All eyes turned to ours, trying to read the news.

Usually whenever I entered the waiting room, I tried to keep my face still and expressionless. I think of my husband at the poker table and how I can never tell when I walk by the game at our dining room table if he's got good cards or bad ones, if he's up or down.

Their eyes were trained on us, first on the doctor, then on me, back and forth. What is the news? Will he make it?

Darryl took a seat with them on one of the couches and I joined him. He put his arm around the patient's wife. He looked directly at her and then at the grown children. He did not avert his eyes as I usually did in these situations.

"It is terribly frightening for you and for all of your family out here, waiting. Waiting and wondering is very hard. Your husband's transplant went very well. He received a good set of new lungs. I know the surgeons have already told you about that. However, here in the ICU he has developed some complications. I think we can sort them out. But I want you to prepare yourselves for set-backs such as this. They are very common. We'll keep you informed every step of the way. We're busy with him right now, trying to help his breathing and bring his oxygen levels up by making adjustments to the settings on the breathing machine. Right now would not be the best time for you to visit unless you feel you absolutely must."

The wife shook her head. "We can wait."

He smiled. "His nurses know everything and will keep you informed. As soon as he stabilizes, we will call you and you can come down to visit him. Is that okay?"

She nodded.

"These must be the worst days of your life."

She nodded.

"We understand what you're going through." He reached over to take her hands in his. "We are with you."

OVER THE YEAR that Darryl Price spent in our ICU completing his fellowship in critical care medicine, I had many opportunities to observe his unique way of using the simplest, most truthful words to convey complicated, painful news to families in the kindest way possible. I recall working with him once and before the shift had even started, I received a strong premonition that a powerful, almost mystical, transformation was about to take place. It was, in fact, brought about in large part by Darryl's words, gestures, and caring soul.

It was night shift. As I stood for a few minutes in the med room staring into my coffee cup before going to start the long night ahead, I could feel powerful swirling, churning waves of energy emanating from my patient's room. Of course I didn't mention this to the others. They already had enough reasons to tease me.

Darryl Price was standing outside the door of the patient's room, in quiet consultation with one of the vascular surgeons. I knew the situation must be serious for him to be here so late at night. Staff doctors had usually gone home by now and left the running of the ICU to the resident on call, who would contact the staff at home if there was a problem.

I lingered in the medication room a few more minutes, delaying entering the world I would inhabit for the long night ahead. At the centre of this world were my patient and his family, each one confronting this crisis in his or her own way. The situation would demand my complete attention and my ability to give myself over to meeting their needs. Over the night ahead, there would be hundreds of facts, details, and numbers to absorb and interpret. At the same time, I would have to remain flexible enough to change as the situation evolved. I thought of the moody piece of music that I loved by Arthur Schoenberg, all dark and dissonant, called "Transfigured Night."

I was ready. I dumped my coffee in the sink, rinsed out my mug, and filled it with spring water from the cooler. I walked over to my room, drinking slowly.

"I'm glad you're on tonight, Tilda," Darryl said. "But it will likely be a busy night for you. We have to talk with the family about what to do in the event of a cardiac arrest. I've reviewed the case thoroughly and I think a 'do not resuscitate' order would be appropriate given the patient's extremely poor prognosis. What do you think?"

I was thinking about how unusual it was to talk about these things before a crisis occurred and how helpful it would be to talk with the family before it was too late.

"Are you in bad form, Tilda?" he asked, peering at me closely. "You look tired."

"Oh, I'm fine," I said, snapping myself out of my reverie.

He looked tired, too, and I told him so.

"It's my son's sixth birthday today," he told me. "I've still got ten more patients here in the unit to see and another few on the floor. I know I won't get home until he's long gone to bed. Anyway, please page me when the family comes in."

The nurse from the day shift had finished tidying up the room as a courtesy to me and stood there, waiting. Of course, I remembered, she's been here over twelve hours. She wants to go home. Me, I've got the whole night ahead. We sat down together at the table on wheels in the patient's room and she brought me up to date on the patient's condition.

Mr. Eagleton, seventy-one years old, had been in our ICU for a week and we all knew his history well. He had been transferred to us from Midland Huronia hospital for repair of a ruptured aortic aneurysm. He had had to return to the OR today for ten hours and was still bleeding internally. His blood pressure was low and his heart rate was fast. Even more troubling was that he was showing no signs of waking up.

"He's not doing very well," the nurse said to conclude her report. She appeared to be finished and stood up to go.

"Is that it?" I asked.

"That's about all I can think of."

"How's the family coping?"

"Oh yeah, I almost forgot. There's a wife and some grown-up kids, but I've been too busy to let them in. You know how it is. I think they're still in the waiting room."

Mrs. Eagleton looked like the kind of woman who, most other times, would be impeccably groomed and well dressed. This night she had thrown on a pair of jogging pants and her husband's bulky old homemade wool sweater before rushing to the hospital. I saw that she had two watches on her wrist and two rings on her finger – her own and her husband's. I took her by the hand and guided her to the ICU. I lowered the side rail a bit so that she could hold his hand, and I encouraged her to talk to him.

"The sound of your voice will be a comfort to him," I said.

She spoke quietly to him and then began to cry when she got no response. "We had our fiftieth anniversary party the other night, the day before he went into the hospital," she told me. "I said to him, 'Alfred, should we go ahead with the party if you're not feeling well?' He'd been working on the boat all day at the cottage and maybe he overdid it. He had a funny look on his face. I gave him two Tylenol, but they didn't seem to help. He said, 'Yes, dear, go ahead with the party, I'll be fine.' And now this."

I couldn't tell if Mr. Eagleton had any pain because he was deeply unconscious and did not respond in any way. We'll never really know if he has pain, I thought, because he will probably die. Even if he did survive this crisis and lingered longer, he probably would not remember. Research showed that most patients report they can't remember the ICU experience. I decided to go ahead and give him more narcotic in case he was having pain even though it would drop his blood pressure further and then I would have to increase the blood pressure medication. I would have to watch him very closely tonight.

I brought chairs for the wife and children and gave them privacy, but hovered quietly in the background. I put in a page to Darryl and returned to do my work. Within minutes he was there. We brought the chairs just outside the patient's door and held the family meeting there. "Mrs. Eagleton," Darryl said to her. He addressed her primarily, but from time to time looked over at the two daughters and the son. "What have you been told about your husband's illness?"

"Our family doctor in Midland said he had to come to Toronto right away for surgery. That was last week. He was nothing like this. Alfred never complained about anything. He just wanted me to ask you to please not put the intravenous in his right arm because he plays the violin. He loves his music. Tell me, doctor, is it very serious?"

Darryl sighed, and then took a deep breath. He pulled his chair closer to Mrs. Eagleton and placed it not so that he faced her, but so that he was sitting alongside her, as if they were going to discuss this case together as colleagues. They could have been two people sitting side by side on a bench on a boardwalk, looking out at the vast ocean. Two friends discussing a shared problem. He placed his hand lightly on the sleeve of her woollen sweater.

"What we have to do tonight is to think of the person inside the body of Mr. Alfred Eagleton. We must think of the things that are important to him as a person and as a man. The brain problem is the main thing, to our way of thinking. He does not have any quality of life and is unlikely ever to have one again. We are all very worried about him. We are capable of doing all of these things, but we don't think these are the right things to do for him, because we don't feel we can bring him back to the good quality of life he had before. We are very disturbed to use these treatments when we don't believe that he can get better. We feel very disturbed when we use these machines and drugs when they are not to the patient's benefit. Yes, it makes us feel we are very clever, fixing all these things, but it's not good for the patient. Good medical treatment, in our opinion, is that we not start any new treatments or add any more artificial means of life support, other than what is already in place. It's okay to lose a bit of dignity for a while, if we can expect a benefit, but I believe, in this case, it's degrading. What can we now do to make his life dignified and comfortable for him? There are many medical things we can do. That part is easy. What is really hard for all the doctors and nurses is that there is no chance of improving his condition."

He let all that sink in and sat there with them for many long moments. Then he continued.

"It is very sad for everyone here, for us, and for you, that your husband is dying. In fact, without these machines and drugs chugging along, he would be dead already. No matter what we do now, the outcome is going to be the same. He will not improve and there is no chance that he will recover from this."

No one could fail to hear the kindness in these harsh words.

"I THINK YOU have a crush on Darryl Price." Morty was teasing me again. "I saw you send him a card in the hospital mail delivery. Was it a fan letter?"

"It was a St. Patrick's Day card that said 'mazel tov' on it. He'll know who it's from and no, I do not have a crush on him. I am a very happily married –"

"Yes, you do. I'm going to call Ivan and tell him."

"I do not. I admire Darryl." I said it in such a way as to show them that yes, I was hot, but only under the collar. "Okay, you're right, I have a crush on him. I'm attracted to his mind."

"Oh, so that's it." Morty smiled knowingly.

"Yes, I like the way he thinks and the way he talks to families."

"Are you sure?"

"Yes, I love his words."

"That all?"

"No, there's more. His courage."

12

THE DIFFERENCE BETWEEN A FOOT
AND A PENIS

Nicole pulled me outside the room, well out of earshot of the patient's mother, to give me a whispered report. I gasped after hearing the first few details.

"You're kidding . . . it's not possible . . . I never had such a patient," I said.

I had just returned to work after a long maternity leave. Ivan and I had a baby boy, whom we named Harry, and I was as happy as could be. That first day back, I was thrilled to see all my old friends and catch up on the gossip. However, what awaited me in my patient's bed that day gave me a shock for which nothing in my ten years of nursing had prepared me.

I think about them still, my patient, Samuel Jürgens, and his mother, Cindy. It makes me wonder if all stories should be told. I'm not sure about this one, but it haunts me, still.

In my patient's chart was a long list. Two whole pages outlined his medical problems, most of which he'd been born with, nineteen years ago. Samuel had a genetic disorder that resulted in severe mental retardation, kidney problems, diabetes, a seizure disorder, major heart malformations (for which he'd undergone numerous corrective surgeries), and severe physical deformities such as a tiny misshapen head with a prominent forehead, misplaced eyes, a severe cleft palate, and webbed fingers and toes.

"But what's he in the ICU for?" I asked, for as serious as his problems were, none was life threatening.

"Pneumonia," Nicole said. "He's here for intravenous antibiotics and mechanical ventilation through his permanent tracheostomy. The mother does just about everything for him. You'll have an easy day. She's moved in with him here and brought in an air mattress that she uses to sleep on the floor beside his bed. His mother does everything for him – and I mean *everything*. Absolutely everything you can think of."

After hearing all that, the first thing I did was wave at the mother sitting in the chair beside her son in the bed and call out to her that I would be with them shortly. The next thing I did was go to the nurse in charge and notify her that for my next shift, I would like a different patient assignment. One day caring for this particular patient would be enough for me. No siree, it's too much to ask. We are a team and we have to share the really difficult cases. They should be assigned on a rotating basis. She agreed and made note of my request. Other nurses nodded in agreement. They didn't like to be in there very much themselves. Take care of him today and you won't have to go in again for a long time, they assured me.

The patient's mother must have sensed my apprehension because she beckoned me over.

"Come on in, Sam won't bite."

I approached them. In the big hospital bed lay a huge, strapping nineteen-year-old body with a tiny, baby brain encased in a distorted, mangled head. From what I understood from the chart, there was something wrong with almost every single part of Sam.

"He functions at the level of a three-month-old infant," said Cindy. She sounded as proud as other mothers I knew who claimed their child was gifted.

I thought of my own son, who was just ten months old. I recalled how at three months, crying, feeding, and sleeping had been the extent of his activities, and at the time I loved every minute of it. But now, at ten months, his repertoire of skills had expanded to sitting up, playing peek-a-boo, and smiling at me in recognition. How much more gratifying and fun was each day that he could do more and more wonderful things! What joy – and relief – we felt as he reached each milestone. Would I love him as much if he couldn't do these things? I hoped I'd never have to find out.

When Cindy left the room for a cigarette break, I decided to get a closer look at what I was so afraid to face. Sam's head was thrown back against the pillow, his neck arched like some science-fiction horror-movie blob, yet he also had acne and hairy armpits, like any teenage boy. He was drooling profusely and was making ugly, raw noises. As he flapped his arms around the bed, his webbed fingers splayed out in all directions. He coughed frequently, and each time he did so, bubbles of green sputum gurgled out and around his trachcostomy.

I could not bring myself to speak to this creature. I could not address him as a nineteen-year-old boy and I wasn't prepared to speak any of the sweet baby talk that I used with my own baby.

But, oh, how his mother adored him!

"Sam loves music," Cindy said when she returned. She slipped a cassette into a tape recorder on his bedside table. It played quacking ducks, ticking clocks, chiming bells, rolling waves, and roaring trains. I watched Sam and could discern no sign whatsoever that he was even aware of these sounds, much less that he loved them.

"See what I mean?" she said. "You love that music, don't you, sweetie? See how he loves it?"

Later when Sam's oxygen saturation dropped a little because of a buildup of lung secretions, Cindy got up to suction him and said, "Come on now, Sam. Stop acting up!" She grinned at me. "He can be a bit of a show-off."

It was exactly what I said about my own baby when he did something wonderful for our friends.

To get through the day, I busied myself with tasks. I checked the oxygen tank and the ventilator, and straightened out the IV tubing. I did everything I could think of to avoid contemplating that face and that body in the bed.

Cindy left his side only to go to the bathroom, or for a cigarette, or for a take-out meal that she brought back to eat in the room beside him. When she returned after even a few minutes, it seemed as if she had missed him terribly during her brief absence. She bounded back into the room and threw herself on him, told him how much she loved him, and asked him had he been a good boy while she was gone? Not giving the nurses any trouble, she hoped?

When Sam slept, she watched him sleep, her eyes rapt with love, just as they were when she watched him drool, groan, or have the occasional seizure. She did everything for him, cleaned his bum, changed his diapers, and cleaned out his mouth, nose, and ears. She gave him his medications, took his vital signs, and suctioned out his lungs.

"How do you do it, Cindy?" At last I had to ask her. "My baby had a cold last week and I was up all night, listening to his cough. I was so worried about him. And you, you've coped with so much. How do you get up four or five times during a night to attend to him? How have you been able to clean him up and talk to him all these years without getting any response in return?"

"He responds to *me*," she said.

"Well, no *meaningful* response," I tried to correct myself.

"To me it's meaningful."

I watched while Cindy massaged Sam's feet, paying full attention to each foot, one at a time. Finally I understood one small thing. Like Cindy, I loved every part of my own baby's body. Sometimes I even put one of his little feet in my mouth, after his bath. When I held one of my baby's little feet, my love for his whole body and the person inside him, swept right through me.

As the day wore on, I kept watching Cindy from the corner of my eye. The expression on her face was serene. She was utterly content. She had no desire to be anywhere else, to be doing anything else, or to have Sam any other way than the way he was.

I watched Cindy give him a back rub. "You like that, don't you, sweetie?" she asked him.

How could she tell whether he liked it or not? What were his signs of pleasure or discomfort? His eyes, askew on his face, opened, then shut, then opened again, but registered nothing.

I would have imagined that Sam's hospitalization would be an opportunity for Cindy to take some time off for herself. I, myself, had such guilty pleasure returning to the work I loved and leaving my baby at home in the care of someone else. Yet child care could be so tedious and draining at times. At least that's how I found it.

Sam didn't sleep much, but when he did take a nap, sometimes Cindy would relax and pull out a book from a plastic bag she kept at her feet. She hadn't gone home to their apartment since Sam had been admitted to the hospital, so she wore the same clothes every day – running shoes, a grey T-shirt that said "Gone Fishin'" on it, and blue jeans. She sat with her ankles wrapped around the legs of the chair, reading an eight-hundred-page paperback that she'd borrowed from the patients' lending library.

"Cindy, may I ask you something?"

She looked up from her book and said, "Shoot."

"Do you ever take a holiday?"

"I could never leave Sam," she said. "I couldn't be away from him."

"What I really want to ask you, Cindy, is this. How do you do it? That's what I want to understand. All the doctors and nurses marvel at you and your devotion to Sam. It's remarkable. I've never seen anything like it."

"He's my son." She shrugged her shoulders. "I love him."

She saw that while I believed her, her answer did not satisfy me.

"I love him as you'd love any child. When he was born, they'd just invented all these life-saving devices and they used every single one of them on him. Boy, did they save him, but *good*! But they told me he wouldn't live to be one year old. Then they swore he'd never make it to two. Would never see three. But here he is, nineteen years old and a fine strapping young man, too. He even has to fill out an income tax return, can you imagine that!"

"It never seems to get you down, taking care of Sam, I mean."

"You know, you go to the waiting room at the children's hospital – that's where we spent the last eighteen years, until we had to come here – and you see parents who are crying. Those are the ones whose kids are having their tonsils out. The others over there, those ones who are laughing, telling jokes are the ones whose kids have cancer but their kid had a good day. Those ones laughing are the ones whose kid was in an accident, but survived."

"I see," I said, and I think I did, a little.

"I remember one little boy, Kevin, who had been a perfectly normal four-year-old. Then – bam – he was in a car accident that left him permanently brain damaged. A vegetable. Now, that's a loss. I never had that, so I don't miss it with Sam. We are very happy together, Sam and I. Happier than most married couples, from what I can tell. I have only one wish . . ."

"What's that?"

"I wish he could have children. I would love to have grandchildren."

I gasped at the very thought. Of all things.

"But of course, I know, it isn't possible. I'm too old."

Was I missing something here?

"Well, I think I'll head out for lunch now. I feel like some Taco Bell. I hope for your sake those refried beans don't act up on me!" She picked up her tattered copy of the Wilbur Smith tome she'd been reading, gave Sam a big kiss on his lips, and said to him, "See ya later, alligator!" and waved goodbye to me.

That evening, before I left at the end of my shift, I changed my plan for the next day. "I want the same patient tomorrow," I told the night nurse coming on. I pencilled myself into the assignment book. "I want to follow up with Sam and his mother."

"CINDY JÜRGENS IS a saint, a philosopher, a hero," I said to the others the next morning at breakfast in the cafeteria.

"No, she's not. She's a nut case," said Laura. "A psycho. You'd have to be crazy to sacrifice your life for another human being."

"I don't think Sam quite qualifies as a member of the species," said Morty. "He's a perfect example of the kind of thing the Church is so bent out of shape about saving," added Morty, a Catholic herself. "We're going all out for this guy when there are people we can actually save who need the ICU bed he's taking up. But we're treating *her*, not him. *She* insists on all this. That's our health-care system for you! Welcome to Canada. You can have whatever you want."

"I thought you voted NDP," I said, trying once and for all to trip her up.

"Being a socialist doesn't mean that I believe in wasting money," she shot back.

"I'm trying to figure out how Cindy does it," I said, returning to the subject that probably only I wanted to discuss. "She never seems to tire, never despairs. I'm in despair every time I take a look at Sam. I can't bring myself to talk to him or touch him." I pushed aside my cranberry muffin.

"Don't feel sorry for Cindy Jürgens. She's getting something out of it, too," said Doris, one of the older veteran nurses who had come over to join us at the table.

"What makes you say that?" I asked.

"Have you taken a look under the sheets?" she asked.

"I don't know what you're talking about," I said, "and I don't think I want to, either."

"I took care of him last week," said Morty, "and there's no doubt in my mind about it. Don't be so naïve, Tilda."

Even Frances nodded in agreement.

Later when Cindy went out for lunch, Doris, the nurse I had spoken with at lunch, came over to my room. She said she wanted to show me something.

"Have you taken a good look at that boy?"

"What are you talking about?"

"His penis. Have you seen it?"

"Of course I have. I did a thorough nursing assessment of him this morning when I started my shift."

"Come over here." Doris closed the curtains around Sam's bed. She pulled back the sheets and there, springing out at me, was the most enormous penis I had ever seen. *That wasn't there before*, I thought. Bulging and bobbing, it seemed to demand satisfaction. It made me think of a stallion, or a German shepherd dog eager and pent-up, springing to attention, urgent for relief. To bring it down would be like felling a tree – and we would have to shout "Timber!" Pushed down, it would have touched his knees.

Without a doubt, it was the biggest I had ever seen in either my extensive professional, or decidedly more limited personal, experience. How could I have missed it earlier?

"He had a diaper on earlier, that's how I missed it," I said.

"I see she's taken it off," Doris remarked.

"For his dignity."

"Or for easier access."

"You could choose to see it either way, couldn't you?"

"Be honest," said Doris, "you can see that *that's* an experienced one. It's been around. It knows what it wants. It's been well used. If it hadn't been in use, it would have been more withered, wasted away. You know, if you don't use it, you lose it. This muscle has been getting a good workout. It's used to getting satisfied. Who else, but with Cindy? She needs it too, she's a single mom on her own, she's not likely to be out meeting guys, at least not one who'd want to come home to *this*." She nodded in the direction of Sam.

We covered it up, but it pushed up against the sheets. Sam, himself, was oblivious, neither in distress nor at rest. He didn't react to anything that I could see, not to cold or hot, light or dark, pain or pleasure, not to anyone's presence, or if they walked away. Strangely enough, it was his extraordinary penis that communicated more than Sam himself ever would.

"Let me ask you something," Doris said. "Just before she left for lunch, did she kiss him? On the lips?"

"Yes, but what are you saying, Doris? That she and Sam . . . ? That a mother would . . . ? With her own disabled son? But she's so devoted to him."

"All the more reason. It's the way they communicate. He gets some tactile stimulation and – who knows if it's pleasure? – I daresay that with that," she pointed, "she does too. They both get off in one way or another and I suppose no one is hurt in the process. The nurses at the children's hospital had their suspicions, too. They called in the Children's Aid Society, but no one could prove it."

I didn't know what to think. I do know that I never saw Cindy act in an inappropriate way.

"OH, WHERE IS Father Szigetti when I really need him?" I said to Morty at the nursing station where I went to think this through.

"Okay, I'll be him for you," she said, crossing herself and making a pious gaze in the direction of Sam's room. "Good Lord, my dear. But Sam is one of God's creations too . . . however, it certainly must have been an *off* day, even for Him."

I had to laugh. I smiled, too, at her choice of earrings that day: tiny silver Greek masks of the theatre – Comedy hanging from one ear lobe and Tragedy from the other.

EARLIER I HAD asked Cindy if she was religious and if she wanted to see a chaplain, but she'd waved away the suggestion. "I have no use for the Church, any more. I mean no disrespect, but my Catholic boyfriend left me when Sam was born and all he gave me was Sam and we're no Catholics."

Now it was time to take Sam's vital signs, and since Cindy wasn't back yet from her lunch, I took them myself. He had spiked a fever and when she walked in I told her.

"No, he hasn't," she scoffed. "Couldn't be."

She took his temperature herself and stared at the thermometer: 38.8°C. I drew blood cultures and the doctor changed the antibiotics. Cindy gave Sam some Tylenol and prepared a basin of water for a sponge bath.

That day Faizel El-Bakshy was the medical resident on duty for the ICU. He was just emerging from his on-call room, straightening his lab coat, a few minutes late, to join us for the short late afternoon rounds. He had been sponsored by a large corporation in Riyadh, Saudi Arabia, to come to Canada to specialize in critical care. "I am ready . . . for to perform arterial puncture procedure on Jürgens, Samuel, the patient," he said in his halting, formal English.

Dr. Daniel Huizinga was the attending staff doctor that week, and he decided that given this new spike in temperature, Sam's intravenous and arterial lines should all be changed to new sites to prevent the spread of a possible infection. Cindy knew exactly what was going on. She'd probably been through it many times before, so I didn't need to explain a thing.

"Did you just finish saying your prayers?" I asked Faizel quietly as he took his place with the team.

"Yes, how did you know?" He smiled. "If I don't pray, I get nervous. I must to pray four times a day, and once during the night." I nodded and he continued, "It is a physical need that I must satisfy, as if my bladder were full, or even, like . . . sexual intercourse."

I had never heard prayer described as an essential need, as if it were a life-saving procedure. We all have strong needs, I thought. Is it wrong to get them met in whatever way we can, if no one gets hurt? Isn't what goes on between two people private, as private as between this man and his God? If whatever goes on between Cindy and Sam brings them closer and helps her to do the yeoman's work of caring for him, day in and day out, who am I, or anyone, to judge?

"Did you manage to get some lunch?" I asked. "It's been pretty busy in the unit today."

"I must not eat until the sun has set. It is Ramadan. I am starving to eat, but I must wait. There is a call in the Emergency department that I must go see."

I knew that there was an untouched lunch tray still in the pantry that would go to waste. I grabbed a slice of banana bread and a carton of milk off the tray and brought it to him. "Here, you've gotta eat. Save this for later, for when the sun sets."

"God bless you."

He told me he had recently received disappointing news. The company was sending him back home sooner than he had expected, as a lowly internist. They would not continue to sponsor him to specialize in cardiology, as he had wished.

"I bet your wife is happy about that." He had told me once how homesick she was.

"Yes, she misses the desert, the sand, and muezzin calling us to prayer. The weather here is difficult for her. She is lonely."

I had never met her, but felt her presence. I pictured Lai'lah, Tabiyah, Ashnoor, their three daughters whom he had told me about and whose pictures he had shown me. I knew of his disappointment at not having a son to carry on the family name.

THERE WERE STILL a few more hours left of my shift. Sam's fever was raging and Cindy looked worried. She knew what it meant when I told her that his white cell count was up: a serious infection, possibly in the blood, and in Sam's case, given all his chronic medical conditions, life-threatening.

After I finished removing Sam's right radial arterial line and helped Faizel put in a new radial art line on the inner aspect of Sam's left wrist, Cindy wanted to wash his hair and give him a shave. I dashed off to the linen cart for more towels. In the hallway I ran into Dr. Huizinga, who looked worried. He wanted to know if I had made any progress in weaning Sam off the ventilator and if his fever had come down. He told me about a twenty-four-year-old woman downstairs in the Emerg who was in a coma and liver failure from a rare drug reaction. She needed to come to the ICU urgently. I knew we didn't have any empty beds.

Later, I stood at the sink and watched Cindy fussing over Sam, cooing softly to him, clucking to herself, staring at the thermometer and fretting over his fever. I was dreading telling her that we might have to rush Sam along so that he could be transferred out of the ICU. She decided she would give Sam yet another sponge bath. Again, she hauled out the large metal basin that we kept under the sink, along with his special soap, shampoo, and conditioner. Then she changed his already clean sheets and smoothed and rearranged them.

Suddenly, I felt impatient with her and eager for my shift to be over. This case was stirring up too many uncomfortable feelings. We had learned in nursing school about being empathetic and non-judgmental but in this situation, I was struggling to do these fundamental things. Did you have to hide all your feelings in order to be a nurse? If so, who out there was so virtuous? And I couldn't put out of my mind that critically ill young woman in Emerg in fulminant hepatic failure. She desperately needed to come to the ICU and there was a chance we could save her, but we didn't have a bed for her. We didn't have a bed for her but here was Sam, with no hope for recovery or real improvement, taking up a bed that she could have. Maybe what Morty had said at breakfast was right, that we couldn't save everybody. Health care cost a lot of money and we had to make choices. Here was Cindy dictating to us what should be done, possibly just to get her own needs met. It couldn't be for Sam's sake that she was doing all of this. *She* was calling all the shots and we were following her orders.

Cindy continued to smooth out Sam's sheets. Sam was grunting and farting. His farting heralded a stream of diarrhea that seemed to please Cindy because it gave her something more to do. His head reared back against the pillow. His eyes were open toward the ceiling, but he did not appear to be aware of anything up there, not the ceiling light, nor the room, nor his mother's constant presence.

On the one hand, what Doris and the other nurses said was mere speculation. It was dangerous and wrong to raise such serious allegations without proof.

On the other hand, what if the rumour were true? I had noticed that Nell, who had been sitting with us at breakfast, had kept quiet. Perhaps she, with all her ludicrous stories and confabulations, was uncomfortable facing a disturbing truth. Anyway, to me it seemed true, or at very least plausible, that Cindy could be having that kind of relationship with her son. The image of it came easily, without effort or strain, full-blown in my mind. It did not require a stretch of the imagination. I thought about how Cindy kissed him on the lips and draped herself across his body. How she wanted him to have children, but said *she* was too old.

But even if it *were* true, it seemed to pale compared to the tragedy of Sam himself. His existence in this world was undoubtedly a tragedy. Or was it? Maybe the failing was in those of us who are unable to accept what we are given and find its meaning. Perhaps that was more important than whatever might be going on between him and his mother.

Oh, but when Sam does die one day, how Cindy will suffer! How lonely and bereft she will be without his companionship, such as it is, and without the pleasure he could give her. Sam was everything to her. Yet, did she love him so much that she was prepared to do everything to keep him alive, or did she not love him enough to let him go?

I turned away from the two of them to face the window. I gripped the edge of the sink and looked out at the dark courtyard below and wondered if Ivan might pick up beer and chicken wings for dinner. Barbecue, Ranch, Cajun . . . I was tired and I wanted to go home. I wanted to see my own baby and make sure he was as normal as I thought he was. As normal as he was when I left him this morning. I wanted to be with Ivan, have fun together, and put all of this out of my mind.

As I prepared Sam's 1900 hours dose of antibiotic, I fleetingly considered labelling the bag with a medication sticker, but omitting the drug. If he were to miss just one or two doses of antibiotics, the infection could overwhelm him, and he would become septic and that would be that. I pushed the terrible thought out of my mind and gave the medication as ordered.

I looked at the clock, waiting for my shift to be over. The minute hand made one complete revolution. Then another. I turned back to watch Cindy massage his feet again and see the way she cradled the heel and held his toes in her hand. It was so plain to see – her hand was full of love for the foot, for the whole person who was her son. Cindy brought his foot up to her face and held it against her cheek. She kissed the sole of his foot and closed her eyes, savouring his taste, his smell. She asked for nothing in return from Sam, just to love him. The way Cindy was holding his foot, the way she rubbed it, kissed it, caressed it against her cheek was exactly what I did with my own little baby's foot. What was the difference? We each had given birth to our sons and loved whatever had come out of us. That my love seemed natural and easy to me, and that hers for Sam seemed impossible, was a failing in me, not in her. If Cindy Jürgens was using her body and Sam's to communicate that love – and what really was the difference between a foot and a penis, anyway? – and if some of that primal, physical love was transmitted to Sam, and if it was perceived in any way in his primitive brain cells, and if maybe, just maybe, it gave him some pleasure or human connection or alleviation of discomfort – we would never know if he had pain or pleasure – during his stay on the planet earth, then who was I – or anyone – to say it was right or wrong, good or bad? If I started deciding all of that, what kind of nurse would I be? What kind of person would I be if my mind were made up about everything? To be the kind of nurse and person I wanted to be, I would have to break through all my prejudices and get beyond all judgment. I decided to have no opinion about the whole matter. The only rule I would have would be compassion.

I went over to Cindy and Sam. She was applying peppermint-scented oil to his feet and moving her hands up his legs.

"Cindy, I'm going to go out to help another nurse who has a busy patient. Sam is stable and the monitor alarms are on. Come and get me if you need me. You and Sam need some privacy."

She looked up, surprised. She had not been alone with him even one minute since he'd come to the hospital. At home he belonged to her, but the hospital had a way of taking claim. We don't own other people, certainly not our children, but Sam belonged to her more than he belonged to the hospital or to any of us. She deserved some time alone with him.

I closed the curtain around them. I shut the door. Then I turned my back on the two of them and gave her time and space to love him however she chose.

13

SHH! IT HAPPENS

I had been a critical care nurse for twelve years. During that time I had written articles about nursing, spoken at conferences, been a mentor to new nurses, and even conducted a research project. However, no matter what foray I made into related pursuits, I always wanted to return to the bedside. For me, it was where I found the greatest challenges and satisfactions. It still is.

Other than two maternity leaves, I had only one extended hiatus from working in the ICU and it was the result of a ridiculous escapade. I had to call work to let them know I would be out of commission for a few weeks.

"Laura, is that you?"

"Tillie! What's up? Why did you call in sick? You sound pretty healthy to me."

"I've had a little . . . mishap."

"Are you okay?"

"Yes, but I broke my ankle."

"What happened?"

I had to tell her. I knew they would never let me live it down. They still remind me of it, whenever the circus comes to town.

"I . . . just hope . . . you had . . ." Laura could hardly speak. She was choking on tears of laughter. "A pink parasol!"

A long-ago pledge I had made to myself to be a "fun" mother when I had my own kids prompted me to do something reckless and foolish. Since my own mother had been an invalid, lying motionless on a couch for days at a time, only to rise up more tired and weak than before, I promised myself I would be different. At a children's birthday party with a circus theme, I watched the kids swinging merrily on the trapeze. I giggled at the clown and even made a few tentative jumps on the trampoline. I decided to ask for permission to try the tightrope.

"Sure," said Boris, the Russian ringleader, with a chuckle. "Go ahead."

It was only a few feet across, four feet off the ground, and surrounded by soft mats. I stepped onto the tightrope and inched along, as graceful and lissome as an acrobat. I executed my aerial stunt beautifully, but upon my clumsy dismount, the loud sound of *crack* was easy enough for anyone to diagnose.

A six-year-old girl looked down at me where I lay on the mat. "Did you break your foot?"

EIGHT WEEKS OFF work with my foot in a cast gave me an opportunity to step away from the bedside and reflect on my profession. It had become a particularly exciting time. The hospital had appointed a new director of nursing who was a brilliant and inspiring leader. She gave dynamic and invigorating lectures about nursing. She believed in the value of the work we did. Not only that, but we knew she would be a formidable presence on our behalf at the corporate table.

When she first arrived, she held a series of informal meetings, open to all staff nurses, and since I had so much free time on my hands, I came to listen to what she had to say.

It was a glorious afternoon in late September. The sun was streaming through tall windows in the auditorium where the meeting was to be held. Our new director would speak and then open up the discussion to all of us to raise whatever issues or concerns were on our minds. No topic was off limits, she assured us. Confidentiality was ensured. Tea and biscuits were served.

First, she showed us a beautiful photograph she had taken on a trip she had made to the south of France. It was a picture of an arched stone bridge and she referred to this structure as a "hermeneutic channel." She spoke about the symbolism of the image, its simple beauty and its union of function and aesthetics. Somehow, she gracefully segued into an entreaty to all nurses to end our long-standing tradition of passive silence in the face of client suffering and injustices in the health-care system. She expressed her belief that nurses are the new "knowledge workers" in the health-care system of the twenty-first century. She called upon each of us to seize and cherish the opportunity to make a difference in our patients' lives. Standing tall before us in a dark suit upon which a jewelled brooch glinted in the sun, she threw her arms open wide with the vastness of her vision of our profession's glorious future.

The nurses sat in pink, white, or blue uniforms, or baggy green scrubs, listening and munching cookies. I was sitting way at the back, wearing my street clothes, having come in from home for the meeting, hobbling in late, still learning how to use my crutches.

I was thrilled that we had a leader with such an exciting vision for our profession. Finally, here was someone at the helm who believed in the value of nursing, and from what I could see, she would fight for the things we deserved – recognition and respect. But still, for me, something was missing. It had nothing to do with our salaries, working conditions, or gruelling schedules. It was something that was never raised publicly. It was something that seemed at odds with her lofty vision of our roles, yet I knew it was an important part of our work.

What I wanted to raise was too wild and too crude for that gentle assembly. It wouldn't sit well with these nice refreshments we were enjoying. I didn't have the courage to raise it. It was an important aspect of our work, yet we hardly ever talked about it, even among ourselves, except to joke about it. It was the underbelly of nursing life.

Many nurses couldn't cope with the dirty work of nursing. Those nurses often chose to work somewhere other than in the hospital with patients, certainly elsewhere than the ICU, where patients and their bodies were the most vulnerable. Some nurses sought cleaner, easier places to work, or took refuge in computers, paperwork, or teaching. Who needs a university degree to give a bedpan? they said.

In fact, so frequently did I hear that bedpan remark that I grew to expect it, like a slogan or a motto of some kind. I had heard it from so many different nurses, in all the hospitals that I had ever worked at. It reminded me of a breed of chimpanzee that I had read about who all have the same habit of wiping their faces with banyan leaves. Who knew how this same behaviour got so widely propagated among unrelated members of the same species who inhabited different continents?

I was dismayed at how nurses reduced our profession to a toilet. They made bedpans our emblem, like the stethoscope symbolized the doctor, and a gavel, the judge. Yet, if we did want to stay at the bedside taking care of patients, this personal, intimate care was an essential part of our job. Sometimes it made us feel unclean and demeaned. We knew that patients who lost control of these functions of their body surely must feel embarrassed and ashamed, but so did *we* at times, for doing this work.

When I had to clean blood, urine, sputum, vomit, or feces (there was a secret hierarchy), I tried to focus on the person, not the bedpan or the basin. I wanted to help my patients keep their dignity, but the trouble was that in those moments, I was struggling to hold on to my own.

Perhaps it was the juxtaposition of hearing those lofty, philosophical thoughts put forth by our new director of nursing, coupled with the opportunity I had around that same time to perform an act of hands-on care for a dying woman in her home that made me reflect on the significance of nursing's dirty secret. I decided that one day I would break through this frontier and expose the scariest, messiest taboo of all.

THANKS TO TV shows like *ER*, it is generally well known that "Code Blue" denotes an emergency – likely a cardiac arrest – somewhere in the hospital (and something of a badge of honour for those chosen to run to attend to it).

"Code Red" is the signal for a fire alarm.

"Code White" means a violent patient, sometimes from the psych ward, who requires the muscles of the security guards.

"Code Green" warns of a toxic spill.

"Code Yellow" is a patient on the loose – someone MIA or gone AWOL.

We nurses coined "Code Brown" for our own purposes. It was our *cri de coeur*, our SOS signal for help – STAT – with a clean-up job.

We called ourselves the Poop Patrol, the Bowel Brigade, the Shit Shovellers, because, at times, that's how we saw ourselves. We all had memorable stories on this subject, and looking back now, here are a few of mine.

One day, Rodney, the hospital assistant, was nowhere to be found, and I urgently needed his help to transfer my patient to the floor. I was under pressure to move this patient out because there was a very sick patient on another floor who had just arrested and needed to come to the ICU right away.

"Okay, Tilda," said Laura, who was in charge that day, "I don't know where Rodney is. You and I will transfer your patient up to the floor ourselves and then swing by the other floor to pick up the arrest patient. I guess we're porters, movers, secretaries, housekeepers, and maids. Whatever. C'mon, let's go."

My patient was all ready. His personal belongings had been returned to him in a big white plastic bag and his meds were sorted into small clear bags. He had recovered from abdominal surgery that had been complicated by a post-op pneumonia, but he had recovered completely. Soon, up on the floor, he would graduate to "DAT" (diet as tolerated) and "AAT" (activity as tolerated) orders.

Laura released the brake of the bed and went to the head to pull and I went to the foot to push. We were barely out of the door when another call came from the floor.

"When are you coming for this patient? He needs to come down to the ICU right away," the ward clerk called out.

"Tell them we're on our way," Laura shouted back.

But just as we were wheeling my patient down the hallway, a dark cloud passed over his face. It was plain to see. Something was bothering him. He clutched at his stomach.

"What's wrong?" I asked.

"I need to, er . . . use the bedpan. Please take me back to my room."

"Wait till we get you to the floor. We're almost there," said Laura, forging ahead toward the elevator. "They may even let you use the toilet, if you behave yourself."

"No, nurse, I need it now. I can't wait."

Laura and I looked at each other.

The insistence in his voice made us turn around and wheel him back to his ICU room. I gave him the bedpan and closed the curtain. Moments later we returned to remove the bedpan and resume our trek to the floor. But something stopped us in our tracks. Laura and I gazed down in the pan, astounded. It was the most massive quantity of feces all in one deposit that we had ever seen. We could see the entire, fully intact imprint of his intestines, sculpted in a multi-layered, coiled mound. We could see the duodenum, the small and large bowels, the cecum, and the rectum. It was finished off with a satisfying (for him, presumably) swirl on the top. We stared at each other. It was a sobering sight. It gave us pause. It was unbelievable that so much stuff could be lodged inside a human's body. But it made us feel small and worthless, too, because of this work we did. For moral support, we carried the bedpan together and while I dumped it into the toilet, Laura flushed.

"I wonder what the Royal Family is doing right now," she grumbled.

"You must feel great now," I said to the patient as I came out and washed my hands at the sink.

"Never felt better!" he sang out.

Like a soldier recounting a war story, or a fisherman boasting about the size of a catch, Laura couldn't help but telling what we had seen to, of all people, Nell, who wasn't the least bit impressed. Handily, she topped our tale.

"Once, when I worked as an outpost nurse in the Australian Outback, I had a patient who pushed out a snake. A live, hissing snake."

"A cobra, I'm sure," scoffed Laura. "Or was it the Great Green Mumbo, by any chance?" She was determined to catch Nell in one of her fabrications, one day.

"Maybe it was a worm. Maybe the patient had a parasite and you thought it was a snake," I suggested.

"If anything, it would be a garter snake," said Frances, who was even more gullible than I, if that was possible.

"Tilda, if you write about this, I swear I'll kill you," said Laura. "But, on second thought, if you do, why don't you start out, 'Dear Diarrhea' . . ." She cackled away at her cleverness.

FOR SOME REASON that none of us could fathom, Nicole never wore gloves when taking care of patients. She thought nothing of plunging her hands into a basin of brown water while cleaning her patient after a bout of diarrhea. She'd even clean up vomit or change an infected, oozing tracheostomy dressing, glove-free.

"Nicky, for God's sake, put on gloves!" we'd shout at her.

"That's gross, Nick," said Tracy.

"Dangerous, too. What about AIDS, hepatitis? The yuck factor?" I asked with an involuntary shudder and tossed her a pair of disposable gloves.

"I prefer to touch patients with my hands," she explained. "I can't feel anything with gloves on. Anyway, I cleaned my own mother when she was dying of cancer and the nurses there used to say the same thing. They were afraid that I'd absorb some radioactive isotopes or traces of her chemo, but I wasn't worried."

Some things we left alone.

MY GANG HAD an annoying habit of commenting on what we brought for lunch when we sat together in the lounge. I hid in a corner to try to keep my meals to myself.

"What have you got there, today, Tillie?" Frances inquired. The others looked up.

I might have had a Tupperware container of leftover stir-fry or a slice of cold pizza, but whatever it was, I didn't wish to discuss it or share with anyone.

"What is *that*?" Laura asked, peering down into my bowl one day. "Your soup looks like what's draining out of my patient's rectal tube."

"Thanks, Laura." I pushed away my lunch, but couldn't push away the thought.

Nicole was known for bringing in huge lunches, sometimes an entire head of iceberg lettuce and a long English cucumber. She proceeded to prepare a salad like some perky demonstrator in a department store, using various gadgets for cutting, dicing, and slicing. She brought in an entire bottle of French dressing that she poured over it all in a huge container that Morty nicknamed the "Jethro Bowl" after the TV show *The Beverly Hillbillies*.

"You could bathe a patient in that bowl," said Tracy.

"Are you going on a safari?" Laura asked her when she saw Nicole's grocery bags.

I had hang-ups about food and I didn't always want to discuss with them what I was eating. My weight was always up and down, then steady, then up again. It was always related to various emotional states. Food was my bugaboo.

"How do you stay so slim?" I once asked Clara, a Polish nurse who had come to Canada to work in our ICU. She spoke a halting, but correct English.

"Zees is vhat I doo." She gave a weary shrug, as if dealing with a slow child. "Eeet's simple. I eat ven I am hungry and I stop ven I am fool."

Imagine. As simple as that.

I WAS FERRETING about among plastic bins in the supply room, searching for a specimen bottle. It was a special one that contained growth medium for testing stool for Cryptosporidium, and for *Clostridium difficile*, and for whatever other mysteries might be growing in the waste products shooting out of my patient's rectal tube.

"What'ya need?" asked Laura, appearing in the doorway.

"I'm looking for a container to collect stool."

"It's commonly called a toilet, dontcha know?"

I shot her a withering glance. "You know what I mean, a specimen bottle."

"Come on, Tilda, surely you can find a better hobby than collecting stool. How 'bout stamps? Or coins?"

"Laura!"

She went right to the drawer, slid it open, and tossed me the bottle. "Here, Tilda. Get a life."

WE CALLED HIM our "tiny dancer," after the Elton John song. He was a diminutive AIDS patient who was a former ballet dancer, originally from France. Now he was unconscious and dying from the fatal pneumonia that these patients so often got. He had constant diarrhea and in order to keep him clean, we inserted a rectal tube. But one alone did not contain it. We inserted another, then another. It took five large rectal tubes to seal his stretched anus. We stood around his bed, shaking our heads, trying to find a better, less invasive solution. It was undignified, crude, disrespectful, probably uncomfortable, but what was the alternative? How else could we keep him clean and his skin dry?

THERE WAS A patient who looked like Jesus. He stretched out his long, thin arms with his hands drooping down. He even had a long beard and soulful, heavenward-looking eyes. He had pancreatitis related to alcoholism and had to have emergency surgery, but remained septic for weeks afterwards. The sclera of his eyes were stark white, his pupils bright blue, like a husky dog. Frances tried innumerable times to convince him to let her shave his scraggly beard. No matter how we positioned his emaciated body, or tried to make him comfortable, he always resumed the pose of the crucifixion.

One night his intestines were so full of infection that they bulged out of his belly, broke open his suture line, and spilled out into the bed. The surgeon came and coiled them back, loop by loop. I helped by pushing the two sides of his wound together like a bulging, overstuffed suitcase, so that it would stay closed. For a time, we had to keep a sterile green towel in place to catch his intestines, in case they popped out again.

He was with us for many months and we all took care of him, but I wasn't aware that he had developed any special bond with me until one day he made a request and it seemed that it was something only I could fulfil.

"Nurse Tilda, clean me out!" he called out.

Frances was his nurse that day and I heard her say, "Tilda has another patient today. I'll do it for you."

"No, I only want Nurse Tilda."

He was chronically constipated and needed frequent manual disimpactions of feces that were jammed up there like hardened clay. With long, extended fingers (double-gloved), we relieved his discomfort.

But what could have been special about the way I did it? Besides, it wasn't what I wanted to be known for!

I CAN STILL see the way the overhead fluorescent light glinted off the shiny metal bedpan that Laura held as she came out of the washroom where she'd gone to retrieve it for her patient.

"This man is going to die," she pronounced about her newly admitted patient.

"Shh. No, you're not," I came over to his side to tell him. "Don't listen to her. You're doing very well."

I don't think he heard Laura anyway, or me for that matter, because moments ago, she had given him morphine for chest pain after a heart attack and he was becoming quite drowsy.

"Why did you say that?" I asked her when we sat down to do our charting. "He's stable, now. He's got a decent blood pressure and is in normal sinus rhythm."

"Whenever they have an acute coronary event and then all of a sudden ask for the bed pan, it's a tipoff. It's usually a vasovagal reaction from a disturbance to their parasympathetic nervous system. I betcha anything this guy's had an anterior infarction," she said, studying his 12-lead ECG.

A few minutes later, something made her glance up at the monitor, seconds before the patient's heart went into a rapid, uncontrolled rhythm. It was a few seconds more until the alarm went off, but by then, Laura had got the crash cart, which she had thought to place just outside the patient's door, and was pushing it ahead of her into the room. We flew into action and there wasn't even time for Laura to say, "What did I tell you?"

"MULTI-SYSTEM ORGAN FAILURE is the highest cause of mortality in ICU patients." Dr. Daniel Huizinga was speaking in the lecture hall, refreshments provided once again. He was usually the absent-minded professor, distracted and whimsical with patients or medical students, or brash and boyish with nurses, but on stage he came to life as a distinguished and commanding speaker.

"In fact, multi-system organ failure is a lot like pornography," he said. "You don't know how to describe it, or define it, but you know it when you see it."

He went on to talk about "stool enemas." It was a new idea in critical care medicine and he wanted to study the benefits of it. The theory was that by returning the patient's own diarrhea to the patient via the rectum, bowel flora that had been eradicated by broad-spectrum antibiotics would be restored. Something new to try. He was enthusiastic about this distasteful plan and eager as a child mucking around with mud pies to try it with patients. "Of course," he added, "I'm counting on the nurses to assist me with this research."

"Thus the coffee and doughnuts," said Morty, looking around at all of us. "Don't touch them. It's a bribe. He thinks if he feeds us he can get us to do his dirty work. Don't we have enough work to do already, without being the doctor's research assistants, too?

Believe me, you're not going to be getting any credit for his
research if you help him with this scheme!"

"Some doctors have a very high disgust tolerance," I said, wrin-
kling my nose at the thought of this procedure and feeling queasy
from the doughnut I'd already eaten.

"Daniel?" Morty waved her hand. "Could you please review the
connection between multi-system organ failure and pornography?"

"WHO WAS YOUR most memorable patient?" I once asked Tracy,
who knew so much, yet said so little.

"Huh! My most memorable patients are usually the ones I try
to forget!" She paused, then said, "Mrs. Powell, without a doubt,
but I can't say I was too fond of her."

I appreciated her honesty because it wasn't something most
nurses would admit, especially ones as conscientious as Tracy.

"I don't know why," she mused, "but Mrs. Powell couldn't –
or maybe wouldn't – control her bowels. It seemed like she enjoyed
making a mess. She didn't care if she was dirty or that she smelled
bad, no matter how many times we bathed her. She enjoyed offend-
ing us and that disgusted me. We couldn't help her preserve her
dignity, because she didn't have any to begin with."

We all remembered Mrs. Powell, but Frances remembered
something else.

"Once I saw her terribly frightened. It was when David Bristol
told her there was nothing more we could do for her. Only that
softened me to her. She was the only patient that I had difficulty
feeling empathy for."

I also remembered how, quietly, among ourselves, we privately
called Mrs. Powell something that rhymed with that name.

She had chronic breathing problems from years of smoking,
and was also obese and diabetic. Her weaning from the ventilator was slow, with many setbacks. Her main interests were
eating and sitting on the bedpan. In fact, rather than choose
between these two activities, she preferred to do them both at the
same time.

She had many habits that revolted us. But we were professionals, or so we kept trying to convince ourselves. We could rise above
it, not allow our personal feelings – even ones of abhorrence, distaste, and disgust – affect the care we gave.

She liked to poke about in her own feces and identify
remnants of foods she had eaten a few hours earlier. She picked
it out and showed us, whole and intact, a long noodle or piece
of banana.

Once I actually found a single pea lying underneath her. It fell
out when I turned her to change the sheets. The princess and the
pea, I thought. *Not.*

"She's a human food processor," said Morty in disgust.

"I can't take it," said Nicole.

Tracy kept her thoughts to herself, gritted her teeth, and bore it
bravely when her turn came.

Mrs. Powell managed to time her farts for whenever we came
near her bed to give nursing care. She opened her legs wide, to
show us her labia and hemorrhoids flapping with each expulsion
of gas. She curled her long bony toes, which were thin and splayed
apart like fingers. They made me think of the roots of a fibrous
tuber. She delighted in her depravity.

The problem wasn't hers, it was ours. By exposing us, by aiming
at us, so to speak, her behaviour spilled all over us. It humiliated
us. We felt shamed.

"Isn't this the most disgusting job in the whole world?" asked
Laura, who kept threatening to leave nursing altogether, to pack it
all in and move to a remote part of northern Ontario or open a
bed and breakfast in the Maritimes, or move to New York to write
jokes for David Letterman. Or, at the very least, she was going to
work in the Cardiovascular ICU, a place that was cleaner and where
people actually, usually, got better.

We equalized the burden of caring for Mrs. Powell by sharing
her on a rotating basis.

Her husband, Jim, came to visit every day wearing what looked
like the same pair of grimy overalls. He stood at the foot of the
bed, hands tucked inside on his chest, under the bib.

"You got lots of gizmos, here, Mother. All the bells and whistles," he said. "Wow, this place is flashing like a casino." He stood there, admiring the ventilator. "Well, Mother, I couldn't make it in any sooner today cuz we had to load the *dunkey* onto the back of the truck, but he wouldn't move. So I says to Barney, get me a plank of plywood and a *pudayto*."

"What was the plywood for?" I asked, listening in. I assumed the potato was to tempt the donkey to move forward, but I wanted to steel myself if there was going to be any mention of cruelty to animals.

"That's to jam in between his hind legs so he don't kick you – you know. And then I give 'em the *pudayto* to coax him on to the truck, but he won't budge. Barney says, hell, no, shove it up his arse. So we did that – shoved it in good, and, boy, did that dunkey take off! Then we had to figure out how we were gonna get that *pudayto* out of his rear end. So I stuck my hand way up there." He demonstrated the shoving and thrusting motions he'd used. "But what wuz we gonna do with the shitty *pudayto*? We gave it to the dunkey to eat. He don't care. He's a dunkey."

Every day, Jim managed to keep his wife amused with his stories, but at times he fretted over her.

"She's not herself, today," he said when he thought she was having a setback and not eating as much as usual. (People often said this about their loved ones, but I always thought that in some ways, illness made people more like themselves than ever.)

"She's quiet today," he said on another occasion. "She's becoming a snob. Too good for us, now that she's in the big city. When I married her, she was white trash just like me, now look at her, all hoity-toity."

Some days she refused to try to wean from the ventilator and begged us to place a lit cigarette at her trach hole so that she could take a few puffs. Jim pleaded with us to let her do it, too.

Morty was the only one to handle the situation with aplomb.

"We've taken care of you all these months when you were so sick and unable to do anything for yourself. You're better now and it's time for you to take care of yourself."

Mrs. Powell motioned that she wanted ice chips and snapped her fingers at Morty as if to say, "Right away!"

"There's no 'right away' around here, Betty! What's happened to your manners? Just because you're sick doesn't mean you can forget all about please and thank you."

If ever I asked Mr. Powell to leave for a few minutes when I had to clean up his wife, he said he preferred to stay and watch.

"That's marriage!" he told me one day. "You start off with a frying pan and end up with a bed pan."

He enjoyed chatting with whichever nurse took care of his wife that day. He bragged about his days as a firefighter and all the heroic rescues he'd made.

"You must have been in a lot of dangerous situations," I said.

"Yeah, they used to say that the rats are leaving and now we're going in."

He warned me one day as he was going home, "Now you take care of my pretty girl there, missy, or this'll be one angry cowboy for you to answer to."

If, for some reason, he couldn't make it in, he'd call and ask about her. If she was eating well (and how!), if she was shitting well (yes sir!), and how was her heart – "Was it doing any of those funny little things?" Had she had one of those "heart o'grams" that day and what in the dickens did those quacks think was wrong with her, anyway?

"You take her today, Morty. You haven't had her for weeks," Nicole said one morning before we started our shifts.

"No way. I'm looking for an unconscious, intubated patient, thank you very much." Morty scanned the patient list board to choose something nice and easy. "Besides, I didn't bring my gas mask. I don't want to breathe in any toxic fumes."

"No, it's your turn. You're the perfect nurse for her 'cause you're such a *shit* disturber, anyway," said Laura.

"Tilda should take her. She won't mind."

"No, I had her yesterday, and last week, too. I've done my duty," I countered, smug and safe.

"How about Frances? She's got allergies. She won't smell a thing."

"Frances has the fresh lung transplant. She's received report already."

"What about –" She looked at Tracy.

"No way, I'm carrying on with the same patient I had yesterday. Ever hear of something called *continuity of care*, Morty? She's all yours! Remember to double-glove."

Morty stormed off but she was never really mad and never for very long.

I heard her later that morning, her voice booming out.

"Three bowel movements already, Betty? It's only ten in the morning. Were you saving it all for me? Well, that's enough poos for you. You've reached your quota for the day. Now, you have to hold it in."

And later in the day: "I'm going to make you a fart chart, Betty. We'll keep track of them. We'll classify them: musical, tooting, ripping, silent but deadly – then the smells – rank, swampy, musty, cheesy, funky, and so on."

Later in the day, Morty pulled a chair out to the hallway and called out to Mrs. Powell, "I'd love to join you in there, Betty, but I'm overcome by your vapours."

Mrs. Powell couldn't speak because she was still on the positive pressure ventilation. I had never heard a patient with a tracheostomy laugh, but I am sure that's what she was doing.

"I'm not going to waste my time trying to help you get better if all you want to do is eat and shit," Morty called out to her. "I'm going out tonight after work and I want to wash my hair." She grabbed a few towels from the linen rack, stuck her head under the faucet in the sink in Mrs. Powell's room, and started to lather her hair with chlorhexidene scrub.

How does she get away with it? I wondered. But whenever I looked in, I saw that both Mrs. Powell and Morty were having a jolly old time, making fun of each other.

Perhaps humour was the best way to deal with a situation like this and the uncomfortable feelings it brought. If only I could find this same lightness in myself.

I FIRST MET Gabrielle Mendoza during one of her admissions to the hospital, early on in the course of her illness. During a lunch break at work, I went up to the Oncology floor to pay her a visit at the request of the family, who were neighbours of mine. Gabrielle was a thirty-three-year-old woman who had breast cancer. When I met her, she had just completed a course of chemotherapy that had left her feverish and weak. But at that moment, when I first met Gabrielle, more than anything, she was distressed at not being able to take a shower.

"I can't stand not being clean," she said softly.

I looked around. It wasn't that there were nurses sitting around at the nursing station doing nothing. There was no one there. I knew how short-staffed that floor was – in fact, I didn't see any nurses, anywhere. Surely they were there, busy in the rooms? It was easy for me to wheel Gabrielle into the shower and help her out. I soaped her up, washed her back, shampooed her hair, dried her off, and then eased her down on to clean sheets. I was proud at how efficiently and smoothly I did everything, talking with her all the while, distracting her with light-hearted conversation during those moments.

One afternoon at home, a number of months later, I received a phone call. Would I come over to help Gabrielle? She wasn't feeling well, her father told me, and he couldn't reach her husband at work. I had heard about the brutal chemo treatments and radiation therapy she had endured and their failure to bring her into remission. Most of all, I had heard of her valiant attempts to continue being a wife and a mother to her two young sons.

When I got that call from her father to come to Gabrielle at home, I said, "I'll be right over." I wondered what I should bring. What did a dying woman need? A stethoscope? A hot water bottle? Herbal tea? I had nothing useful and decided to go with empty hands.

I met her father at the door. He was just returning from the drugstore, carrying a little paper bag. "I bought some milk of magnesia. I think Gabrielle's having a touch of constipation," he explained in his genteel manner.

Gabrielle was lying on top of a rumpled bedspread. She looked pale and weak. A sparkly pink scarf was askew on her head, inadequately covering her baldness. In a jean miniskirt, she still had an admirable figure. Somehow, life must have gone on in that household because there were a few golf balls at the ready beside her husband's electric putting-practice machine in the corner and a scattering of her sons' hockey card collection on the floor beside her bed.

"I have to go to the bathroom," Gabrielle said when she saw me.

With her leaning on us, her father and I guided her to the bathroom and she and I went in together.

"It feels like it's there, but I can't push it out," Gabrielle said in between gasps. "I don't have the strength. I can't do it."

I told her to lean forward against me, so that I could take a look. When I looked down, I saw the biggest, baddest mass of black stool I'd ever seen. It was stretching and widening the opening beyond what I thought was physically possible. That huge mass was causing her shortness of breath. It was why even walking that short distance had been so painful for her and why her abdomen was so distended.

I had no gloves, no instruments, and no one to help me. I knew that I had to do two things: first, get that obstacle out of her and second, ensure that this experience would be one of relief and ease for Gabrielle, with no shame or embarrassment. I desperately wanted something to protect my hands, but there was nothing. I eased my fingers in there and probed around the stool, trying to loosen it up. I held on, tugged just a little and Gabrielle yelped in pain. With my other hand supporting her and holding her upright, I massaged her abdomen.

"Come on, Gabrielle, you can do it," I said as I dug deeper with my fingers and tugged again. She almost fainted with pain as it moved along her rectum. And then it emerged, inching its enormous length out slowly. It splashed into the toilet. She stood up, straightened her shoulders, and shivered with relief. So great was her release from pain that it seemed like a type of pleasure, I think.

The smell filled the room. I tried not to wrinkle my nose. I did not want to take that smell into my lungs, but I forced myself to take deep, neutral breaths, so that Gabrielle would feel my acceptance and respect for what we had accomplished.

I broke up the stool with the toilet plunger so it wouldn't clog the pipes. I washed my hands, then held her up in the shower, then eased her down into a warm bath. The calm smile on her face was my reward.

Gabrielle died at home, a few days later, and I hoped it was in comfort and peace.

14

TIRED, HUNGRY

"Her! That's the one! I don't want that nurse taking care of my husband ever again!"

It was me, standing at the end of the wagging, accusing finger of Brenda Laurence, the ex-wife of Dr. Irving Laurence, who was a patient in our ICU. She was speaking to Sydney Hamilton, our manager – who happened to have stepped out from her office at that very moment – to single me out: a bad nurse. Sydney took it in stride.

"Tilda is an excellent nurse. However, if you have any specific concerns, would you care to discuss them privately with me?"

What happened with the family of Dr. Laurence was that I did something a nurse should never do: I took a dislike to them. Despite my best efforts to conceal my feeling, the family must have sensed it. Apparently, it was mutual.

Dr. Laurence was a seventy-five-year-old man with cancer, diabetes, peripheral vascular disease, COPD*, kidney failure, and

---

*   Chronic obstructive pulmonary disease.

coronary artery disease. He was also hugely obese, which exacerbated all of his other problems, especially his diabetes. It had made him so susceptible to infections that only a few months ago his right foot had to be amputated. We all knew him well from his numerous previous admissions to the ICU. On this particular admission, his main problem was breathing. He was so sleepy that he was difficult to rouse. He was in a deep torpor, snoring loudly and breathing hardly at all. He was not getting enough oxygen and it looked to me like he would need to be intubated soon.

I had already met his ex-wife, Brenda Laurence, that night I had been in charge, and had got to know him and his family well during his many subsequent hospitalizations.

His live-in companion and chauffeur, Howie, brought him to the hospital whenever the naturopathic and homeopathic remedies, along with the puffers and oxygen tank they kept on hand at home, weren't helping him. With his advanced age and many medical problems, the chances were slim that Dr. Laurence would ever fully recover. His will to continue seemed to be weakening with each hospitalization.

I admitted him, and Morty came over like a welcoming committee.

"Hi, Dr. Laurence! You've been picking up a lot of frequent flyer points with us lately, haven't you?" She gave him an affectionate nudge on the arm. He roused briefly to give her a weak smile and then fell back into a snoring stupor.

Laura came over to have a look. "I bet this guy's carbon dioxide level is almost 100," she said. She held a hand over his chest, closed her eyes, and like a wizard, pronounced her diagnosis: "It's 94, I'd say. His baseline normal runs fairly high, but I think he's in hypercapnic respiratory failure."

As far as I knew, Laura's low-tech, old-fashioned diagnostic skills of observing, listening, touching, sensing, and thinking had always proven correct.

"I bet you anything this guy has Pickwick Syndrome," she said, continuing with her own workup. "It's named after a character in a Dickens novel. When I worked in Emerg I saw a patient like this once. It was a hot summer day and this morbidly obese lady came in, hardly breathing – just the occasional grunt – impossible to rouse, just like him. When I got her up on the bed, a grilled cheese sandwich fell out from under her breasts. 'Oh, that's where it went,' she mumbled and took a bite. Pickwick has a very bad prognosis. I swear to you, if he gets intubated, we'll never be able to get him off the ventilator. These patients are impossible to wean."

Daniel Huizinga was the staff doctor on that week, and he came in to talk with the patient in order to ascertain whether he wanted the breathing tube again this time. But by then, Dr. Laurence was so oxygen-deprived and confused that he was in no condition to participate in this discussion.

"Do you want us to put the breathing tube in?" Daniel shouted loudly into his ear.

Dr. Laurence must have heard because he nodded in assent, too taxed to answer in words. Of course he wanted it then, at that frightening moment, but to me, it didn't seem like the best time to put such a question to a person.

"Wake up, wake up, Irv," shrieked Brenda, when she came in later that day. The breathing tube was in and he had been mildly sedated, for comfort.

"Open your eyes, Irv, and look at me." She glanced at me in exasperation and then gazed back at him sweetly. "Oh, why aren't you doing it, you stubborn thing?"

"I'm sure he would if he could," I couldn't help but interject.

She glared at me. "Irv, you can do it. Open your eyes and talk to me." She slapped his cheeks hard, once, then again. She gave a few tugs on his urinary catheter and I jumped up to stop her. "Wake up, Irving, right now! I want to show you the dress I bought in New York to wear to your grandson Mitchell's wedding. Come on, open those gorgeous green eyes."

He opened his eyes, saw her, then closed them, and turned away.

"He's not being stubborn," I explained on his behalf. "He's unable to respond to you."

"Nonsense," she said. "Irving is a very strong man. He never gives up. You don't realize whom you are dealing with."

"He doesn't seem as motivated as usual," I said.

"If you can't have a positive attitude around him, I don't want you taking care of him," Brenda said to me.

I refrained from telling her what the other nurses had been saying.

"He's trying to tell us something," others who knew him better than I were saying. "He's had enough and he's turning away from the family. How much can a man of his age take?"

I kept quiet. Later in the afternoon, for a few brief moments, Dr. Laurence became more alert, and I propped him up so that he could scratch out a note to me in wobbly handwriting on a sheet of paper attached to a clipboard.

"Is this necessary? Do I have any choice in the matter?"

I seized the opportunity.

"Dr. Laurence, do you understand that the breathing tube is keeping you alive right now?"

He nodded.

"Do you realize that if we take the tube out, you will die?"

He nodded.

"Is that what you want?"

He clasped his hands together in prayer, his eyes heavenward. His message couldn't have been clearer, his intention more resolute. Yet, when his family came in later, he closed his eyes and turned away from them. He chose not to express his wishes to them, at least not as unequivocally as he had to me.

We knew from previous admissions that Dr. Laurence and his wife had been separated for many years, but had remained on good terms. She had come in from New York, where she now lived and their son, Sidney, had flown in from California, where he now lived. Dr. Laurence lived with Howie in a huge mansion in the exclusive Bridle Path. On previous admissions, he had been able to tell us something of the travels he had made around the world with Howie. However, it seemed that whenever he needed health care, he was decidedly Canadian. His medical records from our hospital alone took up over five volumes.

Back in the forties, starting with only a dollar in his pocket, Irving Laurence built a vast fortune in the garment industry, manufacturing women's clothing. He later went on to develop a chain of drop-off and drive-through dry cleaning outlets. As it turned out, he wasn't a medical doctor at all. He had donated money for a wing of a medical school in Denver, Colorado. In appreciation for that gift, the university had bestowed on him an honorary doctorate and accepted his older grandson to their medical school. We heard about his father's many achievements, from Sidney, who made frequent references to the family's vast wealth and his father's generosity, often managing to slip in a proud mention of his son, Adam, the one who was slaving away at medical school.

"Is he specializing in moguls or après-ski?" Morty had asked without compunction.

Sid was a filmmaker, a screenwriter, a music stylist, and a movie producer – the story often varied – who lived in Los Angeles. During this admission, Sidney and his mother visited Irving Laurence daily, but always managed to avoid arriving when the other was there. They hadn't been on speaking terms for many years, still keeping alive some old family squabble.

One thing they did have in common was that neither of them believed that the hospital visiting hours applied to them. Neither did they believe in calling in first from the waiting room before they entered the ICU, as we requested all visitors to do. They walked right in whenever they pleased, day or night.

Brenda came in first, early the next morning.

"Sidney probably won't even come today," she said, draping her coat over the computer in the room. "Has my son even been here yet? Did he get here before me?" Then she turned to her mission: she was hell-bent on getting a response from Dr. Laurence.

"Come on, Irving, you can do it!" She slapped him on the cheek. "You look stunning today! C'mon, Irv, you sexy thing. Talk to me!" She flicked her finger on the inside of his thigh. "He needs his glasses," she told me. "Why haven't you put them on him?"

I did as she requested and he closed his eyes behind them.

"You've drugged him!" she cried. "That's why he's like this."

"Your husband has not received any sedation today, nor during the night," I replied.

"He wasn't like this when Ingrid took care of him yesterday. He was better with her."

I looked back in the nursing notes and read that the patient had been unresponsive for over a week.

After an hour of unsuccessful attempts to elicit any response from him, Brenda fled the room, saying she had a luncheon date.

Howie came in later that morning and stayed all day. He was living in the Laurence mansion, taking care of the plants and pets. He wore a cowboy hat and boots and a beautiful shirt, the exact colour of the inside of a cucumber. As soon as he arrived, he put his take-out coffee cup on top of the ventilator and leaned down to kiss Popsi, as he called him, on the cheek. Then he sprayed him all over with Eau d'Homme cologne and gave him a manicure and pedicure. After these ministrations, he sat on the edge of the bed, sipped his coffee, and munched on a chocolate croissant, the flakes dropping all over the bedsheets. Dr. Laurence opened his eyes at the sight of that tempting food. The hunger, the frustration, and the disappointment in the old man's eyes, to which Howie was apparently oblivious, made me unbearably sad.

Howie had other things on his mind, and he shared them with me. He was afraid that his tireless devotion would go unrewarded. He was worried that the family would shaft him when it came to distribution of the estate.

"They're so mean," he complained, "and after all I've done for Popsi over the years! Not only that, but now I'll miss out on those yearly vacations at the villa in the Cayman Islands." He nodded over at the huddle of doctors viewing X-rays on the computer. "What do the big chiefs say? Do you think they're going to pull the plug?"

I looked over at Dr. Laurence to see if he was taking any of this in, but thankfully, his eyes were closed again and either he was sleeping or had completely tuned us out.

I accidentally bumped into the bed as I went over to change an IV bag.

"That's just your clumsy nurse, Popsi." Howie glared at me. "Don't worry, Irv, you're okay. I'll look out for you."

"Has my mother been here?" Sid stood at the door. "Has she been here yet? How long did she stay?"

I didn't like spying for them.

I STEPPED OUT for a few moments to stock up on supplies from the clean utility room and when I came back, I found Brenda had replaced Sid once again and was busy going through the chart.

"That's not allowed," I said, hating to play the role of an enforcer. I put my hand out for the chart.

"I have the right to read my husband's chart," Brenda said in a huff. "How am I supposed to know what's going on? No one tells me anything around here. Irv always shares everything with me."

"I'd be happy to answer any questions you have or bring a doctor in to speak with you." I knew that there were sensitive bits of information in that chart that Dr. Laurence may not have wanted her to know. He had been treated by a psychiatrist for depression, took Viagra on occasion, and had had numerous homosexual relationships over the years, and not only with Howie, his current companion.

"Your husband's chart is private and unless he gives you permission to read it –"

"But he *can't* give me permission," Brenda said. "He won't wake up!"

"Well, then."

I took away the chart, feeling like a child refusing to share her toys.

THE NEXT DAY, in the race to show his devotion to his father, Sid got there first.

"How's Pop doing?"

"Stable," I said. I couldn't say much to these people without getting in trouble.

"Stables are for horses!"

"He's having a good day," I expanded.

"Every day above the grass is a good day!"

"He hasn't changed overnight," I tried.

"Tell him to change already!"

"Heh, heh," I murmured and put on a false smile. His vaudeville act made me bristle. Sid, as a person, made me recoil.

"Say, nurse, do you know how to read all those numbers?" He pointed at the monitor.

"Oh gee, hopefully a doctor will come around soon and explain it to me," I said, hating my sarcasm. I turned away from him as I noticed him staring at my chest.

"What big tits," I heard him comment.

Later, he hung his head and moaned that it had been an extra effort for him to come in today. It had been very difficult because he had a bad cold and maybe I could take his blood pressure and his temperature?

"Rectally, of course," he said with a lewd smirk. "I'm not feeling well. I need some soup. You got any? Can I lie down in the extra bed over here and you can take care of me?"

I busied myself straightening out the tubing on the ventilator and emptying it of condensation that had collected in the coils. I prepared the flow sheet for the nurse coming on to the night shift. I went into the bathroom and flushed the toilet a few times.

Then he asked me to give him a back massage. When I refused that as well, he was visibly displeased.

"It's making me pretty hot, coming in to this place, day after day, being surrounded by all you beautiful women," he said. "Maybe I should bring in a stripper for Dad or one of the pretty, sexy nurses like Julia or Sharon – or – what's the name of that tall, blond one?"

"I don't know who you mean," I said.

"You know, she was the nurse here the other day. The stunning one. The real knockout."

"Karen?"

"That's it! I'll never forget what's'ername! When's Karen coming back?"

"I haven't the faintest idea."

"Bring Karen back. She'll get a rise out of Dad. She'll get him going, whatya think? Dad's got quite the eye for the ladies!"

"I'm sure."

"Maybe Karen could nurse him in the nude."

The whole scene was an enactment of a burlesque melodrama. They were a troupe of travelling actors in a *commedia dell'arte*. The theatre was their father's body. The principal actors were Irving, the aging Patriarch; Sidney, the snivelling, spoiled Son, Brenda, the Jewish Princess Ex-Wife and valiant rescuer; Howie, the embittered, put-upon, long-suffering Servant; and the grand-children, in their bit part for comic relief, off-stage. I could see all this, but still couldn't rise above it and keep to my role as the pro-ducer. I couldn't even seem to stay put in the audience and avoid getting swept up into the dramatic action taking place on centre stage. They annoyed, insulted, and irritated me. They reminded me of my own family. It was all too close for comfort. Worst of all, because of the way they treated me, and because of the way they behaved, I felt, in their presence, ashamed to be a nurse and embar-rassed to be a Jew.

I NEVER FIGURED out how they managed to coordinate their visits so that they rarely had to face one another, but once again, shortly after Sid left, Brenda arrived, this time with another grandchild, Sid's daughter, Melissa, a teenager who spoke to her grandfather in baby talk. After a few minutes she said she was bored and wanted to leave.

"C'mon, honey bunch," her grandmother said, "let's go shopping. Melissa needs shoes for the wedding, Irv," she yelled into his ear.

"Yeah, mention money, that should get him going," said Sid who was back again. "Mother's spending all your money, Dad. Wake up and stop her." He walked to the other side of the bed, where Brenda had been standing, the side toward which Dr. Laurence's head was turned, but as soon as Sid came into his father's line of vision, he turned his face away.

"My mother's nuts," Sid said to me when she left. "Always has been. All she cares about is his money. They've been separated for years, but they still have joint bank accounts. She tries to control everything, but she doesn't love him as much as I do."

I looked over at the father who lay in bed, unmoving, his eyes closed, oblivious to his family, oblivious to everything, really. To me, his big, shaggy face was handsome, despite the baggy skin under his eyes, his bulbous, hairy nose, and sagging features, even despite the endotracheal tube and the heavy-duty plastic tape we used on his face to secure the tube. But his expression was vacant, vacated almost, expressing only the desire to sink deeper within himself and away from us all.

The next day I sat with my friends in the lounge eating lunch, and we all seemed to need to let off steam about difficult families, of which the Laurence family currently topped the list.

"They're driving me crazy," I complained. "They told Sydney they don't want me taking care of him and I can't say I'm too disappointed about it. They have given me an easy out."

"I also had a difficult family last week," said Tracy. "They went to Sydney to complain that I didn't give good 'service.' You know how demeaning that felt?"

"Tell them they should ask for a different waitress, next time," Morty suggested.

"I'm having a hellish day, too," said Nicole. "I've got the twenty-eight-year-old woman who had a baby three days ago and has now gone into acute renal and hepatic failure – it's a rare auto-immune syndrome."

"Did the baby make it?" Frances asked.

"Yes, but it doesn't look very good for the mother. She's septic and that's led to problems with her blood-clotting function. She's dangerously acidotic – her pH is only 6.79 and her lactate is over 12 – so we had to sedate her, paralyze her, the works. Anyway, I'm working my butt off – it's been nonstop in there all day – and the patient's mother, sister, husband are all there, crying at the bedside, asking me a million questions and telling me she's hot, she's cold, she needs a blanket, rub her feet, put Vaseline on her lips. The husband looks at me and says, 'It's our anniversary tomorrow.' What could I say? I didn't want to hear that. I'm getting married next month. I'm planning my wedding. I want to be happy. I feel for them – of course, I do – but I'm tired and want to go home and they're crying their eyes out. I know it doesn't make any sense, but I felt like saying, 'Why such long faces? Come on, it's depressing being around you guys.'"

Morty recalled a funny story. "Remember that patient whose husband kept speaking into a tape recorder? I was taking care of the wife whose name was Louise and he was going, 'I'm talking to . . . what's your name?' he asked me and I said, 'I'm Thelma.' So he goes, 'I'm talking to Thelma, Louise's nurse. Not a bad nurse, but not a great one, either.' He gave everyone a grade. I think I got a B minus."

"We get no appreciation," said Nicole, joining in to this self-pity fest, "and I know we shouldn't expect it, but, remember that hockey coach we had as a patient who gave out gold playoff tickets to the doctors and left a box of stale candy for the nurses?"

"Sometimes you give and give and then get to a point where you feel you can't give any more," sighed Frances. We were taken aback to hear a comment like that from her. She looked guilty at letting us down.

"I don't understand you guys." Laura sat up from where she had been curled up on the couch like a cat, pretending to be having a power nap, pretending she hadn't been listening to any of this conversation. "I *never* have problems with families. I don't get personal with them and I don't expect anything from them. Don't get so emotionally involved. Especially you, Tilda, you're the worst for that. You're sooo *sssensssitive*."

Morty broke into a few twangy bars of Jann Arden's hit song, "*In*sensitive," to bait me.

"Another problem with you," said Laura, surveying me as if she were going to do a complete makeover of me, or at least give me a new hairstyle, "is that you *think* too much. Stop it."

"I suppose you're right," I agreed.

Families never complained about Laura, but Laura also never attempted to forge a relationship with them. She had mastered the art of compassion without losing herself in the process. Families loved her because they knew she gave exquisite care to their loved one, but they also knew to contain themselves in her presence.

"I never have trouble with families, either," mused Nell, who wasn't boasting. In her case it was simply true.

Some nurses had a natural wisdom or an acquired maturity that allowed them to give in such a way that they didn't lose themselves. More than once, I had seen Nell, Frances, Bruno, Ellen, Valerie, or Suman cry with a family over a patient's deterioration. They had been known to occasionally give out their home telephone number to a family member who wanted to speak to them privately. Karen sometimes went to the funerals, visitations, wakes, or shivas of some of her patients and had even made home visits on her own time. For those nurses, none of these gifts they offered seem to either extract or detract from their personal resources.

There were others like that: Julia, Juliet, Murry, Ann, Lisa, Linda, Judith, Richard, Sharon, Anita – and others. The good nurses. The ones who made every patient family's request list, those families who compiled such lists. Then there were all the rest of us. The vast majority of us who struggled to maintain our emotional equilibrium in the presence of so much suffering and despair. All the rest of us who tried to stay open to the pain of others and not be overwhelmed by it.

In school, they'd taught us how important it was to offer empathy to our patients. Sympathy was wishy-washy, sentimental. Empathy was the ability to perceive and feel another's pain. One was supposed to share the patient's "lived experience of illness." One was supposed to get inside the patient, see things from the patient and family's point of view, think and feel like the patient, take on what that person was experiencing. All of this was in order to know them intimately and only by knowing them in this way could the nurse give the greatest gift: empathy, the hallmark of the professional nurse.

What profession other than nursing was defined by this degree of emotional involvement? Certainly not my husband's work selling life insurance, even though it required him to have serious discussions with young, healthy people and convince them of their mortality. Even social workers could keep their distance with words and paperwork. Teachers could choose to get involved in students' personal problems, listen, empathize, and draw them out, but they could also choose not to do so and stick to their subject matter and still be excellent teachers.

However, a nurse who was not sensitive to a patient's emotions, who did not help to assuage bad feelings, who did not offer the ultimate gift of feeling for them – empathy – was simply not meeting a basic requirement of the job.

Did those who taught us ever realize what a demand it was on young (mostly) women (by far the vast majority of nurses) whose boundaries were often so permeable and pliable? Had anyone ever considered the toll such emotional receptiveness took on most of us, both male and female? Why wasn't it covered in the lectures and textbooks of nursing – how one could stay sensitive to the patient's experience, see things from their point of view, be compassionate, and still manage not to get pulled down with them into despair and sadness, or be affected by their anger and frustration? Otherwise, who could do this work effectively for any length of time? Who could sustain it into a lifelong career?

AS MY SECOND day caring for Irving Laurence progressed, he seemed to go deeper and deeper into his detachment from the world. When we turned him in bed, he lay there helplessly and let us do all the work. As the day wore on, he seemed feverish, and sure enough, by the afternoon, he'd spiked a temp.

"He was perfect this morning! What have you done to him?" asked Brenda, throwing off her coat and flying to his side. "He came into this hospital just fine, and look at him now!"

She stayed only a short while and right afterwards, predictably, Sidney showed up. (Was he hiding outside in the bushes, watching her come and go?)

"Before he got sick, Pop was never sick a day in his life," Sid moaned. "He didn't even know what a hospital was."

I tried not to glance over at the stack of old charts piled up on the counter; they spoke volumes. I merely nodded at Sidney as he spoke. His cellphone rang.

Sid had been told frequently to turn off his cellphone while in the hospital, as it could interfere with the electronic equipment, but he kept it on anyway, because, as he explained, he was expecting an urgent call. He was always working on a "million-dollar deal that was about to be put to bed." However, most of the calls I overheard him making seemed to be to his lawyer, to find out the exact details of his father's will, how the estate would be shared between him and his mother, and how quickly the disbursements would take place – would it be days or weeks?

I wasn't assigned to Dr. Laurence's care again, but the questions the experience provoked in me were still very much on my mind a few days later. I had just returned to the ICU from transferring a patient to the floor, so I was free to cruise around the unit, visit patients, and help the other nurses. I happened to walk by the room of a patient who was calling out for help.

I had heard about this patient on rounds. She was a forty-two-year-old woman, a mother of three, who was newly diagnosed with aggressively spreading breast cancer. She wound up in the ICU with a perilous respiratory infection. I knew from having gone over her X-rays with the team that she was deteriorating rapidly and it was only a matter of time until she would need to be intubated.

When she saw my face at the doorway, she reached out toward me. "I'm flailing all around the bed and I can't seem to stop," she said. "My nurses think I'm crazy. Tell them I'm not."

Her nurse, Esmeralda, a petite Philippina nurse with long shiny black hair and a preference for candy-pink scrubs, went over to her. "You're upset, that's what you are, dear," she said with calm authority. "Would you like me to give you medication in your IV to help you calm down?"

As Esmeralda was asking this question, I saw that she was already injecting 5 mg of Valium into the patient's IV line.

"My family were here and now they're gone and I'm scared. I don't know what to do," the woman said. Her breathing was fast and shallow. "Help me! Help me, someone. I'm all swollen up." She held up a puffy, bruised arm to show us where IVs, and attempted IVs, had been.

"Moderate peripheral edema and scattered superficial hema-
tomas," I saw Esmeralda jot down in the chart for her nursing
assessment under the category of "Integumentary System," commonly known as "skin."

She was giving good care and getting her paperwork done, too.
That's efficiency, I thought. That's a nurse who'll rest easy tonight.
She's in it for the long haul.

"I'm scared," the patient said, her eyes beseeching me,
Esmeralda, and then Ruth, the other nurse in the room who was
caring for another patient.

"What's scaring you?" asked Esmeralda, even though we could
think of about a million things.

I noticed that in the few minutes I had been in the room,
uninvolved and merely observing, even *I* was becoming uncomfortable. The patient was so anxious, was moaning so much, and was
so inconsolable, despite the competent efforts that Esmeralda
was making, that it was putting me into a heightened state of alertness and unease. Reassurance wasn't working, the Valium hadn't
kicked in, and this woman's need seemed to fill the room. I could
feel myself getting tense and my own breathing felt a little con-
stricted. I was tempted to shut out the patient's pleading voice and
busy myself with tasks. I could move on to another room, as I
really had no obligation to stay there. There were other nurses who
could use my help.

"I'm upset, I'm so upset, I really am. I hate this place. Get me
out of heerre!" the woman cried out.

Esmeralda patted her arm, a gesture that reminded her at
the same time that it was a good opportunity to stretch out the
patient's other, less swollen arm and take her blood pressure and
then compare it with the electronic read-out of the arterial line
transducer on the monitor. (We considered the high-tech method
more reliable than the hands-on method but we still checked it the
old-fashioned way from time to time to make sure the two read-
ings more or less correlated.)

"How do you do it?" I asked Esmeralda. I saw how emotionally secure and stable she was as she gave good, kind care. She was

compassionate, yet contained within herself. She cared, but she wasn't particularly emotionally involved.

"I come here, give what I can and then I say, bye-bye, time to go home," she said in a chirpy voice.

Ruth, the other nurse, was moody. She had her good days and her bad days. I had seen her give nursing care with incredible skill and compassion and, at other times, be distant and perfunctory with patients. "If you ask me, that patient is a PITA," she said quietly, from her side of the room.

"Not an abbreviation I'm familiar with," I said.

"Pain in the Ass. I know she's dying, but does she have to be such a bitch about it?"

"Ruth, how can you say that?" I asked, acting appalled and self-righteous, with my hands on my hips. But then I stopped myself – hadn't I just had my own *unempathetic* thoughts? Was I any better? I had been in this patient's room for about two minutes and already I wanted to escape. I felt drained of the empathy that I was there to give.

Was this a sign of the "burned-out syndrome" that we had been warned about in school? I had been a nurse for fifteen years, ten of them in critical care. I had read about this phenomenon, studied it in school, and had seen other nurses with severe cases of it. I had always promised myself I would never get that way, but here I was, dragged down by a patient's despair, on edge from her anxiety. I had caught it from this patient as easily as one contracted an infectious disease.

At times, certain people, certain patients had that effect on me: the young ones, the awake ones, the insatiable ones, and the tragic ones. For as sad as some of the deaths were that I helped and witnessed in the ICU, most were not tragic. I felt relieved for the old or very sick people who died; they had managed to slip away and escape. It was sad for those left behind, the family and friends, but those cases were not the ones that caused me to lose my composure. They were not the ones who broke my heart.

A few days later, Laura and Frances returned from a nursing conference that Sydney had sent them on. They reported back to us about the latest products for preventing pressure sores, new techniques for postural drainage of lung secretions, and the latest nursing theory that the hospital seemed eager to adopt, called "patient-centred care."

"Isn't that what our care is already?" I asked.

"Isn't that what we're doing?" Tracy echoed my thought. She was equally dismayed as I was at the deficiency in us that this new title implied. "I mean, how much more patient-centred could our care possibly be?"

Frances explained. "Well, they gave visiting hours as an example. The trend is to let families visit whenever they like, just walk in, day or night, stay as long as they like."

"Haven't you ever seen some patient's blood pressure and heart rate shoot up when their relatives come to visit? We see it all the time. The patient is calm and relaxed. The family comes in and turns to us and says, 'He's in pain. Do something. Give him a pain killer!'" Nicole said. "Sometimes families need to be kept out to let the patient have rest and privacy, too. Sometimes they start asking the patient questions and fussing and within minutes they've got them all riled up and struggling against the tube, oxygen saturations are dropping, and then you have no choice but to sedate them."

Only Morty had the guts to raise the other concern that was on everyone's mind.

"Hey, if the families are in all the time, when do we get the space we need to do our work, too, without them looking over our shoulders, questioning everything? We all know some families who can be more demanding than the patients."

"Oh, yeah, another thing," said Laura with a sly grin. "You're going to love this one. We're supposed to offer families the opportunity to be present during procedures and even during arrests, so that they can see what actually goes on. Maybe if families see what it really entails, they might make more realistic choices. Oh well, food for thought."

It was true. We craved food for thought, as well as spiritual sustenance, physical rest, and time away from this demanding work. We had to take good care of ourselves if we wanted to do the work of taking good care of others. Sure, we were tired and hungry, but it wasn't sleep or food that we needed. What we craved was spiritual regeneration and emotional nourishment in order to do this work properly and cope with its emotional demands. We desperately needed to fill up on whatever the commodity was that became so rapidly depleted within each of us from constantly attending to others' limitless needs. We needed replenishment of the spirit so that we could go on amid all the sadness and despair that surrounded us and not be downed or drowned by it.

We had thrived on the emotional support and understanding that we had received from our former manager, Rosemary, who was a nurse to the core. We felt gratified when our patients improved, or we managed to lessen their suffering, or when we were thanked or even acknowledged. But more than anything, what quelled our longings, restored our souls, and satiated our appetites was the emotional and spiritual nurturance that we received from one another. It was what sustained us.

We debriefed one another after an upsetting encounter with a patient. We shared the horrors of wounds we had seen, patients' discomforts that we were unsuccessful to ameliorate, and heart-breaking tragedies we had witnessed. Who else but another nurse would understand how such things felt? It was through that understanding that we derived the strength we needed to go forward.

We took care of each other. We shared secrets and the intimate details of our lives with one another. We understood one another. The work we did made us open up in this way. In fact I believe that this closeness was the very thing that fortified us to do this emotionally demanding work.

For example, because we knew that Carole had a child with a severe seizure disorder we immediately understood her startled, but then stoic, reaction one night when caring for her patient who was a young man who suddenly started seizing. We knew that Erica was trying to get pregnant, and we took care not to assign her to the critically ill postpartum mother, in case it would frighten her. We now knew of Nell's serious battle with depression and stopped making fun of her sick calls and outlandish excuses. We sent Ellen off for a nap and covered for her in the middle of a busy shift when she was queasy from morning sickness.

Tracy guarded her privacy more than most, yet within our small group she had confided to us that she hadn't seen her mother for years. The mother was a homeless vagrant who roamed the city dragging bags filled with plastic bags and slept in ravines and underpasses. We saw Tracy casually scanning the streets for her when we went out together.

Nicole shared her qualms with us about her engagement to Andrew, a thoracic resident she'd met in our ICU. (Oliver was long gone, as well as a few others over the years.) She was considering postponing the wedding until she felt more certain. She wasn't ready, she said. She wasn't sure he was the one, and she still debated about giving one more all-out attempt to make the pro golf circuit.

Although Frances was single, she yearned to be a mother. She was thinking of going to China to adopt a baby girl. She was also considering going back to school for her degree in nursing and tried to convince Laura to join her, but Laura wouldn't budge.

As for Laura – well, who really knew Laura?

We knew who was in the closet and who was venturing out. We knew about one another's pregnancies and attempts at pregnancy, abortions and miscarriages, weight loss and gain; abusive and happy marriages; problematic and brilliant children; credit card indiscretions, stock market killings, flirtations, and flings.

Some of us even knew Belinda's secret: her husband had died in our ICU of pneumonia from AIDS.

"Frances was the nurse caring for him. I'll never forget it," she told me one day. "I was working at a different hospital at the time. It was such a blur to me that I didn't even recognize her when I came to work here. All I remember was her soothing voice. She was so kind and gentle to me when he died. I just lost control of myself and I think I was wailing and screaming. I'm so embarrassed when I think of it now, but I couldn't help myself. It was then that I decided that this is where I wanted to work one day."

She told me this on the day that she was taking care of a patient who was lying in the same bed in which her husband had died.

NURSES KNOW THE importance of birthdays. No milestone, for that matter, went uncelebrated, nor any loss unsympathized with. For one of my birthdays, Frances brought in a carrot cake covered with a bright neon-green frosting.

"Are there any carrots in it?" Nicole asked.

Frances was known for her improvised recipes. For a potluck dinner at work one night, she had made a lemon meringue pie but, lacking any lemons, substituted oranges.

"How did you know? I *didn't* have enough carrots," she admitted, "so I used sweet potatoes."

Danny Huizinga said he would have just a small slice. "I hope I don't glow in the dark from that frosting. I must say, Frances, it looks a lot more appetizing than that cake with the cherries on top you made last time." He chuckled. "I've performed lung biopsies that looked more appetizing than that."

"Yes, but you did manage to eat two huge slices, as I recall," said Laura, who looked ready to affectionately slug him or else violently hug him, on behalf of Frances, but we managed to restrain her in time.

BUT I WAS beginning to worry about the long-term effects of our constant exposure to suffering. At times I felt that the sadness accumulated in us. At times I saw that it deadened us in certain ways and made us hypersensitive in other ways. More and more I saw that nurses were suffering. Nurses needed hope to go on.

"Who can keep it up for long and remain caring all the time?" Frances asked with a huge sigh.

I looked at her. "If *you* can't keep it up, who can?" I said. "You always say how much you love nursing."

"The passion that drives me to do this work is the very thing that's going to make me leave it in the end," she answered, wearily.

Somehow, of all of us, it was Frances who managed to forge a good relationship with the Laurence family. One day they left a box of Belgian chocolates and a note at the nursing station.

Thank you to all of the staff caring for Irving.

And a very special thank you to Frances (she knows what for).

Brenda Laurence.

I asked Frances what she had done to deserve that special mention.

"All I did was tell her, you do what you believe is right for your husband. Don't worry what the doctors and nurses say. After all, you and your son know him best. That's all."

I marvelled at the degree to which she had conquered herself.

There were many times when we felt empty, bereft, overwhelmed by the demands – the emotional ones much more than the physical ones – of being nurses. Sometimes it seemed that the work asked too much of us, not only as nurses, but also as human beings. Who can give so much, so selflessly? In order to do this work you had to be selfless, because to do it properly, you had to become without a self. You might have a self, but you had to subordinate it, obliterate it in order to meet other people's needs.

We were not supposed to have our own needs. Yes, we were tired and hungry, but who cared? Certainly not the patients, who were mostly unconscious and totally dependent on us. Definitely not the families, who expected complete devotion from us and seemed to resent it when we took a break or even when we got up to leave at the end of a twelve-hour shift and they had to become accustomed to the style and idiosyncrasies of a new nurse.

"Are you back tomorrow?" families often asked as your shift was winding down.

You try to discern from their voice or the expression on their faces if they are relieved or disappointed when you say, no, it's my day off. You know sometimes they ask for you specifically, and sometimes they ask specifically *not* for you, and you try not to care one way or the other.

It wasn't Florence Nightingale they wanted. The real Florence Nightingale was a hard-nosed battle-axe, a military micro manager, and a slave driver. What they wanted was a sweet, altruistic, loving version of Mother Theresa. So few of us measured up.

DR. LAURENCE WAS deteriorating quickly. Decisions would have to be made soon or else things would happen in a wild and uncontrolled way. He was heading toward end-stage respiratory failure and severe biological derangement that could only lead to cardiac arrest. Once again we were faced with the ethical dilemma we faced over and over in the ICU. Either we escalate or maintain the same level of care, or we back off and change our goals. That is, either we continue to ramp up the dosages of the medications and number of machines, jack up the tests and procedures, or we could take another tack altogether: gently and gradually withdraw all these things and turn our focus to the patient's dignity and comfort. Sometimes, the scenario became a showdown. A duel at sundown.

One member of the family chooses to go all out. They tell us not to hold back with any available intervention or treatment. They embark on this campaign because they believe in the miraculous resilience of the patient, or have endowed medical science with the power to bring about a recovery in all circumstances. At times I think this route is chosen because it is the individual's way of showing that their love is superior to that of the other family members'. They will be vindicated in the annals of the family history. "See, I told you so," they must imagine themselves saying one day at a joyful family gathering, "I knew how strong Dad was. You all were ready to give up on him, but thank God, I believed he would make it and I was right."

Another faction of the family feels they have to balance the scales by representing the opposite position. This camp has to oppose the other's aggressive stance in order to declare, "No, it is *I* who loves Dad best. I will show it by doing the unselfish and compassionate act of letting him go in peace. It is I who truly loves him best, because only I am prepared to make that sacrifice."

However, no matter what discussion precedes the course of action, in the end, it is the nurse who puts it into effect.

Morty was taking care of Dr. Laurence and I was in the room with her, taking care of another patient. Brenda arrived but said she could only stay a few minutes because she had left QT, her poodle, in the car and he would be lonely by himself.

"Why don't you send QT in to visit your husband and you stay out in the car?" Morty asked with a straight face, but Brenda was so distracted and distraught, she didn't even react.

The weeks had worn on and we had dealt with crisis after complication after setback and all over again. We were keeping Dr. Laurence going. He kept his eyes closed most of the time, but whenever he did open them, he looked heavenward, clasped his hands together, as if entreating us, pleading with us for mercy.

Howie had stopped coming to visit. He was angry. He called to tell us that he had been removed from the payroll and kicked out of the house.

Sidney became superstitious and forbade any green bedspreads on his father's bed. Green was bad luck, he decided. In fact he insisted we write "No Green Bedspreads" in the chart, like a doctor's order.

"Another thing," he added, "I want nobody mentioning cats."

Someone had mentioned that his father seemed to have nine lives.

"If I hear that once more," he said, "I think I'll scream."

"Are cats bad luck?"

"Yes! I want Dad to have a hundred lives. I can't lose him. Don't you understand that?"

Brenda found religion. She wore a big golden fish on a chain around her neck, which her spiritual advisor told her would bring the healing powers of the sea – her husband was a Pisces – to his recovery. She brought in a New Age rabbi to visit her husband, to pray over him and give him a new Hebrew name so that the Angel of Death would be foiled and not spirit him away.

"We must do everything. We can't give up," she said to Morty, who was taking care of him one day. I heard her ask, "Can he still hear a prayer? If I recite the *Shema* into his ear, will he be able to hear it?"

"Your guess is as good as mine. They say the hearing's the last thing to go, but if you want the truth, Brenda, I think he's right out of it." Morty told it as she saw it.

Sidney and Brenda refused a family meeting in the quiet room. They preferred to stand out in the hallway and pace back and forth, while the doctors talked to them. I offered them chairs but they both said they didn't have time to sit. They had to run off to other engagements and had only a few minutes. When Dr. Leung came over to speak with them, Sid was on his cellphone and Brenda was flipping through the pages of her date book.

"I think we're coming near to the end of what we can offer your father," said Dr. Leung, in her gentle, respectful way. "I'm sorry. I would like to put forth to you the idea that in the event your father suffers a sudden cardiac arrest, we do not believe it is in his best interests to resuscitate him."

"Are you talking about a do not resuscitate order? Do you mean DNR?" asked Sid. "I talked with my son – he's a medical student – and we've changed our minds. We've decided that Dad wouldn't want to have all of this done."

"Oh, yes he would," Brenda countered. "Your father was never a quitter. He does not give up. You, on the other hand . . ."

I decided to speak up from my side of the room.

"On a number of occasions, when he was conscious and able to communicate, Dr. Laurence indicated to many of us that he didn't want to continue with treatment."

Luckily, I had saved some of the notes that Dr. Laurence had written during his lucid moments, a few days ago when I had last cared for him.

Let me go. I've had enough.

Enough already.

I want to die.

Sid inspected the note. "Yup, that's Pop's handwriting, all right."

Brenda looked at me, aghast. "I expected more from you, Tilda! As a member of our community, you should know better. It is forbidden to shorten a life. Only God can do that. The rabbi said that the saving of a life is the highest mitzvah! After all the Jewish people have been through, we must save a life at any cost! Pain and suffering is worth it to preserve a life. The rabbi told me –" but she broke off and sobbed into her silk scarf.

"Not only that," I pressed on, firm in my resolve that I was doing the right thing, the only thing I was there to do: advocate for my patient, "but other nurses also have heard his wishes, straight from him. Perhaps he hid it from you both but he expressed it clearly to us."

Morty nodded to show her corroboration. The doctors listened closely.

"Well, could you just keep him going until Mitchell and Emily's wedding?" asked Brenda. "It's next week and it would ruin Mitchell's special day." She scanned her calendar. "The week after that would work, if you want to do it then."

I was speechless. We all were.

Except Sidney. "You're so shallow," he said to his mother.

"What do we do now?" Brenda said.

"Pull up a chair," I said to them. "Hold his hand. Be with him."

I sat down and showed them how.

15

NARROW MARGINS
AND CLOSE CALLS

We couldn't stop talking about what had happened. When we weren't talking about it, we were thinking about it. When we weren't thinking about it, we were praying it would never happen to any one of us.

It happened in another hospital and we heard that the nurse was being treated for emotional shock. She was inconsolable.

What happened was more than an error or a mistake. It was more than a slip or a moment of inattention. It was an innocent, but fatally wrong action and it accidentally killed the patient. The scary thing was, any of us could imagine ourselves doing the exact same thing, in any number of the rushed or distracted moments we've all had, in any given shift.

"The College of Nurses will probably take disciplinary action against her," said Laura. "She may very well lose her licence over this. One thing's for sure. She'll never work in this town again, you'll see! The coroner will call an inquest and that nurse will be lambasted. That's the end of her."

"Let's be clear about this," said Morty. "A mistake is not necessarily a crime. Let's hope she won't be treated like a criminal."

"I can just imagine her, crying by herself at home," said Nicole. "I bet everyone's coming down on her."

"But not nearly as hard as she's coming down on herself," I said, putting myself in that nurse's place for just a few uncomfortable moments.

Tracy was characteristically quiet, but it appeared she was thinking hard.

"At the very least, there'll be some 'splainin' to do," Laura said with a grim face.

"How will she ever be able to go on? How will she ever return to work?" How can she ever face the others?" I voiced the questions that were on all of our minds.

"How did it happen?"

"Surely she knew that you can't dialyze a patient with ordinary sterile water!"

"Wow, without a buffering agent, a hypotonic solution like that would suck all the sodium out of the cells in a few minutes. A person would practically implode. Geez . . ."

Part unearned smugness, part genuine humility, nonetheless, we were all shaken; no one could rest easy. It could have been any one of us. It could have been me. Easily.

ONE QUIET MORNING, years ago, not long after I had started working in the ICU, I decided to give my patient a bath. Andy was a middle-aged man, a father of two, with acute leukemia. He was in the ICU battling one infection after another, following a long course of chemotherapy. The number of platelets he had in his blood stream – those cells responsible for the body's normal clotting mechanism – was nil: zero. I re-read the lab results. No platelets? Zip? Zilch? How was that possible? I closed the chart and prepared the bath. His temperature was raging. He nodded weakly in assent when I told him what I proposed to do.

"Andy, just lean over so I can wash your back." I helped him reach for the side rail. "That's it, a bit more." He was too weak to pull himself over alone. "Grab on to the side rail," I instructed.

He did as I said, leaned onto the bar for support, and it broke.

The crash, when his body tumbled out of bed and hit the floor, along with the clang and clatter of equipment – IV pole, pumps, and ventilator – that were pulled down with him, reverberated throughout the unit. Everyone came running. I watched the swarming melee. I felt sick.

"Grab his legs!"

"I've got his head!"

"Easy now, let's lift him up together on the count of three."

"Careful," I croaked. "He has zero platelets."

Three days later he died. From infection, from internal bleeding, from cancer itself. He had a lot of reasons to die, but the fall out of bed didn't help. Rosemary called me into her office.

"The bed was old and likely defective. You had the side rail locked into place properly. You did nothing wrong. Because of what happened, we're replacing all the beds in the ICU with brand-new electronic beds. Something good has come of this. I want you to know, Tilda, that you did nothing wrong."

"But he died," I said dully. Perhaps I was absolved, but a man had died and I'd had a part in it. Was there something I could have done differently?

"We told the family exactly what happened. We've offered our sincere apologies and sympathy for what happened. They've accepted it. Now put it out of your mind," said Rosemary. "Go forward. We all support you."

I did as she said. I put it out of my mind. Otherwise, how else could I have gone on working there? Yet every once in a while something jolted me – it was either something I did or something I saw someone else do – and I was humbled and made grateful. From time to time, something would make me stop, check myself, remind myself to take more care, not take anything for granted, and not get sloppy. It all could be otherwise in a single careless moment.

Once, my patient's IV tubing had a cracked connection that I hadn't noticed and the patient's blood leaked out into the bed, along with the medication he was supposed to be receiving. Easily rectified, that one. I cleaned up the patient, changed the sheets, and gave the med again, but whew, I thought – that was a close call.

I WAS CHATTING with my patient's wife. Her husband was sitting up and starting to wean off the ventilator. He was working hard at breathing and she distracted him with joking banter because he often got anxious and short of breath when he was told it was time to work on weaning. Some nurses had suggested I cover up the clock on the wall. He would wean better that way, not counting the minutes the whole time, but it felt devious and I couldn't bring myself to do it.

"I'm going to get you for this – all you've put me through!" his wife told him, giving him a light slap on the shoulder. It was a joke she could make only now that he was on the mend. He smiled weakly.

"You better be good to me when we get home, 'cause I've been through hell because of you!"

He nodded. The road to recovery since his surgery to repair a thoracic aneurysm had been a long and difficult one.

His surgeon came in and greeted him warmly. "Hi, Mr. Trute! How're you doing? It's good to see you out of bed. I've come to discuss the results of your tests."

The wife and patient looked at me in alarm. I looked at the doctor in alarm.

The problem was that this man was Mr. Szabo and he had not been expecting test results. Furthermore, if the doctor got the patient's name wrong, what else might be wrong? If the name was wrong, were the treatments also wrong? Maybe those meant for Mr. Trute (whoever that was) were the ones given to him? What about the surgery, the medications? Worst of all, was the picture the doctor held in his mind not that of her husband, Felix Szabo?

"Excuse me," I interposed and explained the situation.

"Oh." He consulted his notes, apologized lavishly, and fled the room.

Later that day when I told Morty what had happened, she found it greatly amusing. She told us a story and whether it was an

Internet joke or something that had really happened – the way she told it we couldn't tell – it made us howl.

"So, this nurse is taking care of this patient, see, and he says to her, nurse, please check if my testicles are black. What? she says. Of course not! Your testicles aren't black. He asks her again. Nurse, please. Check if my testicles are black. Nonsense, she says. Forget about it. He asks yet again. Are my testicles black? So she throws back the covers and examines him. Holds each one in her hand, moves his dick to the right, then to the left. Nope, she says, your testicles aren't black. Are you satisfied? He looks very taken aback and pulls down the oxygen mask that was muffling his voice. 'Nurse, I was asking if my test results are back.'"

DESPITE ALL OUR checks and double-checks, despite backup systems and safety precautions, mistakes were still made. Before we hung a unit of blood or plasma, we verified five different pieces of identifying information with another nurse. We double-checked each other's doses of insulin, digoxin, dilantin, and heparin, or any drug if we were unfamiliar with it. If we didn't know a drug inside out – its actions, interactions, contraindications, and adverse effects – we didn't give it until we learned everything about it. When Dr. Huizinga told us one night that it was okay to go ahead and give an experimental drug that hadn't yet been approved for nurses to administer, we held fast and didn't give it. How much more careful could we possibly be?

"One day, when medication orders, dosage calculations, and even the dispensing and labelling of the drug are all done by computer, errors will be eliminated," the pharmacist predicted. "It will minimize the human factor."

Yes, but it is nurses' unique role to maximize the human factor. Will monkeys or robots be able to give the drug, explain its side effects, and make adjustments as needed, as nurses do? Will the accuracy rate be higher? Computerizing everything also brings its own set of new problems: it eliminates critical thinking and problem-solving and decision-making skills. What it does – and it did this very thing when all the laboratory orders and reports were computerized – was create new avenues for error.

We nurses checked and second-guessed ourselves constantly. The doctors did too.

Dr. Leung called me one night from her home. I glanced at my watch. It was 0330 hours.

"I was mulling over your patient's renal failure," she said.

In her voice, I heard the pull toward sleep and the opposing pull toward wakefulness.

"I think we're going to have to give him a whopping dose of Lasix to see if we can stimulate his kidneys." She took a deep breath. "Tilda," she said, "I'm going to ask you to give 320 mg."

I gulped. The maximum I had ever given was 80 mg. "That much, Jessica?"

We were both thinking of the many possible toxic side effects of that large a dose.

"His creatinine is 398," I said at the same moment that she asked, "How much is his creatinine?"

"Let's give it a try," she said. "Take it from me as a verbal order and I'll sign it in the morning."

"I don't know," said Laura, thinking it over. "I trust Jessica, but –"

"We'll back you up," said Tracy. Nicole, Morty, and Laura did, too. They all co-signed the medication record beside my signature, as I slowly injected the drug.

By the morning, when the day shift came on, the patient's kidneys were working. Urine was flowing. The only problem was, the drug had made the patient stone deaf.

"It may not be permanent." I stayed late that morning to hear Jessica explain to the family what had happened. "He may regain some hearing. It's a side effect of the drug at that high a dose, but we had to give it a try in order to save his kidneys."

"My husband," the wife sobbed, "is a professor of music."

"PATIENTS ARE DYING from the wrong doses of chemotherapy," Daniel Huizinga announced one morning on rounds, apropos of nothing in particular. He held up his index finger to indicate that a caveat was on its way. "The problem is that patients are also dying from the *correct* doses of chemotherapy. Which is worse? It all amounts to the same thing. We are fallible human beings who know so little about the human body. The public is paying us to be certain, to fix everything, to have all the answers. Understandably, that's what they want. We are all human beings doing the best we can, but they don't care, they just want their loved one better."

If this was the expectation, how could we ever measure up? Of course, the public had the right to be angry when things went wrong, but how could we, as nurses, make sure to do everything right all the time? Even if we did everything correctly, it didn't guarantee that the patient would get better.

Sometimes when patients' conditions worsened, the families would rush in and ask, "Who did this?" or "How could this have happened?" or "What went wrong?" Surely something was done improperly, something was not caught quickly enough, they seemed to say. Someone must have overlooked or mismanaged something, they implied. Yet, in my experience, this was rarely the case. People were sick. Many got sicker. Some got better.

Dr. Huizinga was right when he said that things could go wrong even if everything were done correctly. However, even if everything was done correctly and wrong words were used, that to me seemed like a mistake, or at least a miscalculation that could cause harm. Words could be medicine; I believed that. I had seen them used to heal and to comfort and to encourage. Words could be used in such a way that they were just as damaging as some mistakes I knew of.

On rounds one morning, well within earshot of my patient, Dr. Huizinga speculated about her marked, unexpected improvement.

"Why is this patient getting better?" he demanded.

"Well . . . I . . . I guess the treatments must be working," said the resident.

Daniel shook his head. He was determined to hear everything opposite. "It will be interesting to see a tissue sample report from the autopsy."

"We'll have to wait just a bit for that," I said and closed the patient's door.

"Why is that?" he snapped.

"Well, she's still alive. She's doing better."

"You know what Huizinga's like," Laura said to me later. "I've heard him say to a patient who had made a suicide attempt, 'Did you do it? That was stupid, don't do it again. Get help. But if you are planning to do it again, do it properly next time. No halfway measures.' That's his idea of a psych consult."

Yet I couldn't reconcile his abrasive manner with his supreme dedication and his expertise in action. He was the doctor I would choose if I had a critical illness, yet at times, I could hardly bear to exchange even a few words with him.

ONE DAY DR. David Bristol came into my room to talk to my patient, a forty-year-old Ethiopian woman who was in our ICU with bleeding from internal injuries after her husband beat and stabbed her in a rage because she had not borne him any sons, only daughters. She had also recently been diagnosed with breast cancer.

When I came into the room, Dr. Bristol was already in the midst of the conversation.

"Mrs. Afework, you have a very serious illness and now life-threatening injuries. If your heart stops, do you want us to perform cardiac compressions? In the event that you become unable to make decisions for yourself, someone will have to make them for you. If you require a breathing tube put down into your windpipe, do you want it? It is important that you get organized to ensure that your needs will be taken care of. Where is your family?" He looked around to see if there was a brown-skinned person around to translate his words into Amharic.

"I don't have any family. I am alone."

"Do you have a friend, someone?"

"I have no one."

"Let's suppose you become unconscious. Who's going to make decisions for you? What about your financial matters? Is someone taking care of your children? There is a department of the government that we can contact, and they will make decisions for you or you will have to appoint a substitute decision maker. These are important decisions."

I came to her side after he left. "Did you understand what the doctor said? Some things to think about, in case anything happens, you know, down the road."

She clutched my arm. "Please, nurse," she pleaded. "Don't let that doctor call the government. They will take away my children."

Perhaps he didn't harm her with his words, but he didn't use them to help.

I had been a critical care nurse for many years and was beginning to understand something about these situations that hovered in between what is truthful and what is cruel; what is compassionate, yet wrong; what is correct, yet harmful. I had also come to understand that it is more complicated than merely assigning blame. It wasn't just that many people were involved, or that we were terribly busy, or that there were many distractions though all of these things were true. It was that there were so many nuances, shades of meaning, and interpretations involved, and these things could have effects as serious as mistakes. How could mistakes be avoided or rectified, how could the problem be redressed other than by first seeking to understand from all sides, all angles?

AT LUNCHTIME ONE day in spring, it was finally warm enough to sit outside. We escaped into the sun on a grassy hill at the front of the hospital lawn and leaned against an *outré* industrial brass sculpture of interlocking cubes. Bruno joined us that day, and Belinda, too. Frances thought to bring with her a yellow bedspread from the linen cart and we spread it out like a tablecloth on the grass to eat our lunches. It helped us pretend we were having a leisurely picnic, when we all knew that our circumscribed forty-five-minute lunch break would soon be over.

As usual, Nicole brought a whole head of lettuce and made a salad. Bruno had a spicy chickpea roti he'd bought from Navreen, whose Jamaican take-out business was booming. She kept up her

real job in the hospital's laundry department, but continued to run
her cottage industry from home and supplied our unit. Her menu
had expanded to include rice and peas, meat patties, and curry
goat. We paged her on her beeper if we had a roti or jerk craving
any time during the day. Her number was listed on the blotter at
the nursing station, under "Roti Lady," in between Respirology
and Social Work.

First we caught up on gossip.

". . . Tina's labour went on for three days, and then she had to
be induced. Alexa is having an affair with a married doctor . . .
Erica had another miscarriage, poor thing . . ."

I decided to ask them about what had been uppermost on my
mind, ever since that fatal error a nurse had made with the dialysis solution.

I had been preoccupied with the subject of fallibility ever since
a case was reported in the media of a rock star suing the doctors
who had treated his brother; he had died of a simultaneous cardiac
arrest and a bowel obstruction. It seemed that if people had a lot
of money or celebrity, they could make these public malpractice
allegations. Their way of thinking must be something like this:
*What other possible reason could there be to explain why our
beloved brother died, other than someone must have screwed up?*

The way the media reports these events did not always help
clarify these complex matters, either. I recently read a newspaper
headline: "Drug used to execute death row prisoners was given to
hospital patient who died." That drug was potassium chloride and
I have given it many times to patients. Given correctly, which it
almost always is by nurses every single day in all hospitals, it can
save lives. It is KCl, two essential elements, bonded to make a
third. Sugar can sweeten or kill; morphine, gasoline, and fire can
help or harm, too.

"What's the scariest thing that ever happened to you with a
patient?" I asked them.

Belinda offered hers easily. "That's easy. I was a new grad and I
accidentally switched meds on two patients, but they were both
cardiac patients, so it more or less worked out okay."

"David Bristol came into my room today," said Laura, gearing up for a tirade rather than a confession. "And he says to me, why are your urine totals always listed in multiples of 5? Doesn't your patient ever put out 33 cc or 46 cc? How persnickety can you get? He tells me it's inaccurate to round them off! I told him I'm not a 3 cc nurse."

Morty's story was about someone else's misconduct. "I couldn't believe the nurse who brought down a patient from the floor this morning. He had arrested up there, but she stands there and tells me that she hadn't done his vital signs because she had gone on her coffee break. '*What* did you say?' I asked her. I'm thinking, I'll give you another opportunity to change your story, sister. Let's just pretend I didn't hear that. But she said it again. 'Yeah, I never do my vitals until after my coffee break.' By then they're not *vital* any more, are they? I said to her. She was scary."

"Was she black?" asked Belinda, who was.

"What's the difference?"

"You said 'sister.'"

"As a matter of fact she wasn't, but what's your point?"

"You white chicks don't believe me, but black people are stereo-typed. Everyone thinks we're lazy. I'll be sitting at the nursing station with a white nurse and someone needs help with their patient. Who are they going to ask? Me, because they assume I'm sitting around doing nothing anyway."

The gauntlet had been thrown down to the right person, and Morty rose to the challenge.

"Belinda, the population of Toronto is now more than 50 per cent immigrants. Our profession is well represented by women and men of colour. Maybe at one time nursing had a conservative, white-bread image, but no more. Don't you think you've got a bit of a chip on your shoulder?"

"A chocolate chip, I'd say," said Laura with a snort.

"Is that so?" shot back Belinda. "And how many black nurse managers do you know of at this hospital? Sure, there may be a few token black doctors and lots of cleaning staff, but how many black middle management or nursing leaders do you see? Racism is everywhere. It always will be. Haven't you ever noticed on a news report they don't mention that it's a white guy who commits a crime, but they do mention if he's black."

"What if it's a girl? They'll be sure to mention that!" I said. "What was your scariest thing, Bruno?" I wanted to bring the discussion back to my topic. I had meant his scariest thing with patients, but Bruno blurted out what was obviously on *his* mind.

"Waiting for the results of my AIDS test," he said. "Those twenty-four hours were the worst, the scariest." He looked off into the distance.

"Even scarier than the answer?" someone asked.

"Yup."

Nicole jumped in to deflect the uncomfortable spotlight away from Bruno.

"My worst mistake happened at the last hospital I worked at with a multiple myeloma patient I brought to the ICU from the floor. She had excruciating pain throughout her entire body. She was thrashing around and crying out to Jesus for mercy. The pain had turned her into a raving animal. Her IV bag was empty so I changed her morphine over to one of our bags from the narcotic cupboard. I got busy taking blood work, an X-ray, an ECG, drawing blood cultures, and all the time her family was breathing down my neck. The patient kept on screaming. But then, over a few minutes, she settled down and even fell asleep. Then I realized she wasn't sleeping; she was right out of it. I called her name, tried to get a response, we almost had to call a code. Then I noticed that the concentration of the pre-mixed morphine bag was twice what she'd been receiving on the floor, yet I had been running it at the same rate. Double the dose should have been running at half the rate! I should have cut the rate! Shit, I thought, and ran to get some Narcan! You know what? In seconds, she went from almost being in a coma to rearing up like a horse. Her eyes wide-open, wild. Man, that stuff works! Then I calmed her down, gave her Tylenol for her fever and she said she felt better and was so grateful to me. Should I have mentioned, 'Well, that's nice, because I almost killed you'?"

We all nodded. It was time to go back to work. We threw away our litter in the wastebasket, folded the bedspread, and walked back into the hospital together.

We *were* solid citizens, weren't we?

IT MADE ME recall a party I had gone to once. When people heard I was a nurse, everyone asked me about the case of a young girl who had died in hospital and the two nurses who had been charged in connection with her death.

"I just know what I read in the newspaper, like everyone else," I said, my palms up to show they were empty. "I don't have any inside information."

"How could it have happened?" everyone asked me. "How could a young girl die like that?"

"She had intractable pain. They were running high doses of morphine because she was continually complaining of pain. Maybe she needed closer monitoring or maybe it was a freak reaction, but for some reason, she had a respiratory arrest. She was young and fairly healthy, but they weren't able to resuscitate her. It's tragic, but I can imagine how it could happen. Morphine can be a dangerous drug."

"The nurses wrote her off as a hypochondriac and thought she was trying to get attention," someone said. "The mother was getting on their nerves so they ignored her. That's what it said in the newspaper."

"I can see both sides," I said.

"Why do you always sit on the fence?" Ivan asked, impatient with me. "Surely you have an opinion."

"My opinion is that it is tragic. A young life was needlessly lost. Maybe there were staffing problems. There was probably carelessness, a lack of vigilance; both are human mistakes. There are possible explanations, but no excuses. I doubt it was intentional. I don't think those nurses deserve the same treatment as someone who is accused of assault or murder. I've seen nurses rushed or disorganized or overworked, but I've never seen intention to harm."

Maybe I did sit on the fence, but that was the only vantage point from which I could see both sides and possibly begin to understand the complexity of it all. And it was only from understanding it that there was a chance to find ways of prevention and correction.

I recalled what Laura often said, "It's like when doctors say the cause of some problem is 'multi-factorial.' What they mean is, we haven't a clue."

I HAD BEEN trying to help a nurse who had recently joined our ICU.

"You make me feel like I'm in kindergarten," Vicky said in exasperation. "Do you think I don't know anything? I've been a nurse for nine years. I've worked in palliative care, in obstetrics, psychiatry."

"Yes, but you've only worked in critical care for two weeks," I said.

Not only that, but you have a lot to learn, I refrained from adding, when I saw the embarrassment I was causing her. Vicky was a recent graduate from the critical care course and had been buddied with me to help ease her into the ICU.

"You hung a drug without a label on it. How would anyone else know what's in that IV bag? You stuck a needle in the patient's pillow –"

"I meant to remove it," she explained.

"But you forgot and it's a dangerous habit. You didn't transcribe the doctor's orders and see, now the patient has missed her 1400 hours dose of ampicillin."

Frances walked by to see what was going on. My face flooded red with shame. Frances, who had been so patient with me when I was new, had caught me with the tables turned.

"It's time for your break, Tilda," she told me with a wink and a shove in the direction of the door. "I'll work with Vicky."

ON ANOTHER OCCASION, just as I was getting ready to leave at the end of a shift, my patient, who had been extubated and had improved over the course of the day with me, called out.

"Nurse, I'm dying. You gave me the wrong pills. Are you trying to poison me?"

I pulled up short. There had been a time in my career when a comment like that would have made me defensive, but not any more. I looked over the medication record, reviewed the drugs I'd given, matched them against the doctor's original orders. I kept in mind that the patient was still confused from his chronic liver failure and also claimed he was making a tea party for his friends on the ceiling of the antique shop in his kitchen. I looked at the bottles and vials I'd used that day. I recalculated the dosages of drugs I'd given. Mentally, I went through all the motions of my day.

"Good night," I said to him. "Sleep well."

When I was driving home or just as I was dropping off to sleep at night, of all the many good, helpful things I had done in any given shift, the one thing that always would pop up in my mind was a medication I forgot to sign off; a volume of bodily fluid I had neglected to add to the tally; the blood work I'd sent off in a green-top test tube that should have gone in a red top.

"It happens to me, too," said Frances, "all the time."

MARIANNE SORENSEN WAS one of the sickest patients I'd ever taken care of. She had undergone a lung transplant for pulmonary fibrosis, a serious condition that in her case had no known cause and was likely terminal. Both during and after her surgery, Marianne experienced many complications: bleeding, pneumonia, an acute rejection reaction, and poor oxygenation. A drastic measure had to be implemented on the day that I was taking care of her. It was called ECMO – extra corporeal membrane oxygenation. It was an advanced, highly technological procedure, usually performed only in the operating room during open-heart surgery, to bypass the heart and lungs and take over the work of these essential organs. In Marianne's case, it would be used until her own heart and her new, but fragile lungs recovered.

That afternoon, Team Canada was in the final game of a hockey tournament against Team USA in the Olympics in Nagano, Japan. The broadcast was playing softly on the radio at the nursing station and in a number of patient rooms throughout the ICU. On and off throughout the day there were ripples of cheers or groans.

All the while, in Marianne's room, we were participating in a far more fateful Olympics. We kept our eyes on the numbers, wave-forms, and oscillator screens that helped us navigate through her body. I didn't dare look at Marianne's face because I didn't want to see a certain expression that I've seen on some patient's faces. When I see it, it sometimes makes me lose faith that we will be able to turn things around. I didn't even have a moment to glance at Marianne herself, her exposed, stretched-out body, much less her grey, ashen face, so busy was I fighting to get oxygen into her blood cells, working with the medications to increase her circulation, bal-ancing her fluids so that enough was going in, and coaxing more to come out.

Out of the corner of my eye, I glimpsed the anxious faces of her husband, mother, father, and sister, who were hovering in the background, but I had no time to answer any of their questions or offer any words of reassurance.

Toward the end of the day, Team Canada lost and we were afraid we were going to lose Marianne's life, too.

"We'll try ECMO," Daniel Huizinga told the family. "It's a last resort. Some centres have modest success with it. It may help, it may not. The next twenty-four hours will be crucial."

In one hand I held a thick tube of the bright cherry-red blood that was being returned to Marianne's body, saturated with oxygen molecules. In my other hand, I held a slightly cooler, darker tubing of blood that was flowing out of her body. It was the spent, venous blood that had been used by her body to sustain life, moment to moment. There had never been a time when I felt more literally that a patient's life was in my hands.

"I suggest you get some rest," I told the family, whom I knew had been up all night and all day. I offered them blankets and towels. "You can lie down in the waiting room. Take care of your-selves. Whatever happens with Marianne, it will be a long haul for everybody."

"Will she make it?" The mother clutched my arm, my hand – at straws.

"I don't know. We're doing our best . . . she's hanging in there." They needed more from me than that. "She's critically ill and we're fighting for her life. Right now, it's all about heartbeats, oxygen, blood pressure." Then I thought of something useful to say. "I have seen other young people who were this sick get better." That gave them some hope, I could see.

"Do you think it's safe to leave her for a little while to get some rest?" they asked.

If I said yes and something happened, they would never forgive me. If I said no, they would exhaust themselves and be of no use to themselves or Marianne. They saw my hesitation and didn't press.

For the rest of that day, I worked nonstop. Frances, Laura, Tracy, Justine, Nicole, and many others were also there, helping.

Frances tried to pull me away to take a break, even ten minutes.

"No, I can't," I insisted.

I was high on this powerful drug. It was the most thrilling thing in the world to be working so hard to save a person's life.

When my shift came to an end, it was time to hand Marianne over to the night nurse who was coming in to replace me. My heart sank when Pamela walked into the room. She was a competent nurse, but I didn't trust her to give the extra vigilance required, the extra tender touch, the kind words I wanted for the family. I toyed with the idea of staying for an overtime shift. It would be twenty-four hours and I'd be on my feet constantly, but I was pumped for action. Maybe I could do it.

"You can't do that, Tilda. It's crazy," said Frances. "You'll be exhausted. It's not safe for the patient or healthy for you. No way. Go home."

So, reluctantly, I handed over my baby to another mother, Pamela. She didn't look happy about it.

"I didn't want a busy patient," she grumbled. "I'm tired. This is my fifth night in a row. I should have called in to ask for an easier assignment."

"Why are you working so many shifts?"

"We just bought a new house and want to take the kids on vacation this winter, and I've gotten way behind on my bills. Man, I'm beat and the night hasn't even started." She took a sip from her cup of coffee.

"Maybe you'd like to switch with another nurse. Marianne is very sick. You'll definitely have a busy night. She's on ECMO."

"Shit! I've never had an ECMO patient before. It's a lot of work, isn't it?" She surveyed the huge complicated machinery and the thick tubes of blood going in and out of the patient's arteries and veins. The perfusionists were responsible for the machines, but Marianne was very unstable and would need constant, unrelenting, unwavering nursing care every minute of the night.

The next day, I couldn't wait to get back in there with Marianne and her family.

"I got her through the night, but I didn't get a break," said Pamela when she saw me. She yawned widely. "Thanks for coming in early. I can't wait to get out of here."

My worries were for nothing. Marianne had improved during the night under Pamela's care. All the work was neatly done. All the blood work drawn, vital signs recorded accurately.

"How about the family? How are they holding up?"

"What family? They called in to come see her, but I don't let families in at night. She doesn't need visitors now. The patient has to rest. The nurse too."

Marianne spent many difficult weeks in the ICU and experienced even more complications – a bowel obstruction, internal bleeding, blood infections, and briefly, kidney failure that required dialysis. Each time, we thought it was the last thing, but she made it, over and over again.

Her mother spoke to me during one of the crises. "For months now, we've had to keep preparing ourselves for the possibility that she's going to die and, at the same time, pray that she'll make it."

Marianne's body and mind made it intact, but her spirits were very low.

A photograph on the wall in Marianne's room of her beloved golden retriever, Hugo, gave me an idea. I conspired with her husband, got our nurse manager's approval, and obtained clearance from the infectious disease specialists. (I had brought a patient's dog in once before and it had definitely cheered up the patient. Unfortunately, it was the only time I ever saw a dog cry. I am certain that the boy was crying.) Some nurses were wary of my plan, but most supported me. Marianne's mother was unsure. Marianne's husband, Rick, was excited and believed wholeheartedly that bringing Hugo in would delight Marianne and lift her mood. But Pamela happened to come up in the elevator with Marianne's mom and they discussed the dog's upcoming visit.

"I wouldn't let a dog in if *I* were sick," Pamela said to the mother. "Dogs have germs. Their mouths are full of bacteria. You can get all kinds of diseases from animals and Marianne is already immunosuppressed. That's all she needs."

The mother forbade the dog to visit.

THE WORST MISTAKE I ever made is one that still fills me with regret. I saw it over and over again and didn't do anything about it. No one did. My biggest mistake was Pamela. Pamela was not lazy or stupid or disorganized. She was not bad or evil. Pamela was indifferent. Pamela was completely cut off from her patients' suffering. Perhaps that degree of apathy and disconnection from human beings – the quality that is the exact opposite of empathy – in a nurse, is a form of incompetence.

On a day when the hospital's hot water was turned off for plumbing repairs, most nurses boiled water in kettles to heat up their patients' baths. Some decided to skip the bath for that day altogether. Not Pamela. She gave her patient a bath with tepid water.

Once Pamela called a Code White – violent patient. Her patient was recovering from a drug overdose and was frightened and violent as the chemicals in his body were wearing off. He was kicking and lashing out and security guards had to be called to the ICU to help us restrain him.

"I'll tie your arms and legs down if you're not careful!" I heard her shout at him in exasperation. Later, even after he was securely restrained and sedated, it seemed to me that she was just a bit rougher with him than was necessary for her own protection.

I should have reported her. We all should have. I should have taken her aside and talked to her, nurse to nurse. I should have tried to reach out to her and make her see how hardened she had become. Perhaps I should have documented some of the things she did. We all knew it was going on and looked away, not wanting to report one of our own.

THE DOG NEVER came for a visit but I did get an opportunity to offer Marianne another pleasure. After having the breathing tube in her throat for such a long time, she had to learn to swallow again. A speech pathologist worked with her and progress was slow.

"Swallowing is crucial," she explained to Marianne. "Not just to get food in, but to protect the airway, the passage into the lungs."

One day, it was decided that we could start with a small ice chip, see how she managed with that. I sat her up in bed and placed the ice chip on Marianne's tongue. She swallowed it. Then another, and another.

"Let's take a break, now," I said.

Later, we tried again. She swallowed the ice chip eagerly, proud of her achievement.

"How was it?" I asked.

"Delicious," she sighed.

"She's doing great," I reported to the team. "I'm going to try a Popsicle."

"Okay," agreed Jessica.

"How about a Popsicle, Marianne?" I asked her.

Her eyes opened wide. "Do you think I'm ready? Do you think I can do it?"

I was confident, yet I knew that if she aspirated, it would be a mistake, another setback. I would be blamed; it would be an error of judgment. However, if it worked, what a triumph!

"Let's give it a try. Shall we?"

"Bring it on!" She pulled herself up to a sitting position.

The kitchen sent up a cherry Popsicle on a paper plate, labelled with Marianne's name.

I broke it into little pieces, let it soften and mashed it up a bit. My heart was racing.

I placed a chunk, the size of a ruby jewel, into her open mouth and her tongue carried it back.

"That's . . ." She closed her eyes.

I had to look away. She deserved privacy to experience this simple pleasure.

"That's . . ." She fell back against the pillow.

"Are you okay, Marianne?"

For a moment, I thought she had fainted. I glanced at her oxygen saturations on the monitor. I reached for my stethoscope.

She opened her eyes. She smiled a dreamy smile. "It's an orgasm."

16

A DOSE OF PHOTO-REALISM

Oh! The charms, trinkets, icons, *objets d'art*, knick-knacks, and assorted bric-a-brac I have seen at patients' bedsides over the years. I have kept a list of what I'd observed:

A filigree guardian angel; a Mario Lemieux bobble-head doll; an unopened bottle of tropical Boochoo juice from the Philippines (to have a sip of it was a dying man's unrequited last wish); West African juju charm; kirpan – a Sikh dagger – and special wooden comb and stainless steel bracelet; wreath of plastic flowers and a friendship candle (unlit); a laughing jade Buddha; hand-shaped *hamsa* with a blue-green centre (to ward off the evil eye); a cassette tape of Anne Murray's greatest hits ("If I ever hear 'Snowbird' again, I'll barf" – Morty's comment); three oranges and a clay bowl of rice; a discarded dialysis filter still containing a patient's blood, saved so that it could be buried with her; a battery-operated plastic fish that sang "Don't Worry, Be Happy"; a pair of deer antlers from a hunting expedition; vials of holy water and miniature plastic

Madonnas; laminated prayer cards of assorted saints, especially St. Jude, the saint of extreme causes; a Native Indian dream catcher and a canoe paddle; tiny scrolls in foreign calligraphy; marble rosaries and olivewood crosses; two goldfish (Pebbles and Bam-Bam) swimming in an IV bag of saline; single eagle feather; Buddhist mala beads; small jar of Long Life Rejuvenation Powder with the price tag still on – $395.

Family or friends brought these small objects to the patient's bedside. Sometimes they were taped to the wall, hung on an IV pole, thumb-tacked to a bulletin board, or pinned to a pillow (and occasionally, accidentally, bundled up and thrown out with the dirty laundry). I regarded them as salutes to the memory of the patient's former life as a healthy, ordinary person. (It was health that had conferred their ordinariness, in contrast to the extraordinary state they were in now.) These placements at patients' bedsides were like altars, the focal point for families' prayers. I marvelled at the sincere and steadfast faith of people in these desperate situations, trying to invoke the healing powers attributed to these objects.

My nursing practice had evolved in such a way that the technical tasks and skills I had worked so hard to master had long since become second nature to me. My goal had become to perform those tasks in such a way as to convey the loving kindness I felt for my patients. I wanted to minister to their mind, spirit, and emotions as thoroughly as I did to their bodies. Over the years, I have managed to create positive and healing relationships with many patients and families. However, in order to do this, it has always been imperative to me to know at least something of my patients as the people they truly are.

I have become somewhat of a detective, always prowling or sleuthing for the hints and keys that could help me solve the mysteries. In many cases, those precious objects were all that I had to go on to help me in my quest. As I looked at those mementos and held them in my hand, I pondered their meaning to the patient. I examined them for clues to the identity and personality of my patient – a person who often remained hidden, obscured and unknown. Those little objects connected me to the patient and family. They spoke to me when the patient could not. And if the patient was conscious enough to be at all aware of the surroundings, then these objects had another purpose: perhaps even a glimpse of these familiar talismans was a comfort. Maybe they would serve as an encouraging beacon or signpost along the way to the patients' desired destination: home.

However, as fascinating and poignant as I found these personal items and as much as I was touched by them, nothing affected me nearly as much as when a family member brought in a photograph. It was only then, gazing at that photograph, that I began to learn the story I longed to know. A missing puzzle piece was suddenly slipped into place.

Photographs, placed lovingly, wistfully, but above all, with great hope, at patients' bedsides always stopped me in my tracks. It was usually a picture of the person before becoming a patient, enjoying a characteristic activity. A father at a family cottage, standing on a Georgian Bay dock, holding up his big catch; a young woman glancing up from a telephone conversation to smile at the photographer; a joyful wedding day, family all around. Often, there was a picture of a grandchild or a beloved pet.

Families told me that they put those pictures there as a goad, to motivate the patient. I could also see that sometimes they served as a kind of mnemonic device to jog a patient's confused or clouded mind. Whereas the personal mementos brought to the patient's bedside were intended for the patients, I believe that the photographs were placed there for us – the nurses, doctors, and all the people caring for that person – to see. In one sense, it seemed a family's way to put us on notice: to let us know that their expectation was a return of their loved one to the previous robust state preserved in that image. Additionally, the photograph was placed there to remind us that the patient we saw in the bed looked nothing like the person they really are. "This is who they *really* are," the photograph was put in place to announce.

A stew was beginning to simmer in my mind. The meat, potatoes, onions, and carrots were incidents collected over the years in the ICU:

I LED A man to his daughter's bed. She had just returned from the OR after emergency surgery for a perforated ulcer that caused stomach contents to leak into her abdomen. She was swollen with sepsis, intubated and strapped down with all our trappings. I guided him with my arm around his shoulder.

"This is not Kelly," he said, visibly relieved that this horrible sight, whoever this was laid out in the bed that I had mistakenly brought him to see, was not his daughter.

"Yes," I said as gently as possible. "It is."

"But she's so bloated. That's not her. Kelly is slim and beautiful."

"It's called edema, or third-spacing. The tissues fill up with fluids when there is this amount of infection. It will go away in time."

"It can't be," he said, turning to leave. "It's impossible."

I showed him her hands, her fingers, and then her name band.

"Kelly," I called. "Your dad's here."

Only when she squeezed his hand did he recognize her.

COLLEEN LOOKED TERRIBLE. Emaciated and yellow, her skin was sloughing off in sheets. She was in kidney and liver failure and was so weak that she couldn't even lift her arm up off the bed. Worst of all, she'd suffered strokes that made her unable to express herself. She looked at us with helpless, frustrated eyes. We'd pulled her through pneumonia and many subsequent complications, but had mixed feelings about our "success." We'd brought her through to this?

Over her bed were pictures of her three children and one in which she was wearing a mini-skirt, skipping rope with them in front of their house.

"It was taken just last year," said her husband. "That's what Colleen *really* looks like. Not that." He looked over at the shrunken, drooling woman in the bed and made an involuntary shudder.

SOME NURSES SHARED with me their experiences with patient photographs.

"Remember the young man with the pancreatic cancer and that picture of him in his chef's hat working in that fancy restaurant?"

"How 'bout that wrinkled old lady who kept a picture – a fairly recent one, too – of herself in a sexy halter top and a pair of Calvin Klein jeans?"

"I'll never forget a patient so disfigured by a skin disease that she pinned a picture of her former self to her hospital gown. 'I was not always as you see me now,' she told me quietly."

"When I worked on the floor, I had a patient who kept a photograph taped to her hospital gown. It was a picture of her son who died over twenty years ago. He was wearing an Afro and bell-bottoms and a jean vest. 'She must have kissed that picture a million times,' her husband told me."

THE MEDICAL RESIDENT presented a case during rounds. "Mrs. Tanaka is a twenty-five-year-old woman, previously healthy, gave birth last night, full term, C-section delivery. Had a cardiac arrest, was resuscitated, is now in septic shock."

I stepped forward. "She's been improving overnight . . . vital signs are normal, good pain control, but oxygenation is still a problem."

"Let's review her X-ray," said Dr. Leung.

We discussed the details at length. Then, just as we were about to move on to the next patient, something caught my eye. A passport-sized photograph taped to the cardiac monitor. It was a petite woman in a kimono and geisha makeup, holding a pink sunshade over her shoulder with clasped white-gloved hands. Could this be her? I looked back and forth between picture and patient, patient and picture, trying all the while to picture the *person*.

"What did she have, boy or girl?" I asked.

"Girl," the resident said. "A healthy baby girl."

"REMEMBER THAT CHINESE mother who made us give those twigs and sticks and desiccated reptile organs to her son? We had to grind it all up with a mortar and pestle like in some medieval apothecary!" said Laura.

"What I can't understand," said Tracy over whom common sense always ruled, "is why people don't realize that even something natural can have side effects and drug interactions. How can we give these things, without knowing what's in them?"

"Remember how some of us refused to give the mystery mixtures and she gave the concoctions to her son, herself, down his nasogastric tube?" Laura went on. "And when he got better she believed it was because of her medicine, not ours! Can you believe it? Thousands of dollars of drugs and equipment and she thinks she cured his meningitis with her potions of eye of newt and ox balls!"

"Let her think that, what do you care?" I asked.

Morty remembered that case, too. "Daniel Huizinga told me to go ahead and give it but use lots of water to dilute it. I told him that considering all the chemicals in Lake Ontario, I'd need a prescription for that water!"

"WE HAVE TO help Ellen," said Laura, pulling me along. "She's having a meltdown."

Ellen was not a new nurse but she hadn't been there as long as we had.

We found her leaning against the counter in her patient's room, sobbing. Other nurses had taken over the care of her patient. Cardiac and thoracic surgeons had appeared out of nowhere and were swarming the room. Like high-tech carpenters, they carried with them all the instruments they needed to do the job, which in this case was open-heart surgery, right there in the patient's room. Every second counted and there weren't enough seconds available to transfer the patient to the operating room.

"Christopher learned sign language in preparation for his lung transplant," Ellen said through her tears, "so he could communicate while he was intubated. He kept signing 'thirsty,' 'thirsty,' but I couldn't give him anything to drink. Then he started it again." She showed us the "t" and "h" with her fingers. "I said to him, 'Yeah, yeah, I know you're thirsty, Chris, but you can't have anything to drink right now.' I was too busy to even talk to him. But it turned out he was going 'th' for 'thank you' and it just about broke my heart!"

Tears dripped down her cheeks, and she stared at me blankly. She was in shock. I put a blanket around her shoulders and Frances brought her a cup of juice.

I had to wonder what made an experienced nurse suddenly seize up and react as if it were her first time dealing with a tragedy. Ellen was an excellent nurse but she prided herself on never getting emotionally involved with patients.

We heard the buzz of the electric saw and looked over as the surgeon cut into the sternum and then heard the resounding crack as they pulled apart the rib cage. The bed was drenched in red.

"I was having a conversation with this guy an hour ago and now, look! They're opening his heart!" she cried. We looked closer and got a glimpse of the pulsating heart amid the sterile green towels that covered the rest of his body.

"My own brother is the same age, twenty-four," Ellen went on, needing to tell the whole story. "This young guy is a math whiz. He'd been doing so well after his surgery. His dad came in earlier this evening and showed me photographs of him. One was of Chris playing with his dog, and another was of his graduation from university. When I saw those photographs, something changed in me. For some reason, this time, I decided to make a new decision: I would open my heart to it all."

Ellen shivered, took a sip of juice, and continued. "Chris was weaning off the ventilator but around midnight, his pressure started dropping. His father had gone home and I didn't want to call him back, yet. But by 0230 hours Chris' pressure was in his boots and he was in bad shape. By 0245 hours I called the parents to tell them to come back. At 0300 he arrested. All I could think of was those damn pictures! My heart ached for the patient and his parents. Actually it felt like my heart was being ripped out of my chest. I'm telling you, I nursed this guy with my whole heart. I crossed over the protective walls that I'd always put up. Suddenly I reversed that decision and when I knew that this poor, great guy, someone's son and someone's boyfriend – I kept seeing those images in the photographs – was so sick, that he might even die, I couldn't handle it. The room was suddenly black and spinning. Thank God Tracy and Laura showed up to help me."

I was on to something. It was something I wanted to understand better. I wanted to explore, measure, test, and describe it.

"That sounds like research," said Sydney, our manager, eagerly.

"DO YOU GUYS ever take a look at some of the things people keep by their bedsides? What about the photographs the families bring in – do you notice them?" I asked my friends.

"I swear, the more paraphernalia the family hauls in, the worse the prognosis," pronounced Laura. "That's the research you should do, Tilda. Figure out the relationship between the amount of stuff they bring in and the patient's mortality rate."

She kicked a defective cardiac monitor stashed under the counter at the nursing station, ready to be sent out for repairs. "This place is really getting to me. I hate this hell hole. This place is the House of Horrors."

"Why are you still so negative? Your attitude is like poison." I rose up against her in sudden anger. "Why do this work if you hate it so much? I don't believe you, anyway. Someone who's as good a nurse as you are can't possibly hate it."

"That's what you say," she retorted. She was busy making a stuffed voodoo doll of Dr. Bristol. As he walked by she asked him, "How's your back feeling, David?" and she jabbed in a pin and chortled in a maniacal way. "Having any strange aches or pains, lately?"

He looked at her, bemused.

She'd been busy with more and more bizarre antics lately. Going from room to room, she put Hannibal Lector or Jack Nicholson's

face from *The Shining* on everyone's computer as a screensaver.
She filled Sydney Hamilton's leather briefcase with laxative pellets,
just as she once threatened she would do. She ordered a party-size
pizza with ten toppings and had it sent to Dr. Huizinga's house.
She stuffed our knapsacks with items that took us by surprise when
we opened them at home: a Foley catheter, an enema bag, or a
rectal tube (all unused!). She plastered the walls of the residents
on-call room with pictures cut out from a calendar called "Cutesy
Kitty Cats": a white Persian with a pink bow, a fluffy calico in a
basket, a tabby kitten playing with a ball of yarn. Over the years,
it seemed as if her imagination was carrying her farther and farther
away from us.

"You're going through a second childhood," I said.

"I'm reacting sanely to a mad, mad world," she cackled.

"You have a comeback for everything."

"I've applied for a job in the OR. I won't have to talk to anyone
over there and I'll just yell back at the surgeons if they give me a
hard time."

She was bluffing, but I feared one day she would follow through
on one of her threats and leave the ICU or even nursing. What a
loss that would be.

"DON'T YOU BELIEVE in miracles?" asked Gloria, one of the religious nurses. She was pinning a gold-coloured medallion engraved
with an image of hands, clasped in prayer, onto her patient's
pillow, at the family's request. She knew I was a heathen, an apos-
tate, a heretic, but there was still a chance I could become a
believer; it was never too late to be saved.

"Of course I do," I said. "Well, to be honest, I'm not sure."

"When patients get better, isn't that a miracle?"

"I don't think of it that way. When patients get better, I think
that what we did worked. That they had the resources in them to
respond to the treatments. I believe in God, but that's not how I
think God operates, granting or withholding miracles."

Gloria tried to smile. "The patients I feel saddest for are the
ones with no faith. What comfort can they have? Where are they

going when they die? I can't think of a worse or more frightening feeling. Those are the ones I feel sad for. The nurses, too," she added slyly.

"The patients I feel saddest for are the ones where we humans interfere long beyond the call of duty and prolong their earthly suffering," I said. "I feel we are torturing them."

I was ready to leave it at that, each of us holding our different views, but I caught the expression in Gloria's eyes: pity for me, clearly a lost lamb.

I DIDN'T EXPECT the reaction I received from some of the nurses in response to my research project.

"Do you think that my nursing care is any different if there's a photograph at the bedside or not?" they asked, angrily.

"*All* patients receive the best care with or without a photograph!" others insisted.

"Photographs? They're there, but I never even notice them," a few reported.

"I can't bear to see those photographs. They break my heart, especially when I realize that the patient may never look like that again, or return to that happy life."

"There's no need for a photograph when it's an organ donor! It serves no purpose!"

"Get real, Tilda. Photographs are not the cure for cancer! Why are you wasting your time with such a trivial question?" This was Morty's comment in response and she made a point of signing her name to my survey.

I explained myself first, to those who asked. "I need to get to know the patient I'm caring for. I can't just care for a body or body parts. Our patients so often can't speak for themselves and they don't even look like themselves, so I need clues, a glimpse into their world. It makes my work more meaningful."

"For me, it makes my work harder," said Tracy with a sigh. "Once I start getting too personally involved, then I know it's game over for me. You see them like they are in the bed and then the contrast in the picture of what they were like before, and it's too depressing, especially if you know they might not get back to that picture of health again."

"But some do," Frances reminded her.

There were many sacred cows in nursing. Things we did just because they had always been done that way. If nursing was to be a science, we needed reasons and rationales for what we did. Did a patient need a bath every day? Was it better to alleviate a fever or let it run its course? What were the best methods to contain the spread of infection? Was a temperature more accurate taken orally or rectally? What was the best way to care for different types of wounds to foster healing? Were we adequately alleviating our patients' pain? Were we doing enough to understand patients' experience of critical illness? What helped people get through their ordeal and what wasn't helpful? What should we tell them when family ask to bring children visitors? Was it possibly traumatic for the children? To my mind there was so much to study, questions to raise, ground to break.

THE RESPONSES TO my survey kept pouring in.

"Those pictures – I avoid them! It's disturbing to see the way the patient was before, compared with now."

"The photographs that families bring in are so depressing. I never look at them. You can still give good care without getting emotionally involved with patients."

"But," I reasoned with the ones who came to discuss the subject with me, "don't you find they help you get to know the patient? I mean, if the patients can't speak for themselves, how do you know the patient? What were they like before they got sick, what were their interests, hobbies, and professions? Who loves them? Whom do they love?"

"What do I care about all that? I can give good care to patients without getting into all of that personal stuff. They're not here for us to get to know them," someone said.

"But if you don't get to know them," I said, "aren't you just doing just technical tasks? Don't you feel a need to connect in some way with that person underneath all the tubes, wires, electrodes?"

I wanted to show them how I felt, yet I was beginning to see their point of view. These comments were coming from nurses I regarded highly. From nurses whom I would choose to take care of me or someone I loved. Was it just an idiosyncratic trait of mine, that I craved that personal connection? Perhaps knowing the patient as an individual wasn't a requirement of the job. I could see how it could be an impediment and how for many nurses it made their work more difficult. Who could blame those nurses who tried to minimize that emotional cost?

But I had always noticed how touched families were when a doctor or a nurse became emotionally involved. When a nurse cried, or a doctor had difficulty giving bad news, when our expressions of sadness began to approach theirs and met them somewhere in the middle, however briefly, I believe they felt more cared about, listened to, and comforted, regardless of the patient outcome. Yet I knew the price that these emotions exacted of us.

"I'm like you, Tillie," admitted Nicole, and Frances nodded in agreement. "I love those pictures and always look for them. Sure, they make me sad, but I still love to see them. Remember that picture of the grandfather with his grandson? The one where he was showing the little boy a bird perched on his finger? How about that elderly couple and how the wife made a collage of their life in photographs? Hiking in Arizona, snorkelling in Montego Bay. I loved the one where they were sitting intertwined. His arm was flung back against her face in a caress and one of her arms was draped across his knee, the other across the back of his shoulders. You had to look closely to be able to tell whose body was whose. He died, you know . . ."

"A GOOD RESEARCHER should be aware of any personal bias," the statistician told me. I had made an appointment with her to go over the raw data and analyze the findings. "You seem surprised with your results. Are they at odds with your original hypothesis?"

I nodded. I was guilty of doing research to prove what *I* believed.

I couldn't explain how the majority of nurses saw those pictures and needed to look away. How could I reconcile that most nurses,

82 per cent of them, reported that photographs helped them to get to know the patient better and at the same time 86 per cent stated that they found the pictures upsetting?

I presented my findings at a national critical care conference and as a result, another opportunity opened up for me. I was invited to participate in a large nursing research study, this one to determine the effects of nursing care on patient outcomes. Its purpose was to generate concrete evidence of the value of nursing care to patients. It would provide the proof needed to lobby the government for more nurses by substantiating that professional nursing care can decrease length of hospital stays, reduce complications, and improve patient satisfaction. But something in me resisted taking part in this project, even though I knew it was important work and that it was an honour to be chosen. The truth was, I was reluctant to stray too far from the bedside. I wanted to work with patients and their families and, of course, nurses. What I had discovered was that the more I did it, the more I enjoyed it and the more there was to learn – because at the heart of it all was a mystery.

ONE MORNING, AS I was still mulling over this new career opportunity, I had a conversation with a patient's wife that gave me ample proof – if I'd ever needed any – of the value of nurses' work.

Helen Fisher came to see us. It was unusual for patients' families to come back after we had transferred them out, almost unheard of if the patient died, as her husband had. He had been a patient in our ICU after a liver transplant and had developed an abdominal obstruction that required surgery, and then had numerous infections. He survived the ICU and made it up to the floor, but died a few weeks later.

"Every day when I came in, I found him in such a terrible state. He was left in such a mess," Mrs. Fisher cried. "One day I came in and his colostomy bag was so full it had exploded. There he was, lying in his own feces. It was pouring into his wound! I called for help, but it took an hour before a nurse came and she said she wasn't his nurse and she wouldn't help him!"

It was appalling that a patient could be so neglected. Yet while I commiserated with her, I could at the same time envision the nurses' situation and my heart went out to them, too. I knew the conditions on the floor and what the nurses' workload was like. There were two or three nurses for as many as forty patients who were just as sick and needy as John Fisher had been. Nurses were running ragged in all directions, trying to meet everyone's needs, handing out medications, changing dressings, taking vital signs, having to chart every single thing they did – all their efforts a sort of piecework marathon in a factory sweatshop. They were overworked and exhausted. No matter how much they tried, they could never master the work. They were Sorcerer's Apprentices: each one filling buckets of water to empty an endlessly overflowing fountain.

What Mr. Fisher had needed was good nursing care and if the conditions had been right, he could have received it and it would have made all the difference, whether he had lived or died.

Privately, Helen Fisher confided even more to me. It was a moment so intimate and precious, and that she chose to share it with me is a gift I will always treasure.

"So I cleaned him up myself. Then I wanted to get him up to walk around the ward. But first he drew the curtains around and pulled me behind them. 'Come here, Helen,' he said, 'I want to touch your breasts.' There he was, so sick, so debilitated, and with a shit bag hanging from his belly, and he could still think of making love to me. Oh, how I adored that man!"

She cried in my arms, and other nurses who had also got to know her gathered around to comfort her as well. What research would capture that?

Perhaps I was foolish to dismiss the opportunity to participate in the research project, but I was loath to do anything that would put me at a remove from patient care. And I balked at the notion that we still had to prove what was obvious to most of us: nurses helped make people better. When could we just get on with doing our work? Why did we still need validation of our worth?

Even Florence Nightingale had done a similar research study during the Crimean War. She documented the work that the nurses

did, the rate of infections of the soldiers and the number of their
wounds that healed. She proved the effectiveness of professional
nursing care by measuring outcomes way back then and here we
were, over two hundred years later, still doing it.

"You don't know what a nurse does until you need one. That's
the only way people understand it," said Laura when I told my
friends about the research study.

"They think going into research is the only way to advance your
career," said Morty. "Why is leaving the bedside always regarded
as a step up? It's because shift work is seen as demeaning. What
do these administrators think goes on in this place 'after hours'?
Do they ever notice all the nurses streaming into the hospital when
they walk out the door at the end of the day? Do they have any
idea how marginalized we feel working during odd hours – nights,
weekends and holidays, with no support staff, no places to rest or
study during breaks, no place to get a healthy meal, no educational
in-services or workshops, no administrators, teachers or nursing
leaders during those off hours?"

"Hey, Morty! Would you get off your platform or soap box or
bandwagon, or whatever it is you're on, and get back to work?"
chided Laura.

OVER THE YEARS, one by one, all the nurses who had teased me
about my university degree and even those who had scoffed at
the need for a nurse to even have a degree in the first place,
were registering for university programs in nursing. They are
completing their degrees – some even going on to do graduate
work in nursing – and at the same time they're juggling having
babies, raising kids, finding child care, supporting a household,
and working their fair share of nights and weekends as nurses.
They do it because the pressure is on and they know they have
to, to ensure their marketability. But once there, I see how they
love learning and how higher education is transforming them
into even better nurses.

"You don't want to end up like another Laura or Frances, do
you?" a nursing instructor asked me one day, after she heard that

I had turned down the prestigious research job offer. "Nurses like them aren't going anywhere. They're staying right at the bedside. They're going to be stuck there forever. Without a degree in nursing, their options are so limited. You have a degree, and if you go on to do a Master's you could teach or do research."

End up like a Laura or a Frances? Did I hear her correctly?

Did she know what I would give to be a nurse of their calibre? To have an ounce of their intuition, their skills, their wisdom and compassion? Did she have any idea how those nurses went by the book and followed all the rules and knew just when to abandon the book and the rules in order to save the day – and the patient? Sure, they could update their knowledge or learn new theories, or become teachers or administrators – but what a loss to patients *that* would be! I stood there, dumbfounded and dismayed that this teacher didn't know this herself. How far removed some of our leaders were from patients.

THOSE SMALL SOUVENIRS and the personal photographs I come across at patients' bedsides continue to intrigue me. Sometimes I think they are the only gifts our patients can bear. Even patients who are known music lovers can't listen to a sonata if they are in pain. Nor do they seem to wish to be read or sung to. Their pain and discomforts overwhelm them and require their full concentration. No poetry, no music, no TV or radio for the critically ill. It is only when patients start to recover that they begin to tolerate these things, just barely and gradually. Beauty was too much for seriously ill people. There was even a sign at the front door of the ICU that prohibited it.

"No Flowers."

"Why?" I had asked Laura once. "Surely bright colours –"

"They're a source of infection and many people are allergic. Then there's the old wives' tale that flowers gobble up too much oxygen, especially at night. Those scavenging tulips! Down, you nasty nasturtiums! You greedy roses!" She barked at an innocent potted plant sitting on the desk at the nursing station, to the amusement of the ward clerk sitting by the phone.

"I had no ideas flowers were so dangerous. And violent, too."

Frances nodded. "Don't you remember on the wards how the head nurse used to go around on evenings and take the flowers out of the patients' room and put the vases on the floor outside their door?"

"Sounds creepy," I said.

"Yeah, and then in the morning, they'd bring the flowers back."

Morty began to sing the old ballad about where have all the flowers gone, a long time ago.

"But isn't there more we could do to make the ICU a more pleasant place?" Tracy asked. "What if we had beautiful paintings, wall hangings, and quilts on display? What if we had a waterfall in here or a source of sunlight, or an indoor garden? Not everything has to be functional, does it? Maybe being around art could help people feel better."

"Yeah, why don't we get some feng shui happening here?" said Nicole.

"Florence Nightingale wrote about this, too," I said. "She said that the main thing a nurse could do was to put the patient in the best condition for nature to do the work of healing. She wrote about nutrition, fresh air, rest, light, cleanliness, privacy, a pleasing atmosphere, peacefulness, comfort, a cheerful environment."

"Yeah, well, all that's gone out the window," said Laura. "If there was a window for it to go out, in this place. No windows allowed. We're sealed in here like in a mausoleum. No fresh air. Why do you think our clothes and shoes are so tight by the end of the day? Why do you think we're all stuffed up and sneezing when we come to work? There's no circulation in here. Why do we have so much sick time? Why do you think we get headaches, especially in those rooms?" She pointed over to a few particularly poorly ventilated rooms that were rumoured to be migraine producing. "This is a sick place. Look at what we're dealing with now."

She pointed to our isolation room, where we had recently admitted a patient with a mysterious pneumonia. SARS (Severe Acute Respiratory Syndrome) had arrived and it was changing the way we did almost everything. Everyone was terming it the "new normal," but how would things ever be normal again? There were many inconveniences and discomforts, but far worse than all of that was that now, each time we walked into a patient's room, we were afraid for our lives.

In our hospital, we treated many SARS patients and suspected SARS patients. A few of them worsened and had to come to our ICU. It was terrifying to go in to the room and know that each time we did so we were putting ourselves, each other, and our families at risk. We coped by taking turns sharing the responsibility of caring for these patients. We offered one another words of encouragement and covered one another generously for breaks. Every time we went into a patient's room, we helped each other don the bulky protective gear. First, we tied on long gowns and strapped a hefty negative pressure filter machine to our waists. Then we put on two or three pairs of gloves – taping them down tight at the wrists – bonnet and booties, and then goggles that fogged up and masks that pinched our noses raw. On top of all this equipment, we pulled on a full-length space suit that puffed out with the blowing of the negative pressure machine. We looked like roly-poly astronauts. It was unbearably hot and cumbersome as we worked silently and alone in the room, caring for a patient who could only see our eyes looking back at them over our masks. Somehow, once we met the patients' eyes and saw how terrified *they* were, we found the courage to offer the care and comfort we were there to give. In many ways it was our shining hour. We congratulated one another and tried our best to keep up the morale.

But it was a frightening, chaotic time and many nurses were angry. Every day the information changed as the experts were learning about this new disease. It seemed as if almost every day that we came to work there was a new set of rules about the appropriate gear needed to protect ourselves. The lengthy screening process of every patient, staff member, and visitor was oppressive, but unavoidable. The stringent precautions we had to take for all patients slowed us down. There were many troubling questions that were left unanswered. Infectious disease experts and public health officials did their best to keep us informed, but nonetheless, new and contradictory information surfaced on a daily, sometimes hourly, basis.

Our work felt overwhelming and we were afraid. When I mentioned where I worked to a neighbour, he jumped ten feet away and continued our conversation at that distance. Some people I met during that period praised me for my work, yet refused to shake my hand or come near me. Even though only a few of us were actually exposed and had to be quarantined, we all knew of many nurses and other professionals who were quarantined, and a few who did in fact contract SARS.

Many nurses and other staff continue to feel angry and resentful about the dangers our work exposes us to. Yet I believe that during the crisis of SARS, we received the most up-to-date information that was available under the circumstances. There were problems and inefficiencies due to the sudden, excessive strain on the health-care system, but within my limited experience, I don't believe anyone is to blame.

Others feel differently. I heard one nurse preparing to go into a SARS patient's room and while she was undergoing the time-consuming suiting-up process, assisted by another nurse, I could hear her from where I sat at the nursing station.

"I haven't seen a doctor all day," she said. "I heard one resident tell another, 'Minimize how much you go in. Let the nurse go in.' They're basing their treatment solely on my assessment and my observations of the patient." Her tirade continued when she came out of the patient's room, after she stripped off all the gear. I saw her flushed face and the sweat dripping off her arms and darkening the back of her uniform. "They should pay us danger pay," she grumbled as she scrubbed her hands at the sink.

"This isn't the time to be asking for more money! The public's health and safety are at stake. We all knew there were risks in this line of work when we went into it," Laura said.

"Don't we have the right to refuse unsafe work?" she shot back.

"Come on," said Laura. "Dealing with infection is nothing new for any of us. We've all had needle stick injuries, splashes in our eyes with all kinds of fluids and we've all cared for patients with AIDS and hepatitis. Don't you remember when Tracy got that scare with the tuberculosis patient and had to go on medication when she was pregnant?"

"Remember that time we were giving that experimental drug and you had to sign a waiver that you weren't pregnant, allergic, wearing contact lenses, or on steroids before you went in there? Now that was scary!" Nicole said.

"How about last year with that 'flu epidemic and we all had to be vaccinated before coming back to work here? This is a hazardous place. Enter at your own risk," Tracy said.

"Yeah, but this is different. SARS can be fatal," she reminded us and that gave us a moment's pause. "Don't you think we should be compensated for this new danger?" She continued, "The managers all got vouchers for fancy hotels and a night on the town. They got bonuses. What did we get? A movie coupon and a T-shirt! Oh, and a certificate of 'thank you very much, for risking your lives' from the management."

"At least be glad we're spared the exposure to the real dangers: flowers and ferns," I said and at long last, one of my jokes got a rise out of them.

"IN CONCLUSION," I said looking around from the podium, "we need to find ways to support nurses in the emotionally dangerous work we do. Many nurses found these photographs upsetting. This finding attests to the emotional price our work exacts of us. We know a lot about the looming nursing shortage, workload issues, burnout, the hazards in our working environment, and the moral distress in our institutions. However, this research documents another kind of stress that is equally infectious, risky to our health, and difficult to treat. We have to recognize that nurses are affected by the sadness of our work. The constant proximity to this degree of suffering is eroding our emotional health. Nurses are suffering. We need to find ways to assist nurses to cope with these perils of our work."

The audience clapped politely. What I was saying wasn't new. It was well known that nurses' work is difficult and stressful. Sometimes even depressing and now, more than ever, dangerous. But nurses have always taken on the sorrow and suffering of the world. Most of us are proud to be nurses, but reluctant to speak publicly about these challenges, since those in helping professions aren't supposed to complain.

The audience turned their attention to the next speaker, who would speak about a topic with which everyone was more familiar and comfortable: Guidelines for Nursing Care of the Patient in Fulminant Hepatic Failure.

17

A PRISONER OF WAR

Tracy bounded over to me as I was starting my day and she was coming to the end of her night shift. We didn't work together as much any more because she'd had to change her schedule in order to accommodate the early-morning university classes she was taking.

"How can you possibly listen to a lecture now?" I asked, scanning her face for signs of fatigue. "You must be exhausted."

"No, I'm not at all." Her eyes were lively, but something was troubling her. "This course I'm taking has got me thinking. Do you remember Mr. Kerr's death? I wanted to talk to you about how we could have done it differently."

We all remembered the details about our patients, especially their deaths. Even when a patient died when we weren't at work, we sought out the nurse who had been there, to tell us what had happened so that we could put it to rest in our minds.

"His death was terrible. The son was so upset with us. Remember how we left the tube in because we thought it would be too upsetting for the family to hear the sounds of his last breaths? But that just made it go on longer. We gave him morphine to make

him look better and make the family feel better. The narcotic was
for the family! They couldn't bear to see anything that looked like
he was struggling. Who were we serving?"

"I know." I remembered this and much more. We had increased
the rate of the morphine drip as the father gasped his last breaths,
but even with morphine, he'd opened his eyes and looked around.
Perhaps it seemed to the son that his father wanted to say something, but couldn't. The mother was sobbing, the daughters were
clinging to the mother, and the son was furious. "You promised he
wouldn't suffer," he had cried.

"Sometimes it feels like we are orchestrating the whole process
to make the families feel better. It doesn't feel honest. We didn't
want to hasten it or prolong it, but remember how the family kept
asking how much longer it would take? They wanted it over quickly
and they assumed we could arrange that," said Tracy, who suddenly
did look weary. "Which we can, of course. They were shocked
when I turned off the monitor, but we weren't using it any more."

We had all seen this reaction time and time again. Families rely
on the monitor. They become so glued to it, sometimes for weeks,
and then when the time comes and we pushed the "off" button, it
is as if that is the moment of death.

"I know. They looked like my kids look at me when I turn off
the TV and tell them to go to bed. It's like they can't believe I'd do
this to them!"

We laughed uneasily.

"Mr. Kerr's death has been haunting me," said Tracy. "We
didn't handle it very well."

I agreed. "The way a patient dies in the ICU is the nurse's responsibility. Decisions are made – or not – in the family meeting, but in
the end, the care of the dying patient is left to the nurse."

I thought for a moment. "Trace, how would you have done that
death differently?"

"I don't know, but the son was so angry at us," said Tracy. "I
can't stop thinking about it."

"But the real reason the son was angry was that his father was
dying."

"I know," she said and suddenly looked deflated. It was as if the fatigue, from having worked all night, suddenly occurred to her. I watched as she came to a halt, let down. But a second wind kicked in and she rallied to continue our debriefing.

"Then remember how afterwards we brought the family back in, as we always do, after we tidied him up, removed the IVs, tubes, and machines, and freshened the room. We made sure everything was nice and neat. We wanted to show them that he looked like himself again. Exactly how he would have looked if he'd died naturally. Sometimes, how we handle death feels dishonest."

"I know," I sighed.

"You know how sometimes we joke around afterwards?" Tracy continued. "I hate myself for it, but can't seem to stop. Once I leaned over a corpse I was wrapping with another nurse to turn up the radio to catch a song I liked. I guess I had to make a disconnect with what I was really doing."

"I know what you mean," I said. "Just the other day, I was wrapping a body for the morgue and Morty was going on her tirade again about the shrouds and how they're an occupational hazard. 'Why do they make shrouds from this toxic plastic stuff?' she was saying. You know how when we open them up they have that industrial chemical smell that we all try to avoid inhaling? 'They're going to make us sick,' she says. 'Why can't they make biodegradable shrouds? You know, dust to dust. Eco-friendly shrouds! There's a market for that!' So, to the tune of 'Born Free,' she starts singing, 'Die Green'!"

Oh, how we howled at things that were not the least bit funny, but the fleeting pleasure of the intoxication was rarely worth the queasy hangover of discomfort.

WE CLAIMED WE had seen everything, done everything. We were unshockable and unshakable. We boasted that nothing fazed us. We were seasoned veterans and felt confident that we could handle anything. After all, we'd dealt with the worst-case scenarios. We'd seen every drastic, catastrophic thing that could possibly happen to a human being. We were wrong. One day a patient rolled in that changed everything.

I received Mr. Bellissimo from the OR. He had cancer of the prostate that had spread to his bladder. But cancer was the least of his problems. He arrested on the floor and then developed a pulmonary embolism after a long cardiac resuscitation. Most troubling was the finding on the CT scan of his brain damage due to prolonged oxygen deprivation. However, nothing about any of that was unusual to us. We had seen other patients like him before; patients like him, and worse.

"We've managed to stabilize your father, right now," I told his two grown-up daughters, Maria and Theresa, as I brought them into the ICU for the first time, "but he's still critically ill."

"Up on the floor, they worked on him for hours," Maria, the older one, said. "But maybe, if they had gotten to him sooner, things would have been different?"

"I don't know," I said, "but sometimes it can be difficult to resuscitate a seventy-six-year-old heart."

Wait, I wanted to warn them. *Stop, for a minute. Don't let us do all of this. If you let us, we'll go too far and then it will be harder to stop than not to have started at all.*

Mr. Bellissimo experienced no major crises or setbacks in the first few days, but even Dr. Huizinga and the surgeons looked uncharacteristically grim. They didn't paint their usually optimistic picture to the family. I tried to be positive when I spoke to the daughters. After all, it was too soon to predict that a man this ill couldn't get better, even though my intuition told me otherwise.

"We're doing everything we can for him," I assured his daughters, who were busy setting up camp in the waiting room, determined to stay for the duration.

For some reason, in case I might have thought otherwise, Maria said, "Dad's a real fighter."

"That's good," I said. "He will have a long road to recovery."

"He loves to dance," she said, and I was pleased she wanted me to know that about him.

"Bring in a picture of your dad, if you wish. We'll put it up on the wall for everyone to see."

"Unfortunately, he never danced with our mother," I heard Theresa mutter.

"Mom died last year," explained Maria, glaring at her sister to be quiet. "Dad lives with me."

"How was he before he got sick?"

"Plays bocce ball every Saturday! Drinks a double espresso before bed every night."

"Plus a grappa or two," murmured Theresa.

"Dad has a great sense of humour," Maria said and looked over at him with dutiful adoration. "Don't you, Dad? Nurse, I'll give you an example of just how funny he is."

"When he's sober," interjected Theresa bitterly.

"If anyone ever asked Dad if he had any children, he used to say, no, but my wife has two."

Maria shook her head in amazement at her father's extraordinary wit.

A week later, Mr. Bellissimo developed an intestinal blockage and needed emergency surgery. Even Dr. Huizinga, famous for taking on challenges that no one else would touch, looked worried. When I came into the room to visit Morty, who was taking care of him that day, I found Daniel with his hands deep in the muck of the patient's bleeding intestines. He took the patient back to the OR but when he returned he was still bleeding. We hung unit after unit of blood (we stopped counting at sixteen) and just as we pumped it into his veins, it oozed back out through his incision. Blood flowed onto the mattress, dripped down off the sides of the bed onto the floor. I went to get a mop.

"I'm going to bring the Red Cross in here so they can see where their precious resource is going!" Morty announced, looking down at her blood-splattered running shoes. "What a waste!"

Theresa was fidgety and tended to come and go while Maria was stalwart and sat in the room for most of the day, watching the cardiac monitor. I remembered Tracy's comment and saw how Maria was watching the monitor exactly like it was a TV, with her eyes glued to her favourite program.

"I'm keeping an eye on Dad's heart," she explained when she noticed me watching her watching.

When I bent over him, to listen to his lungs and heart with my stethoscope, Maria regarded me as if I might, if I chose to do so, invoke the miracle they were praying for. The intensity of her gaze and the expectations it held, were unbearable because I had come to the realization that in her father's case, I didn't believe in what I was doing. Even worse, I had come to the conclusion that what we were doing was wrong, because it was causing suffering for no benefit.

"We've talked about it and decided we want to have everything done," Theresa said when she joined her sister in the afternoon.

"Is it what your father would want?" I asked.

I decided not to wait for the family meeting to be called, arranged, and endured. I took the initiative to tell them what I knew. "It doesn't look very good. The CT scan shows massive brain damage. He's still critically ill. Have you thought at all about the possibility that he might not recover?"

"Yes, but that nice female doctor, you know, the pretty Chinese one? She said he might not recognize us. That he might get the words, but not know their meaning. That's okay with us." Maria spoke for them both. "We'll take him like that."

"Even before all this happened he sometimes thought it was 1950 and he was still in Italy," said Theresa with a giggle.

Oh well, at least the war is over.

"She said it might be like he'll be one of those people who see the golf club and the golf ball, but can't bring the two together. That wouldn't be so bad, would it?" Maria reasoned.

"That would describe a lot of beginning golfers," said Theresa with a grin that looked to me, at that moment, positively goofy.

Two and a half weeks later Mr. Bellissimo was still there and the daughters chose to interpret his "survival" as evidence of his innate fighting spirit. However, their father was now full of a raging blood infection and pneumonia, too. We had him on three different inotropes at maximum doses to maintain his blood pressure, the systolic hovering only around 85.

"His X-ray looks like a snowstorm," Nicole told me when I went in to cover for her break. "It's a total white-out. Take a look at it. The daughters haven't a clue how to interpret what they've been told about the CT scan of his brain," she said. "They say it's like if he'll see a coffee cup, he might put his hand into the coffee, rather than grasp the handle. He's got global cerebral hypoxia, for goodness' sakes. He's going to be in a vegetative state, if he even recovers from everything else wrong with him. Why doesn't someone spell it out for them in terms they can understand?"

"Go for lunch," I urged her.

Since Mr. Bellissimo couldn't move by himself, we repositioned his body every few hours to make him comfortable. I called for Lola, the hospital assistant, to help me. At first she wasn't paying attention, but all of a sudden I saw her eyes fill with tears as she looked down at the patient's swollen face, ballooned out and straining tightly around the breathing tube, his black fingers and toes, his skin, dripping with infected sores.

"Your father, Lola. Where is he?" I asked.

"In Bosnia," she said quietly.

"Sarajevo?" I asked because I didn't know the name of any other city.

"No, Banja Luka," she said. "This man is the same age as my father. I would hate to see my father like this. Why are they doing this to him? Don't they see how cruel it is?"

"I don't know."

All the nurses were aware of Mr. Bellissimo's case, and it was to his room that our gaze turned with mystified curiosity and incredulity when we arrived at the beginning of each shift. We were all checking to see if he was still there.

Another week passed and Mr. Bellissimo was still hanging on, after yet another cardiac arrest and a few more complicated setbacks: infections, intestinal obstructions, and more organ failure.

Morty called in the night before a shift and requested to be his nurse the next day.

"I've decided what I'm going to do," Morty told us when she came in. She was wearing her "No Whining" sweatshirt and dangling earrings in the shape of tiny inukshuks. There was a determined, devilish look in her eye that I had never seen before. I decided to keep a close watch on her.

On rounds, Dr. Huizinga put forth a pathetic case for continuing treatment.

"What I mean to say," he said and pushed his glasses up to his head so that he could rub his eyes, "is that I am attempting to determine the extent to which, by that I mean the extent to which I, and hopefully in conjunction with Mr. Bellissimo's daughters that is, but this may or may not be the case, and with all due respect to Dr. Dejenni," he gave a deferential glance to a visiting colleague, "who's come here at my request to offer a second opinion – notwithstanding the hospital's exorbitant parking fees . . ."

"He's floundering," I said, embarrassed for him.

"What a ditherer!" exclaimed Nicole in astonishment.

"He's a coward." Laura was disgusted.

Yet we were all so fond of him. We knew he was kind and caring, and a brilliant and daring doctor.

"He's an idiot," Morty blurted out.

Daniel overheard her and looked crushed.

"Go apologize to him, right now," I told her. "You've hurt his feelings."

"No way." She folded her arms across her chest.

"Justine, I have a sense you're in disagreement with the treatment plan," Dr. Huizinga said.

"Don't you disagree, too? Be honest, Danny! You can't even defend what we're doing. You can't even come up with a convincing case for it."

"No. I have to admit . . ." He hung his head. "We are bound by the family's wishes. Say, are they perhaps motivated by religious beliefs?" he speculated. "Are they Catholic?"

"If these people are in any way religious," said Morty, glaring at him, "their father is in purgatory."

Later, Morty read out loud to all of us gathered at the nursing station the note that Dr. Huizinga had scribbled in the patient's chart:

" 'The severity of the situation was explained, along with the possible limitations of escalating treatment. My view is that his survival is not guaranteed and the most likely outcome is non-survival.' "

"*Non-survival!* Isn't that the richest euphemism you've ever heard?" Morty said. "What bullshit! This is the crap he writes on a patient who is practically dead?"

No one rose to her bait. We'd heard it all before, so many times, and we needed a break from talking about it, thinking about it, and most of all, from doing it day and night. The hundreds of versions of this same conversation had finally left us exhausted.

As soon as the daughters walked in the door later that morning, Morty was ready for them.

"Maria. Theresa. Today I'm going to answer all your questions. I will tell you everything you want to know. Would you like to see what we're doing to your father? Good. Here goes." She grabbed the curtain, pulled it around the bed, and flung off the blankets that had been covering their father. Morty stripped back his gown and showed them his bloated body, the mottled limbs, the necrotic fingers and toes, wrinkled and black as prunes.

"Dead tissue," she said.

The sickening smell of his exposed, rotting body quickly filled the room.

"These fingers and toes will fall off, any day now," she said evenly. "These too," she said as she showed them his testicles, the size of two bulging cantaloupes. She pointed out how they were leaking rivulets of clear yellow fluid all over the soaked, folded towels upon which they had been propped. She allowed them to register these sights for a few minutes.

I kept my eyes on the daughters' horrified faces and took a mental note of where the chairs were in case I had to catch them if they fainted.

"I'm now going to suction the secretions out of his lungs," said Morty, evenly.

They watched him strain and cough and choke as she pushed the plastic catheter into his lungs and then as it sucked out strings and clumps of green sputum. Morty suctioned his black mouth, which was full of sores and blood clots.

As she prepared to clean around his tracheostomy with swabs dipped in hydrogen peroxide, something caught Morty's eye. She looked down, leaned closer, and what she saw there made her reel back in horror. With a pair of tweezers she picked out two long white wriggling things.

"Maggots!" She gagged and dropped them on the floor.

I retched, too, and looked about for a garbage can I thought for a moment I might need.

"Maggots fester in dead tissue!" she practically shouted at them as the two daughters ran out, sobbing.

"This is a corpse. I have never been so disgusted in my whole life." Morty peeled off her gloves and threw them in the garbage. We both went over to the sink to wash our hands.

We went outside the room to get as far away as allowed and possible from the situation.

"A corpse doesn't disgust me, but *nursing* a corpse does," she said. It was the first time I had ever heard her voice go quiet.

"If he was really a corpse, I wouldn't feel as bad, but he's a living human being that we are heaping this indignity upon," I said. "Who knows what he's feeling?"

"They treat prisoners of war better than this," Morty said.

"We're torturing him, whether he feels it or not."

"ARE YOU SUGGESTING that our treatment of Mr. Bellissimo is *futile*?" Dr. David Bristol asked me on rounds when he heard my complaints.

"Please don't put words into my mouth," I said. "I didn't say that."

"You – and many of the nurses – have been implying it."

"Okay, yes, I'll say it. What we are doing is futile." It felt so strange to say that word. It was a word I'd never said before. I'd never tasted it in my mouth before. It was so concentrated and bitter.

How could I do this work if I thought any of it futile?

"Futility." David spat out the word. "Can you define it for us?"

He waited and the team listened closely with him.

He'd trapped me into doing something that was against my nature. Futility meant there was no hope, and if nursing had taught me anything, it was that there was always reason to hope. If one knew what to hope for. Not always hope for a cure or a complete recovery, but hope for peace, comfort, and dignity.

"Futility? I can't define it exactly, but I know it when I see it," I said lamely.

"That's not good enough," he said, amused at my discomfort. "Give me proof."

"It seems to me, David, that we're being devious here. Families see all the technology we have to offer and they want to believe it can help their loved one, too. They don't know enough to decide whether or not it is warranted. They don't want to have to make those decisions themselves. Who can blame them? We all know that someone of Mr. Bellissimo's age who has this many serious medical problems cannot survive. Yet we act as if it's a possibility. We expect the family to help us choose – do they want inotropes? Compressions? Dialysis? Shocks? All of the above? We make it like a Chinese menu – one from column A, one from column B, and they have to place the order all by themselves."

"No *sub-sta-too-shuns*," said Morty, but for once, her interjection didn't break the tension.

"And," I said, "we're not doing enough to interpret these situations for families so that they understand the implications of their decisions. The public is informed by pop culture, television, and sensational stories in the press. People hear about miracles cures, overnight recoveries, and unexpected successes. They have no idea what's really in store for them when they come here and they're in no state to make rational decisions. They're worried that someone will accuse them of not doing the right thing or they worry that they won't be able to live with themselves afterwards. Their decisions are based on fears of possible regret. The responsibility is too much for them to bear."

I stood there recalling another discussion on the subject of futility. It was a terrible argument I'd had once with my husband, the most positive, optimistic person I know. I told him how angry I was and how I had tried so hard to get along with him, but that it was no use.

"I have tried and tried to communicate with you," I said. "I can't try any more."

"There can never be enough trying," he yelled back at me.

As angry as I was – and, thankfully, we eventually made up – even in those heated moments, how I loved his hope, in the face of my temporary loss of faith.

"Tilda, if you can't handle this situation, I suggest you not take care of this patient."

"David, you're right. I can't handle the situation. Do you want to know why? Because what we're doing to Mr. Bellissimo is wrong."

Most doctors just couldn't make the switch. To them, even an artificial semblance of life was preferable to what they saw as the worst possible outcome, the failure of all their efforts: death. Something preventable, diagnosable, or treatable must have been missed. Perhaps it was born out of a fear that some family member would come forward and accuse them of an oversight, or of not trying hard enough. But perhaps because of our immediate, first-hand proximity to our patients' suffering, most nurses felt differently.

"When it comes to doing deaths, you guys are like Wayne Gretzky trying to figure skate!" said Morty and finally managed to get a weak semblance of the reaction she wanted out of them.

THE FOLLOWING WEEK, Dr. Huizinga was the attending staff physician, and he was the next to have to face an unruly insurgence of the rabble. We accosted him with our outrage and indignation.

"Talk to the daughters about withdrawing treatment!"

"Enough is enough!"

"It's time to let nature take its course!"

"We've gone too far this time!"

"It's refreshing to hear the nurses' perspectives," he said, stepping back from us. "Frankly, it's one I've tended not to pay much attention to. A physician has to be optimistic. It's difficult to be the bearer of bad news. Perhaps we avoid these conversations with patients because of our own discomfort. Perhaps we don't take the time to explain everything thoroughly."

"We lead people to believe that we can cure everything," I said.

"You're probably right," he conceded unhappily. "Ah, medicine is an art, but patients expect doctors to be scientists and know everything," he said.

Spoken like a true scientist.

Later that day, Mr. Bellissimo's daughters came to me with a suggestion.

"If Dad's brain is damaged, could he have a brain transplant?" Their eyes were bright.

I looked at them, stunned. I didn't say anything. I didn't know where to begin.

"And another thing," said Maria, "my daughter read on the Internet that breast milk can help people fight infections."

"What?" *Were they prepared to offer some?*

"Yes," she said, "breast milk boosts immunity."

"Where are you going to get . . . it?" I inquired.

"Isn't there a maternity ward in this hospital?"

"No, there isn't any more." It was true. Our "general" hospital had become so specialized that something normal like the birth of a baby or even the routine removal of an inflamed appendix was not performed. "There is no maternity ward here," I said unhelpfully.

"You think because he has cancer that he's a lost cause," Maria said to me as a warning. "Don't give up on him so easily. He'll surprise you."

THE BELLISSIMO CASE made me recall a patient I'd once taken care of who was a survivor of Auschwitz. I needed to insert an IV and the best vein I could find was a beautiful thick one running right through the concentration camp number tattoo on her arm. Perhaps this place now will give life, not remind her of near death

and total evil, I rationalized, as I slid the angiocath into the com-
pliant vein and received my reward of the red flashback of blood
to tell me that I was in the vein.

I couldn't help myself but ask the husband to tell me about what
his wife had been through.

"They called her Christine," he said. "They changed her name
from Esther and hid her. She was lucky one, see? Blond and blue
eyes. But they found her and sent her to the camp."

"Which is worse," I had to ask, "this or that?" I shuddered.

"That," he said without hesitation and stared at me, unblinking.

Together, we took a look over at her. Her hands, contracted into
hardened claws, scraped at the air as if trying to escape. Her face
was frozen into an anguished, contorted grimace.

"She survived that horror . . . hasn't she been through enough?"
I guess I gave myself a certain licence to be familiar in this case, to
push my questions past a barrier I had never crossed before.

"She survived that, she'll survive this." He sat down to read
a Yiddish newspaper, one that looked like it had survived the
war, too.

BETWEEN THE TWO of them, Mr. Bellissimo's daughters kept up the
round-the-clock vigil. However, eventually Theresa had to return
to her family and work, but Maria was there when I came in one
morning. I encouraged her to tell me about her father. I listened to
how he had tried in vain to persuade her daughter not to marry a
boy from Trinidad and how he had loved the delicious lasagna she
made. Maria trimmed his beard, smoothed the blankets, and
exchanged the blue one for the yellow one. She rubbed his feet and
put mineral oil on them.

"We're not religious," she explained, "but we were brought up
Catholic, taught to respect our father – even if he doesn't exactly
respect us."

"What do you mean?"

"He's a tough son of a – excuse me. He's very . . . strict." She
pursed her lips. "Anyway, we're hoping for the best, but trying to
be realistic."

"Do you understand the situation?" I asked.

"Yes, but we believe he'll make it. I asked Dr. Bristol if there was any chance he'd make it and he said that there's less than 1 per cent chance. But even if that's the case, we're willing to take it. All we're asking for is a 100 per cent effort. It's worth it for a human being, don't you agree?" She pulled a Blue Jays baseball cap out of a plastic bag she'd brought with her and then a Maple Leafs cap and put one on either side of her father's swollen head. Diagonally across his body, she draped a banner that said *Forza d'Italia* in red, green and white.

"REMEMBER JOAN HOUSLEY? Why can't more families be like hers?" the nurses asked one another.

When they realized that a cure for their mother's advanced cancer was not possible, Mrs. Housley's husband, Jim, along with their three daughters, Jill, Janet, and Jenny, all agreed when I suggested we turn off the cardiac monitor and focus our attention on her comfort and dignity, on Joan herself. But I had had to make my case before the team, beforehand.

"It's not as if we're going to treat an arrhythmia, are we? We're not going to do CPR, right?" I argued. I saw Daniel considering this radical move I was suggesting. "I've heard you say it yourself, Danny, 'Don't do a test unless you're prepared to treat the results.'"

I saw how difficult it was for him to shift his thinking, how hard he had to work to restrain himself, to do nothing and not feel the ensuing sense of defeat.

The night Joan did arrest, Tracy and Nicole sat with her until her family arrived. The resident on that night was young and hesitant. He hadn't got to know her as we had.

"Don't you think we should give it a try?" he said. "Just one round of CPR?"

"No. We know her wishes." I stood firm. "She told us, herself."

"But no one documented it," he whined.

"Trust me," I said.

After six weeks, the Bellissimo daughters hardly visited any more. Even Maria called only occasionally or sent a fax of her questions or suggestions. A lone granddaughter came a few times.

"He's leaking on me," she said, holding up her scarf to show me.

"His skin is falling off," I said. "It happens when the person is . . ." *Dead*, I wanted to say . . . "Terribly sick."

"What would happen," she ventured – and I knew exactly what she was going to ask – "if everything were turned off?"

She wouldn't dare ask this question if her mother were there, so I answered quickly, in case she arrived. "Your grandfather's condition is so fragile, so close to death, that if even one thing was turned off, or turned down even a little, like this oxygen dial," I pointed to it and circled my fingers around it gingerly, "he would probably die in a few minutes."

The nurses charted extra-carefully. Not only the fluids in and out, numbers up and down, but also what was done and not done, what was said, and not said.

"Defensive documentation," our nurse manager advised us.

"A family meeting," I said to the granddaughter in a staccato short form that this desperate situation seemed to warrant. "We need one."

"My mother and my aunt Theresa don't want any more meetings," she said.

"Not a big meeting, a little one, here in the room. Not in the quiet room. Not sitting down, standing up. A short talk, here in the room."

The daughters had been eluding us. They had stopped answering the phone or returning our messages. One day they sent a fax with a series of requests, including one that their father was to be treated only by senior staff physicians, no residents or interns. The room was to be kept at precisely 22°C. There were to be no cool drafts or glaring lights. They requested that only "the cheerful nurses" be assigned to their father's care. "We do not want people with negative thoughts caring for our father."

On the day when Mr. Bellissimo's heart rate slowed to a sluggish 50 beats a minute and the few drops of urine that he put out were black and full of sludge, Dr. Leung was the attending staff physician and I was the nurse in charge.

After all these years, three children, numerous scientific research studies, and hundreds of academic papers, Jessica showed no signs of aging. She was still so beautiful.

"I guess we'll have to offer them dialysis," she said firmly, but I saw by her averted eyes that she was not exactly at one with this additional intervention herself.

"But Jessica," I said, "what will we gain by offering dialysis?"

"The daughters are representing his wishes. These are his wishes." She shrugged her shoulders as she added, "Apparently."

"But they're not acting in his best interests! They're not rational."

"I have spoken with them at length, and I'm convinced they believe this is what their father would have wanted. It would be presumptuous and arrogant of us to move to a paternalistic approach and assume we know what is best for patients. Not only that, but in this case it could become highly adversarial." She sighed wearily. "Tilda, think about the situation it puts us in if we override them. You have to understand where we, the doctors, are coming from."

She saw my skeptical expression. I could feel it on my face.

"I don't know!" She held up her hands. "We don't have all the answers."

"No, but neither do the daughters and they're making bad choices," I said. "How can we protect the father from his daughters' bad choices?"

"Tilda, *you* presume that *you* know what's best for him, even better than his own family?"

"Jessica, this poor man is rotting in the bed. I'm merely stating the obvious! It's common sense!"

"How can you know for sure that Mr. Bellissimo wouldn't want this done?"

"Do you know anyone who would?"

Jessica took a deep breath and composed herself.

"The thing I value the most, the thing that is most important to me in my practice is to be completely transparent and honest in everything that I do. Constitutionally, I am not able to tell a lie. That is who I am, and the day that changes is the day I get out of this profession. It is our duty to carry out the patient's wishes. Therefore, I have no qualms about this situation. I'm here, along with the nurses, to support the decisions the family has made. Let me remind you, Tilda, that we are not here to pass judgment. This is our job, whether I agree with the family or not. It is not about our beliefs, it is about the patient's beliefs."

Then it was my turn, and Jessica listened to me with equal patience and respect.

"To me, Jessica, the thing I value most, the thing that is most important to me in *my* practice is kindness. Nothing is more important to me than doing work that is kind. That's why I'm having such a difficult time with this case. It is cruel."

"This is not an assault and battery. Let's remember that," she said, bristling slightly at my intimation that she would be a part of anything that was cruel. "We are all motivated here by a desire to do good. Please keep that in mind, Tilda."

"Yes, but what we're doing isn't benevolent. Anyone can see that . . ." I was losing steam.

"How would you handle it then?" she asked. "Pretend it's you now, Dr. Shalof."

"I wouldn't offer one more medical intervention, certainly not dialysis or CPR in the event of another cardiac arrest. I would immediately insist on withdrawal of treatment and turn the focus over to comfort of the patient and support of the family. I would bring in second, third, fourth opinions, for the professional corroboration. I would bring in legal advisors, if necessary. A judge. A court injunction. An appointed guardian."

"All that could take weeks in itself," she said, smiling at my simple-mindedness. "In the meanwhile, we're not harming him."

"Oh, yes, we are," I said. "I guess it's different for the nurses than for the doctors. We're right there with patients, minute by minute, day and night. We *do* these things to the patients. We see them in the state they're in. We see the family's suffering and how we are prolonging it. The doctors come and go. Have you seen how Mr. Bellissimo's skin is all dripping, open sores? Have you watched how he grimaces in pain with whatever we do to him?

We keep giving him little boosts of epinephrine to keep him going all day. We can't even give him much morphine because it drops his pressure too much."

"I hope you don't feel, Tilda, that my word prevails over yours," Jessica said.

I knew she was trying to be conciliatory and draw this unsettling conversation to a peaceful close. She didn't need to do that. She and I had become friends as well as colleagues, and I had grown to love and respect her. We had worked together for years. I remembered when she started out as a resident, then as a senior fellow, and I was such a neophyte nurse, just trying to keep up with the basics. Our argument was not personal or acrimonious, even though it was vociferous and emotional.

"We are a team," she insisted.

"Yeah, but why do the daughters prevail?" I could hear myself whining like a child.

"They're the next of kin. You know the law, Tilda. I am simply following the law."

"The law cares nothing about compassion or the dignity of real people! We're making him into a freak, and allowing him to become grotesque. What we are doing has no purpose other than to mollify the daughters, to avoid confrontation, possibly even litigation –"

Laura came over to us, carrying something in her hand.

"How did you know there could be a lawsuit, Tilda? One of the daughters just sent this fax. It says her father deteriorated while under your care yesterday, and she thinks you caused it. She's threatening to bring in a lawyer to review the chart. She's got it in for *you*, baby!"

"That's fine. I have nothing to hide."

"Are you on a mutiny?" Laura looked amused. "You know you're becoming a drama queen."

"No," I answered, "I'm refusing to take care of this patient. I am a conscientious objector, a peace activist, and a front-line soldier. I'm going on a work-to-rule campaign."

That was that. For now.

"IF YOU GUYS are going to talk about Mr. B., I'm leaving," Laura said after work that evening. We were in a bar near the hospital, having drinks. "I don't want to hear another word about that case."

"No. There's nothing to talk about. I simply refuse to take care of him," I said.

"Are you on strike?"

"Kind of." I knew I wouldn't last.

"You won't last," Laura said.

"There's no way I'm going in there again either," said Tracy. "I'm with you, Tilda."

"Every human being deserves nursing care," said Frances. "I don't like it either, but I'll take care of him. I agree with Jessica Leung. It's our duty to carry out people's wishes. As nurses, we can't just give up on a person because we have a disagreement with the family. We have to put our personal opinions aside and do what is right for the patient."

I decided to boldly take the lead with an idea I had been cooking up, privately. I was ready to spring it on them. "Listen guys," I said. "I've figured out what we have to do to make sure this never happens to any of us."

"I thought we said we weren't going to talk about work!" protested Laura.

"I've been thinking of getting a tattoo on my chest that says 'Do Not Resuscitate,'" said Nicole. "After this case of Mr. B.'s, I'm not taking any chances. When the time comes, who knows what *my* family will do with me? Oh yeah, and one more request, make sure Murry takes care of me. I know he'll pluck my chin hairs and touch up my grey roots before my family comes to visit."

We all knew she took her mortality more seriously than her light-hearted words indicated. For some time we'd all known that Nicole had been preparing photo albums and storing away treasured keepsakes for the children whose names she'd already picked out and whom she hoped to have one day. Frances sipped her beer quietly. After all, it wasn't the first time we'd had one of these apocalyptic conversations.

"Dump my carcass in a garbage can," Morty said. "I don't believe in graves or funerals and I certainly don't want my liver going to some drugged-out alcoholic."

"We have to draw up living wills, decide on our advance directives, and write everything down," said Tracy. "We have to make our wishes known. Sign our donor cards. What else is there to do?"

"I'll tell you what I'm proposing," I said. "A pact. We'll appoint each other – our group – to be the decision makers for one another if any of us gets critically ill. We'll communicate clearly to one another what we want done in various scenarios – make our wishes known – as well as putting it in writing. We can't leave these decisions to our family. They won't know what to do. Who would know better what to do than us? Who's in on this with me?"

"What about the last remaining one?" asked Morty, thinking this over.

"I don't know, I guess she'll be on her own. I haven't worked out *all* the details, yet."

We fell silent. We'd had enough talk of death. But it was something worth considering, they conceded. Perhaps some other time, on another day. On another occasion. Not now.

18

SHIFT CHANGE

The ersatz Chinese buffet offered everything imaginable, from pad Thai to cole slaw to egg rolls to lasagna – fortune cookies and apple pie, too – and we stuffed ourselves, drank silly cocktails, and stayed, talking until the restaurant cleared out. Then Frances brought out a cake for Nicole's birthday and for once it was made of the proper ingredients – butter, sugar, flour, eggs – she didn't cut any corners. We were celebrating so many things that night, but most of all, our abiding friendship, bonded in the work we had been doing together for almost fifteen years.

That night we were in mourning, too. Just a few days ago we had heard the shocking news that Nell Mason had been found dead, the cause unknown. Frances, and others, had tried to stay in contact with her over the years, but she had drifted farther and farther away from everyone and now, this.

"It's tragic," said Frances. "What a fabulous nurse Nell was. Daniel Huizinga used to say, if Nell says there is something wrong with the patient and if he couldn't find it, he'd stay all night if necessary, until he figured out what was wrong. He trusted her completely."

"We all did," said Laura, who was choked up. "Maybe I shouldn't have made such fun of her. But all those crazy excuses and – let's face it – far-fetched stories! Some of them *were* pretty amusing, though," she said with a chuckle.

"Could any of them have been true? The pet camel? The elevator cutting loose? The wild dogs on the beach and how she poked" – I made the motion with two fingers jabbing the air – "and then pulled" – I yanked down the imaginary head of the dog under the pretend ocean surface – "them and drowned them to save her life?"

"Did she ever tell you about when she ran a medical station on a native reserve all by herself?" asked Laura, who couldn't resist just one more. "One day a man and a woman were brought in, stuck together. Yes, after sex, they couldn't separate themselves. 'So, how do you treat something like that, Nell?' I asked her. I thought, finally, I'll catch her. Without missing a beat, Nell said, 'Chlorpromazine, 50 mg IV, does the trick.'"

"To the man or to the woman?" I wondered aloud, but no one answered.

"There was always an element of truth in those stories," said Frances. "Nell was such a wonderful nurse and such fun to work with. I learned so much from her. I imagine that if an alien from another planet came to Earth and said, bring me your best nurse, everyone would agree that it would have to have been Nell."

"I'll miss her," I said and then added guiltily, "and her stories, too."

IN THE WARM glow of a candle in the middle of the table, I looked at the faces of these women and felt a sweet wistfulness. I wanted us to go on working together forever, but I could sense restlessness in each of them and we all had known for some time that changes were in the works.

It was time for cake. Nicole was just about to raise the knife, but for some reason hesitated and passed it along to Tracy, who also couldn't make the first cut. Tracy moved it over to stop in front of Morty, who had recently gone back to calling herself Justine.

She said she'd had enough of the old prank. Even her earrings had changed: she was wearing simple gold studs.

"Sure, I'll cut it," she said.

Justine grasped the knife, steadied the blade with her index finger, and pulled it down smoothly, first through the air, then through the frilly pink roses and the white blanket of icing, down as neatly and cleanly as a golf swing, the skill she'd just learned under Nicole's tutelage. Justine was looking forward to playing with her new husband (she had divorced the first one, Tom) who was an avid golfer. They had met co-starring in lead roles in a local amateur production of *Grease*.

Justine passed the cake to Frances, for whom cake cutting was not as straightforward a procedure. Her hand wavered. She was on Weight Watchers once again and had been good all week, in order to allow for this treat. She widened, then narrowed the angle for her intended portion, and then changed her tack altogether.

"How about I cut you a slice, Nicky, seeing as how you're the birthday girl?" Nicole, newly pregnant and a bit queasy, still could be accorded a generous slice. Frances brought down the little caloric guillotine.

For her own slice, Frances dragged the knife down slowly, like a senior citizen doing the crawl in a Miami pool. She took her time and did it as if against resistance, as if she'd cut many, many cakes in her day and knew all too well the complications and implications involved in cake cutting.

"Pass that cake down here," growled Laura. "What's taking you guys so long?"

In Laura's hand, the knife came down swiftly, causing the roses to spring back in surprise. We looked at one another and smiled. Laura slapped a hunk of cake and icing to her plate, sat back in her chair, and brought the plate and fork to her mouth as if she were ravenous. No, it wasn't possible – we had just finished a huge meal – but she craved the sweetness.

"You need to get laid, Laura," said Justine, across the table from her. "You're horny and you need a good –"

"Good, bad, or indifferent, I'll be eating cake until that happens."

"Maybe what you need, Laura," I suggested, "is a break from the ICU. Why don't you take some time off and go on a long vacation somewhere?"

"I *am* going somewhere," she announced, taking us by surprise.

"So where are you off to, Laura?" Nicole asked.

"Medical school," she said calmly.

"No!" I said in alarm.

"Yes."

"No!"

She smiled.

"What a sellout!" I said.

"'You're too smart to be a nurse, Laura, why aren't you a doctor?'" Laura said in a mocking voice. "People are always telling me that I'm wasting my talent as a nurse. I tell them it takes a lot of intelligence to be a nurse, but they don't get it. I say to them, aren't you glad there are smart nurses like me, caring for people? They still don't get it. Well, I've had enough! I'm going to be a doctor. I'll make decent money and maybe get some respect."

"It's very hard to get accepted to medical school," I warned her. "You might not get in."

"I'm in already," she said. "I got my acceptance a few days ago. Nurses know to go where the need is and I told them I'm prepared to go to a remote, under-serviced area and I think that helped get me accepted."

"Are you?"

"Of course."

"What a loss!" I said.

Of course, I could see how a solitary, isolated medical practice would suit Laura well. She could be the surly, self-reliant maverick that she was and probably do a lot of good for people who really needed it. They would love her. She would make a wonderful doctor.

No one noticed Tracy taking a modest slice of cake. We still so often overlooked soft-spoken, unassuming Tracy, yet I had come to understand that she wasn't withdrawn or remote, just quiet, thoughtful, and lately preoccupied with her father's health. About

a month ago she had called us at work, and the number on the telephone display was an internal hospital extension.

"Where are you?" I asked her.

"I'm downstairs in Emerg."

She was always calm in any situation, but now I could hear her
voice tremble.

"What happened? Your kids okay? Ron?"

"It's my dad. He had a heart attack."

"We'll be right down."

Pang-Mei took over my patient for me. "Of course, go down
and see Tracy's father. I know what it's like. My mother had
severe abdo pain the other night and I had to take her to Emerg.
'No, no,' she told everyone who came near her – she barely
speaks English, she's worse than me – '*I a DNR. I a DNR.*' I
told her, no, Ma, we're not there yet, the doctor just wants to do
an X-ray!"

"She's lucky, Pang-Mei. She's got you and you've prepared her
well."

Tracy's father was okay, but Tracy was a mess. Her eyes were
bloodshot from staying up all night with him. She had not left his
side for a minute. However, the biggest hurdle for her had been
just getting into the hospital. With a second wave of SARS threatening to spread like an epidemic, even stricter control measures
had been put back into effect throughout the entire hospital. No
one other than staff giving direct patient care was allowed into the
hospital. Somehow, Tracy had managed to sneak in and get to her
dad. He was lucky; all the other patients were on their own, with
no visitors to keep them company or give their loved one that
special attention.

Tracy's dad had been kept in the holding area of the
Emergency department, lying on a stretcher, for two days,
waiting for a bed. Finally they found one for him on Cardiology
and he was being transferred there, just as we arrived. He was in
stable condition, but would be kept for a few days more until a
heart catheterization could be done to determine if he had
any blockages in his coronary arteries and see if bypass surgery
was an option.

Frances had helped him wash himself, gave him a shave, and then went down to the drugstore to buy him a toothbrush and toothpaste.

Laura had joined us, took one look at him, and marched off to find a resident and point out to him that Mr. Smyth's right leg was swollen and painful, possibly indicating a deep vein thrombosis – and "how could you have missed that?" I heard her accosting him. She also managed to convince the doctor to increase his dosage of pain medication as he was clearly in discomfort but was the stoic type who never complained.

"The patient under-complains, the doctor under-prescribes, and the nurse under-administers – it all adds up to pain control worth diddly-squat," she said to us, as if all the responsibilities of the world had come to rest on her shoulders. "Do they really believe that patients in pain are at risk of becoming drug addicts? Is that what they're afraid of? Honestly! How many times have you guys ever seen a case of over-shooting *pain* medication?"

Nicole had helped Tracy's father to change into a fresh hospital gown. I told Tracy to step out for a minute so she didn't have to help put the urine bottle in place so that her father could pee.

"Get out of here for a sec, Tracy. Just be a daughter now, not a nurse."

I knew the difference. How well I knew how hard it is to be both. Better to be one at a time. I pulled up a chair and sat beside Mr. Smyth's bed and asked him what he thought about the war against Iraq.

"I've seen a lot of war," he said, "and I've been thinking about my grandchildren. War isn't good for children, you know."

He told me about his experience in the British Navy. He had been a submarine gunner off the coast of Normandy during World War II.

"You girls are angels," he said, looking not quite as grisly as before Frances's beauty treatment.

"No, we're not," said Justine, shaking her head vigorously.

"Speak for yourself," said Laura, who was leaning up against a low-lying window ledge. "*You* may be a devil, Justine, but *I'm* an angel."

"No, nurses are ordinary human beings, professionals doing a demanding job. All we're asking for is fair working conditions, a decent wage –"

"That's enough, Justine." I poked her. "This isn't the time."

"If anybody is to be praised," she continued in a calmer vein, "it's these nurses who work on the floors. You haven't seen a nurse yet, Mr. Smyth, because your nurse has eight other patients who are in worse shape than you. The entire hospital has become one big intensive care unit. The typical hospital patient is being sent home now to be cared for by whoever is available and willing. Patients who are now in the ICU are ones that not too long ago were unsalvageable altogether. Hospitals have to change."

She hardly stopped to take a breath and continued.

"Can you imagine working here on this floor, running around all day, never feeling that you can master the work, never feeling in control over your time, or the demands made on you? Never feeling like you can do a satisfactory day's work? You know exactly what the patient needs, but your hands are tied. The institution takes away all our creativity, initiative, and power and turns nurses into stones."

Tracy's dad was listening closely. "You gals deserve more respect."

"No," Justine railed on, "nurses have to respect themselves first. We can't expect respect from anyone else until we have it for ourselves and we have a long way to go on that score."

I had been watching the nurses on that floor. I saw them rushing around, answering phones, setting up lunch trays, taking a blood pressure, and dashing off every so often to record everything in the charts. All the while, with this new and frightening virus, nurses were having to don masks, gloves, gowns, and goggles, and change out of all that and scrub their hands, and then put on a new set of everything all over again before going to the next patient.

"You know what's the hardest thing about these masks?" said Frances, pulling hers down briefly for a gulp of air.

"Breathing?" I asked.

"I don't know, but they're playing havoc with my makeup," said Nicole. "I have to keep reapplying my lipstick!"

"That, too," Frances said. "The worst thing is you can't read patients' facial expressions. And you can't smile at them."

"Only with your eyes," I said, making mine smile at her.

"Can you imagine how patients are feeling these days, being isolated, only occasionally seeing a nurse appear at their door? Two eyes over the top of a mask?" Frances asked.

"You've all been so good to me," said Mr. Smyth. "How can I ever thank you gals?"

"It's nothing," Frances told him, eager to relieve his sense of obligation. "I give 100 per cent to my patients. Why wouldn't I give *110 per cent* to one of our own?"

How many people can say that about the way they do their work? How many nurses can say that about their practice, that they give 100 per cent? How many nurses can say it and have it be as true it was as in Frances's case? Was I a giver like that? Had I managed to conquer myself to that extent? Not quite, I knew, but I was still in it, with no plans to go anywhere else.

It used to be that I gave what I could, yet at times had felt so depleted, resentful, and bereft. Now, I know what it is that I give and I have learned to value it. I've learned how to take care of myself and know now that I can find compassion for other people's pain only when I've first found room in my heart for my own.

THERE WERE MORE reasons to celebrate that night.

Justine had just graduated with her degree in nursing and as the class valedictorian, she had given a thought-provoking speech about the perilous, but promising future of nursing. She delivered it with the new, more sober attitude she'd adopted lately. Still, she managed to keep the crowd entertained and, at times, had them laughing uproariously.

"If you ever want a break from nursing," I joked, "you'd have a bright future in stand-up comedy."

"Funny you should mention that," she said. "I've decided to leave nursing."

"What?" I gasped, thinking for a moment that my comment had jinxed her, but as soon as she said, "I've applied to law school," in a flash, I realized what sense that made.

"Maybe through legal channels or politics, I can make a contribution to nursing. Let's face it, my strength isn't patient care."

It was big of her to admit that, but I didn't entirely agree. She had kept many patients in stitches and wasn't laughter the best medicine? She intimidated some families, but they all respected her intelligence and knew her heart was in the right place.

"Everything changed for me that night that I was totally out of line. I lost control of myself and was lucky I didn't get caught and that no one reported me."

The incident she was referring to had happened a few weeks ago and I had been in charge. Justine was caring for an elderly woman. When I came in on rounds I saw that there were ten IV pumps running and six IV lines in various parts of her body, and tubes and drains everywhere. The ventilator was on maximum settings and the patient was thrashing in the bed so wildly that we had to restrain her hands in order to do what we were doing, which naturally made her even more upset. But what was the alternative? We still didn't know. Our response when the family kept asking for "everything to be done" was to try to impress on them that "everything *was* being done." For them, it was not enough. There was nothing more we could offer, but they wanted nothing short of a miracle.

But there, in the meanwhile, lay Justine's patient, a helpless old woman, straining at the tube in her mouth and grimacing with every single thing we did to her. For me, the worst part was seeing the terror in her eyes. What could I do but look away? But not Justine. Not that night. She chose to see everything.

The family had left for the day and suddenly Justine jumped up.

"I'm going to call them," she said, "I've had enough of this."

"What are you going to say to them?" I trailed after her toward the telephone. There was no stopping her – I didn't even try – and soon I heard her talking to the patient's son.

"Look here, this is your mother's nurse, Justine Fraser. What? . . . Is everything all right? No, everything is not all right. . . .

You'd better get in here right away. We've got the ventilator going full blast and your mother is on every known drug, running at industrial-strength doses. Unfortunately, we cannot cure old age! If your mother arrests tonight, I want you to be here to watch me pound on her chest and crack her ribs to try to get her heart started up again! You guys are not thinking clearly. This is cruel. You're doing it for yourselves, to put *your* minds at ease. It's not for your mother."

Unbelievably, from what we could gather, they were thanking her over the phone.

"I was way out of line," Justine now admitted, "and I know it. But that night I decided to be guided by what I believed was right for the patient. The place finally got to me. It pushed me right over the edge! I'm ashamed of the way I behaved. The way I spoke to the family was wrong. They could have reported me, but they didn't."

Shaken by Justine's harsh words, the family had rushed in and faced the realization that there was no point in continuing treatment. Perhaps Justine had made them see the situation differently and that helped them to make different choices. Or maybe they had felt coerced or shocked by her words. Perhaps they were relieved that someone had made some of these fateful decisions and they didn't have to bear any of these onerous responsibilities. At any rate, they came in, and we gradually, slowly, brought the battery of machines and drugs to a grinding halt. We pulled out the tube and stripped away the equipment and listened to the room becoming quiet, except for the deep, rasping, irregular sounds of the mother's last breaths and the family's sobbing. We pulled up chairs alongside the bed and stayed with the patient and the family until the end.

I watched the straight backs, the outstretched arms, the kind, attentive faces of the nurses around me, as we did this sacred work. I looked around at their faces and their eyes met mine. I think I had an inkling that night that it might be the last time we would all work together as nurses.

WE HADN'T SEEN much of Tracy lately, who was still taking university courses to complete her degree in nursing, and was busy with her young family and taking care of her father who was recuperating at home. She had switched to permanent nights and weekends and that was apparently taking its toll, too.

"My neighbour says to me 'have a nice weekend' and I'm thinking what weekend? My weekend is Wednesday and Thursday. I don't know how much longer I'm going to be able to keep this up," she said with a weary sigh. "It's too hard on my family. I overheard my kids talking the other day," she continued. "Matthew was saying to Jake, 'Stay away from Mom. She's crabby when she works nights.' "

MY HEART WAS sinking. They were dropping like flies.

I looked over at Frances.

"Don't worry, Tilda," she reassured me. "I'm not going anywhere."

But I sensed reservation in her voice.

"At least not for now," she added.

I searched her face for clues, for assurances she'd stay, but she wouldn't commit.

"Promise me *you're* not going anywhere, Frances."

She kept quiet.

"C'mon, Jabber Jaws," said Laura. "You'll be here forever. You'll never leave this place."

"I can't go on without you guys," I said.

"This is not the *Titanic* going down, Tilda. I'm sure you'll survive," said Frances sternly. "The manager of the OR called me and asked if I'd like to work there. He promised to send me on the course next month, but when I took a look at the textbook, I had my doubts. It's all about retractors, ratchets, and forceps. The advantage is it's straight days, and just the occasional on-call duty for nights or weekends."

I looked at her in dismay. "How could you?" I guilt-tripped her.

"I'm turning forty-four this year, Tilda. How much longer can I keep doing all these nights and weekends? Christmas, New Year's?

Nursing is for the young. Besides, all the suffering and death – it chips at you after a while, the sadness of the work we do."

"But Frances, you always said you could handle the emotional demands. Remember how you told me you believed that our work was good, that we helped people and that was what always kept your mind at ease?"

"Yeah, I still feel that way, but being around so much sadness is making me sad, too. It creates more sadness than there was in the first place. I'll give you an example of when it really hit me. Do you guys remember that young girl, only twenty-four? 'It's not fatal, is it?' the mother asked me, but I was too busy to talk to her, her daughter was so sick. But even when I finally got things under control, I found myself putting off going out to the waiting room to face the mother. I never used to do that.

"They were East Indian; I remember the mother's red sari and the gold bracelets along her arm. Surely they had been told how serious pulmonary fibrosis could be. She had cared for her daughter for years, and now she had to turn her over to us and stand by and watch. We were the mothers, now. Later when I was on lunch, I could hear someone calling for the arrest cart and I thought to myself, *Just stay put and eat your lunch, Frances. It's your break. Other people can take care of the situation.* But I couldn't sit there and eat my lunch while my patient was arresting and so I went back to her room. There was a crowd in there. They didn't need an extra pair of hands in there right then, but I knew where I *was* needed. I went out to the waiting room. I didn't even have to say a word. She saw my face and I had to practically carry her like a newborn baby down to the ICU. Anyway, the daughter was arresting and they were still working on her and the mother kept asking me what was happening and all I could say was 'It doesn't look good.' I didn't say much more but she couldn't have taken much more right then, anyway. She collapsed onto the floor. Belinda, Ellen, Pang-Mei, and Bruno were all on that day and they helped me carry her into the resident's on-call room where we tried to lay her down on the bed. But she didn't want to go on the bed. She threw herself back onto the floor and started writhing around. I sent someone to get a crash cart for the mother, just in case.

Belinda thought she'd fainted, Pamela thought for sure it was a seizure, but I could see it wasn't that. Someone else thought we should give her Valium. I gave her oxygen and took her vitals. Her blood pressure was okay, but meanwhile she had lost consciousness, so I slipped in a bite block to protect her airway. Someone brought her a blanket from the warming cupboard, and we stretched her out on the carpeted floor and covered her. Everyone was speculating about the problem and what could be the cause. Then I figured it out. I knew the diagnosis. Grief. That's what it looks like and that's what it was. There was no other diagnosis and the only treatment was nursing care. I have always prided myself on giving that kind of care, but it sure takes its toll at times. Now, I don't know any more if I want to spend all my time around such sadness."

"Yeah, it's not only that, it's the politics, too," said Laura. "The last straw for me came about a month ago. I was in charge and I had to double up nurses in two different rooms and it was very unsafe because both patients were very unstable. To top it off, I was short-staffed for the next shift and had to spend every spare moment on the phone trying to call in overtime. I didn't have enough nurses, so we had to close the ICU and we ended up turning down a lung transplant and the ruptured aortic aneurysm had to go somewhere else. The lungs went somewhere else and I hope to God the aneurysm made it. I had to bed-space another patient in the recovery room, but they were stretched to the limit over there so I had to leave the unit, go over and take care of the patient myself, for a few hours. That morning, I said to myself, 'That's it. I've had enough.'"

So now Laura and Justine were leaving nursing and Tracy and Frances were having second thoughts.

It was no surprise to us that Nicole was leaving. We had known about it for some time. She was moving to Atlanta, Georgia, for just a few years only – she'd be back, she insisted – with her husband, Andrew, who was now a thoracic surgeon, and they had a baby on the way, too. Andrew had been offered a staff position at a big medical centre. Nicole had been looking so classy lately in the pearl necklace he'd given her – she'd taken to wearing it with her green scrubs.

"Lots of great golf courses down there," she said. "You'll all have to come and visit. Right, *y'all? You come on down, you hear?*" she added, practising her Southern accent.

"Andrew is looking forward to not having to wait weeks for his patients to get their CT scans and MRIS. He won't have to scramble to book procedures and OR time for his patients and won't have to scrounge around for research money. It'll be a nice break for him and I'm *sure* we'll be back one day."

"Who can blame him?" Laura said.

"The MRI, the MRI," said Justine in a mocking voice. "That's all you ever hear about these days – how long you have to wait for an MRI. You'd think MRIS were saving so many lives. Why is the MRI always trotted out as the gold standard of our health-care system? For God's sake, when will people realize that it's not more MRIS we need? It's more nurses. The ratio of nurses per capita is a far better indicator of the standard of our health-care system than the number of MRIS to go around. If you're sick, you need a nurse, not an MRI."

"And whatever happened to the doctors who went into medicine for the love of it?" I asked. "Because it's their passion? Medicine is becoming a business, and if people choose medicine as a way to make money, they should go to the States because there, health care is a commodity for sale and you can shop around for the best product. Patients are the customers and if you're rich you get better health care than if you're poor. In Canada, health care is a basic human right, a service that every human being deserves. Tell me, have any of you ever seen someone get preferential treatment? A Canadian over a non-resident? A white person over one of colour? A VIP over an ordinary citizen?"

"Can't we have one night out together without talking about work?" complained Laura. "We've talked enough about work. Well, what about you, Tilda? What are your plans?"

They would all laugh at me if I told them how much I still loved nursing. How I appreciated the opportunity it afforded me to work equally with my hands and mind, my body and spirit. How I still had so much to learn. How I enjoy the rigour of the shift work, the immediacy of helping people in crisis, the privilege of accompanying people through some of the most difficult moments of their lives, the challenge of the complex cases, and the energizing capacity of this work. I have never wanted to leave the bedside, only now to step away momentarily, take a look around and see it all.

"I'M SO FULL," said Frances, loosening her jeans as we rolled out of the restaurant after midnight.

"Me, too," groaned Laura.

"Yeah, but the problem with these all-you-can eat buffets is that a week later you're hungry again," Justine quipped.

Yes, finally, we were full.

As we went our separate ways that night of celebration, commemoration, and farewell, I knew we would always be close in heart, if not at hand.

IT WAS JULY and time for a brand-new set of residents, fresh from their intern year to join us in the ICU for a few weeks. One of them, Kendal, had just returned from a mission with Médecins Sans Frontières. Kendal, with her clogs, rumpled chino pants, Sherpa wool sweater, black mailbag across her chest and resting at her hip, and tight curly hair, had just returned from Cambodia and had brought some visiting doctors on a tour of the ICU. They joined us on morning rounds.

"They feel disheartened," she translated for us. "One of them is saying to me that seeing all that we have here, he doesn't even feel like a doctor any more. I am telling him that if I went to his country, I wouldn't know how to treat malaria, land mine victims, malnutrition, dysentery, and leprosy. I don't have their skills to face what they deal with."

She listened more and then reported back to us. "They say that it's not doctors – what they need more than anything is nurses in the Third World countries." She looked at us.

"Yeah, we could go over there as bedpan teachers," someone joked.

Still with that! I thought. *Have we made no progress?*

"Not exactly," said Kendal. "They need nurses to teach the people, nurses to organize and run clinics, develop immunization programs, offer primary care, teach other nurses there how to do work as skilled as yours."

THAT DAY I was working with Tikki, one of the nurses who had just joined the ICU. I was supervising her during her last few days of orientation to the ICU. She had a tiny nose ring and spiky purple hair. I'd seen her once early in the morning, dressed in black clothes, coming to work directly from an all-night Goth rave at The Docks. Tikki was a university graduate, new to nursing, even newer to critical care, and she seemed full of confidence and skill. I had no worries about her coping with the ICU.

"How are you doing?" I asked her.

"Great, thanks. No problem."

"What's your impression of this place so far? Do you think you'll like working here?"

She looked thoughtful and paused for a moment before she spoke.

"This is an extreme place," she said. "It's very harsh in here, what we do to people . . . and some of it seems, rather . . . *unwise.*"

I nodded. Maybe so, maybe so. After all these years, I'm still trying to sort it out. We all are. But I believe that there *is*, in fact, a great deal of wisdom in the way we take care of sick people. One thing I know for sure is that at times when our wisdom falters, compassion always abounds. That is what nursing has taught me above all: compassion is the greatest wisdom.